The *BACK STAGE*® Handbook for Performing Artists

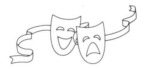

Compiled and Edited by
Sherry Eaker

BACK STAGE BOOKS
An imprint of Watson-Guptill Publications/New York

Sherry Eaker is the editor of the theater section of *Back Stage*, the national trade publication geared to the performer in both the commercial and non-profit theater arenas. She is Vice President of the Drama Desk, the organization of New York theater critics, editors, and reporters, and chairs its Program Committee. Ms. Eaker is both a Tony Award and Drama Desk Award voter, and is a member of the Manhattan Association of Cabarets and of the National Theater Conference, an association of leaders of noncommercial theaters. She frequently serves on panels focusing on the working actor.

Senior Editor: Tad Lathrop
Project Editor: Darrel Irving
Book and Jacket Design: Jay Anning

Copyright © 1989 Billboard Publications, Inc.

First published 1989 by Back Stage Books, an imprint of Watson-Guptill Publications, a division of Billboard Publications, Inc., 1515 Broadway, New York, NY 10036

Library of Congress Cataloging-in-Publication Data

The back stage handbook for performing
   artists.

   Includes index.
   1. Acting—Vocational guidance—United
States—Directories.   2. Performing arts—
Vocational guidance—United States—Direc-
tories.   I. Eaker, Sherry.   II. Back stage.
PN2055.B27   1989   792'.028'02573   88-34446
ISBN 0-8230-7508-7

Manufactured in the United States of America
First Printing, 1989

1   2   3   4   5   6   7   8   9   /   94   93   92   91   90   89

*To my father, who raised the curtain for me and made it all possible,
and to my mother, who's been coaching me along the way*

A special thanks to Claire Dorsey and Toni Reinhold for their assistance on this project. Thanks also to staffers David Sheward and Thomas Walsh, and to Dan McNally, Michael Hofferber, Geoffrey Johnson, and all the free-lance writers who have made valuable contributions to *Back Stage* over the years.

Contents

Introduction

by Sherry Eaker

Although Broadway may be the ultimate goal of many performing artists, there are places other than the Great White Way where more realistic opportunities exist. Discovering where these opportunities are, defining them and learning how to make the necessary contacts in order to pursue them is what this book is all about.

This is also the focus of *Back Stage*, the weekly trade paper geared toward the entertainment industry. Each week, aside from carrying audition information for productions going on in New York and across the country, *Back Stage* features "how-to" articles designed to help working actors, singers, dancers, directors, and playwrights move ahead in their careers.

The idea of putting all these articles together in book form was the result of countless requests I continually receive asking for specific back issues. In response to these requests I've chosen for this handbook over 30 feature stories that have run in *Back Stage* over the past year. Where relevant, these articles are accompanied by trade lists, in keeping with the traditional format of *Back Stage*. Every single list has been updated right up until presstime, to assure the greatest possible accuracy.

Let me emphasize at this point, especially for those performers who are first entering the profession, that there's a whole lot more to an acting, singing, or dancing career than just training and performing. You're going to spend at least half of your energy just *finding and getting the work*. This is a fact that should be stressed in university theater departments, but it rarely is. Sure, there are plenty of talented people out there, but unless you as a performer become adept at the business side of the entertainment industry—skilled at setting up shop, making contacts, and learning the art of auditioning, etc.—your talent will be as useful to the industry as having a degree in physics.

The first two chapters cover, first and foremost, resumes and photos. Since your resume is your number one marketing tool, this chapter details how to put one together to make it most effective, and shows you the most efficient means of sending your resume out. Because a resume is always accompanied by a headshot, learning how to choose the right photographer is the focus of the second chapter.

The third chapter is about temporary employment services. Let's face it, most performers don't make a decent living from their performing careers when they first start out. And for those who don't want to work in a restaurant, this chapter describes the kinds of temporary jobs that are available and how the employment services operate.

As an actor just starting out you'll need a telephone answering service. You might say, "What do I need a service for, I just bought a telephone answering machine." Well, from a survey taken by *Back Stage*, we found out that agents and casting directors would rather leave a message with a service than on a tape, so how to go about selecting an answering service is the concern of the next chapter.

Play scripts, sheet music, monologue collections, and playwright anthologies are also basics for performing artists, and a complete rundown of performing arts book shops make up another section under the "Basic Tools" umbrella.

There are hundreds of acting schools, dance studios and voice teachers in the United States. So, how do you choose one that's right for you? The chapters grouped under the section called "Training" set up some criteria for selecting schools and teachers, and are accompanied by lists that show where to find them.

Now that you've "set up shop" and are busy taking classes, your next step is "Finding the Work." Hopefully, you're already reading the trade papers every week to find out what's being cast. You'll also need to make contact with agents and casting directors since it is they who can help you land a role. Keeping in touch with them on a constant basis, via sending professional postcards, is necessary, *especially* when you're performing somewhere. They need to be reminded that you are a working actor. Included under "Finding the Work" are lists of New York- and Los Angeles-based SAG, AFTRA and Equity franchised agents, New York- and Los Angeles-based independent casting directors and network casting directors, as well as a list of casting heads at all the major motion picture and TV film studios on the West Coast. There's also a chapter on tips on TV commercial acting, accompanied by a list of the casting directors who head up the casting departments at the various New York-based advertising agencies.

Personal managers function differently than agents. Exactly what these differences are is explained in the chapter on managers, which contains a list of these professionals on both coasts and their areas of specialty.

As we've noted, auditioning is an art in itself; nowadays many acting schools offer classes on audition technique alone. One of the chapters in this section offers advice on auditioning for the musical theater.

Suppose you're a playwright or director or actor and have your hands on a wonderful property and don't want to have to be dependent on others to move it along. What do you do? Produce it yourself! Producing your own show can be a tremendous learning experience, and the chapters designated under "Getting a Show on the Road" tell you specifically what you need to know and do—from creating a budget, to hiring a cast, from renting a space to rehearse and perform in, to hiring a publicist or, if finances dictate, doing your own publicity.

I mentioned "realistic opportunities" earlier on. And there *are* lots of opportunities for performers at all levels of experience on stages all across the country. The section titled "Working in the Theater" features chapters which describe in detail types of theaters, theater companies, booking agents, producers, and complete contact information.

Listed are theater companies in New York and Los Angeles, nonprofit resident theaters across the country, nationwide Equity and non-Equity dinner theaters, and Theater for Young Audiences companies.

"Off the Main Stage" focuses on other great opportunities. Theme parks, for example, can offer intense and varied experiences for the beginner. Where these theme parks are, the kind of performers they're seeking and where and when they hold their audition tours is detailed here.

Cruise lines are another outlet for performers, especially those who want to see the world and escape the tensions of the city. Since there's more involved than just being "an actor aweigh," the advantages and disadvantages of cruise line work is discussed along with a comprehensive contact list.

Performers, as well as staff and technicians, may also take stock in summer stock. Once a year, hundreds of theater producers gather at various sites across the country auditioning performers and interviewing directors, technicians, and staffpersons for the spots that are available at their summer theaters. The chapter on summer stock combined auditions informs as to who, when and where these auditions are held, gives application procedures and deadlines, and tells how to prepare.

Fairly profitable outlets for performers are the industrial shows and industrial films. Coined "business theater," an industrial show is usually a big-budget production using the most advanced technology and offering valuable training and experience for performers. And, growing by leaps and bounds are opportunities for actors in the quickly expanding field of industrial films. A list of producers of live industrials is included here, but the list of producers of industrial and corporate films is so long that it warrants a book by itself. You may want to refer to *Back Stage*'s yearly *Film and Tape Directory* which lists production companies in all the major cities in the United States.

Think you've got what it takes to make people laugh? The chapter on comedy deals with the growing field of stand-up and what booking agents look for when auditioning acts. And, whether you're a stand-up comedian or cabaret singer, you'll need to know how to build an audience for your club act. Included in these chapters is a step-by-step approach that will just about guarantee a full house.

There are lots of opportunities out there, but not every opportunity offered is a realistic one. Just as phonies and con artists exist in the business world, there are plenty of them around in the show business world. Unfortunately, in such a competitive market, many novice performers fall prey to promises of "stardom" and many end up losing more than just their pride. Based on the many letters and calls that *Back Stage* has received from performers over the years, we put together a comprehensive report on what performers should be aware of and situations they should avoid in the chapter called "Actors Aware."

Show business *is* a business and if you, the performing artist, want to succeed at it you must treat it as such. No one is going to do it for you at the beginning, and the earlier in your career that you start dealing with the business aspects of the business, the greater are your chances of succeeding artistically. Whether or not you get to Broadway, there are audiences waiting for you. There are theaters everywhere, and they have stages where you can act, dance, sing, entertain, and derive the satisfaction that comes from performing.

PART ONE

The Basic Tools

Resumes

by Jill Charles

The Picture/Resume is the performer's business card, reference letter, portfolio, and certificate of professional standing all rolled into one. It is the marketing tool that will get you work. Putting it together, making it effective, and getting it out should become part of your daily work and should be given the kind of preparation you would give to an audition for an important role. Without a good picture/resume you may not even get to audition for that important role, so this aspect of the performer's craft must be given special attention. While a good photo is essential, remember that it is usually the resume stapled to its back that clinches the audition once the picture gets the casting director's attention.

There is no standard format for the resume itself. Each resume is as individual as the performer it represents. Certain data, however, should always be included in a resume, and some information is better left out. The guidelines below will help you determine what to include and what to exclude in your resume.

When organizing your resume, pay careful attention to its overall look. It should be pleasing to look at, well structured and easy to understand. Imagine how many resumes casting people and directors receive. If yours is hard to read and digest, your credits and skills simply will not register with them. One way of making sure that your resume is easy to understand is to organize it into parts or sections. It should contain top, body, a training section and a special skills section.

THE TOP—VITAL STATISTICS AND CONTACT INFORMATION

The top section of your resume should generally include vital statistics and contact information, such as your name, contact phone number, union affiliations, and talent agent's name. It is not necessary, and not necessarily wise, to put a home address or home phone number here. Once you send out a resume, there is no way of knowing what will happen to it (some even turn up on city sidewalks) and for your own protection it is best to list only a service number.

The important vital statistics include height, weight, and the color of your hair and eyes. This information is essential for a casting person. You may include or omit such items as age, vocal range, and measurements. A general rule of thumb is to include information that will help make you stand out, or underscore a special ability. Omit data that will confuse, mislead or somehow create false impressions.

Measurements need be listed only in modeling or commercial resumes. For their own protection, many actresses prefer to leave measurements to the costume designer after they have the role. You may want to include your social security number—some agents prefer that their clients do so—but this is not essential since it is not needed until you are hired for a job.

Many performers dislike putting an age range on a resume because they do not want to be typecast into a narrow bracket. They theorize that the casting person should decide whether they appear to be the appropriate age for a role. This is an acceptable approach if a photo is a true representation of a performer. If, for example, an actor appears to be a young 20s in a photo and actually looks 30 at the audition, the casting person will more than likely not be pleased. If you do put an age range on your resume, make it realistic—few can successfully play ages 15 to 40.

Listing vocal range is important if you can sing. If there is no mention of vocal range, and no musical credits on your resume, the assumption may be made that you cannot sing at all. If you can carry a tune, and could sing in a chorus or handle a song in a nonmusical play, list your vocal range on your resume. Show anything you have done that may be pertinent to singing ability, including musical roles and training.

THE BODY—EXPERIENCE

In the body of the resume you will list your experience. This is usually organized by genre: theater, film, television, and commercials. You do not have to list the categories in this order though. List the categories according to the emphasis *you* place on them. If you do more work in one area than another, it is a good idea to compile two or more different resumes, so that your "film" resume lists film credits first, while your "theatrical" resume lists theater credits first. Those who have sufficient experience, may wish to break theater down into subdivisions, such as Broadway, national tours, Off Broadway, showcase, stock, regional, musical plays, and so on.

A variety of approaches may be used when listing your credits, but one basic tenet holds—include the information that makes you look best, *but don't lie* or stretch the truth. Most people who look at resumes see a lot of them and know the tricks performers use to fatten up slim credits. The phrase "representative roles" is a transparent camouflage for "roles I did in scene-study class" or "roles I would like to play." Your resume should represent your actual experience and should show the role, the play, and the theater where you performed it. An understudy role should be listed as such, with a notation ("performed twice" or whatever) if you actually performed the role. Whether you list all the directors you've worked under or just those who are better-known is a choice you should make based on the impressiveness of the list and the overall look it will give to the layout. Don't crowd the credits with names that probably will not be recognized (the name and location of the theater company is sufficient), but if you have worked with well-known directors, say so. It is not necessary to list playwrights' names, unless you performed a new play and you want to emphasize that.

If you are entering the professional world from a training school, your credits will probably be limited. Make the most of what you have done, but don't try to stretch things too far. List professional credits, like summer stock, before school credits. Try to give a positive (but honest) picture of whatever experience you gained in school, and list any guest directors you worked with who might be known outside your school.

TRAINING

The purpose of the Training section is simply to show where and with whom you have trained. This will help those who see it determine the areas and extent of your training in acting, voice, dance, and related theater skills. If you have trained with well-known teachers be sure to include their names. If, however, the names are not well-known and their inclusion makes the resume look cluttered, do not list them; the type and duration of training should be sufficient.

SPECIAL SKILLS

The Special Skills section should list those talents that might be useful in commercial work, or that a theater company might find especially interesting. Start with theater-related skills such as stage combat, acrobatics, the ability to play musical instruments, and accents and dialects. Then include athletic abilities, and whether or not you drive a car (standard and/or automatic). You can add to this list almost anything you do well, such as photography, graphic design, sign language, carpentry, or electronics; these skills can also generate conversation at an interview or audition.

UPDATING

Part of the nature of resumes is that they continually need to be updated, and this can create time and money problems. If you do not get around to updating your resume until the handwritten additions threaten to take it over, you might try exercising this option—design your resume with a heading at the bottom titled "Recent Credits." Leave space under this heading to describe your latest projects. Not only will this keep your resume looking neat, but it will also project the idea that you are constantly working. Of course, you will always want to have something written in this space, so when you have your resume printed, exclude your most recent credit and then jot it down in the open space after the resume has been printed. This is also a good way to call special attention to upcoming readings or workshops you will be doing.

TYPING AND PRINTING

Once your original is prepared, the resume can be printed in quantity. But first you must decide whether to have the original typed, word-processed, or typeset. There are three factors to consider in making this decision: the look of the resume, the ease with which it can be updated, and the cost.

Typeset resumes look wonderful after they have been copied, but typesetting involves greater expense. You might then find yourself using the same resume longer than you really want to because you are hesitant about spending the money to have it updated. Some typesetters keep resumes on file for relatively inexpensive updates, but this still generally costs more than the word-processing method.

Probably the best buy for your money will be found at word-processing resume services. And copies that have been word-processed no longer need look like "computer type," or "dot matrix type," in which the letters are actually comprised of a series of small dots printed close together. Resume services using word processors now run their copies on "letter quality" printers. These provide copy that is indistinguishable from that of a typewriter; they can also boldface to highlight headings and other captions. This gives an appearance that is very similar to typesetting with less expense. Some word-processing services now offer laser printing, which presents the option of a variety of type styles. Many of these services can store your resume on a file in a computer, so that updates can be made at a reasonable price.

If you have access to a good typewriter it can be cost-effective to type your own originals, retype them whenever necessary, and have them copied by a copy center. These resumes should be printed by the offset method, not run through a Xerox machine. Even though some of the most sophisticated copiers make excellent copies, offset printing will give you completely clean, absolutely consistent copy, and the difference in price on 100 copies is negligible.

If you have a computer, you can run off your own originals, and keep your resume on file for easy updating. Be sure your printer is capable of turning out high-quality originals. If you are thinking about buying a computer, this should be a major consideration. Letter quality printers generally cost $100 to $300 more than dot matrix printers, but if you intend to use the computer for your resumes and cover letters, a good printer is well worth the extra investment. Boldfacing, which can improve the overall appearance of your resume, is possible with almost any printer and word-processing software.

Resumes should always be trimmed to 8×10 size sheets. To accommodate this, the layout of the resume must fall within an 8×10 inch space. An 8×10 resume is essential—otherwise it will overlap your photo and look unprofessional.

MAILING PICTURE/RESUMES

Now that you have 100 newly composed, attractive, cleanly offset-printed resumes, it is time to put them to work. It is important to organize a system of sending out resumes with cover letters and postcards on a regular basis to a targeted group of theaters, casting directors, and agents. Letters should look businesslike and professional while reflecting something of yourself.

You can select your targets from such sources as *Back Stage*, the *Ross Reports*, the *New York Casting & Survival Guide*, and other lists. There are also a number of sources that provide mailing lists on peel-off labels. If you have your own computer, you can put lists from any of these sources into your data base and run off labels to targeted groups at given times, such as regional theaters in the late summer, or summer stock theaters in March. If you are working with a typewriter, labels can still save you the time of hand-addressing each envelope. Lists are available for casting directors in every area of theater, modeling, film and TV, theaters with summer and winter seasons, talent agents, and personal managers—just about anyone you would ever want to send a copy of your picture/resume.

MAILING OPTIONS

Sending out picture/resumes and postcards, keeping track of who should get them, and when and how often, can become an organizational nightmare and a stumbling block in a performer's career. There are, fortunately, alternatives. Shakespeare Theatrical Mailing Service in New York City (they serve performers anywhere in the country), for example, was created to help actors with this process. This company will send out letters, picture/resumes, flyers, or whatever a client wishes, to any number of names in their extensive up-to-date data bank. Prices vary, depending on the number of pieces sent out and the frequency of mailings.

Choosing between the "do-it-yourself" approach or the "hiring a mailing service" option should be done after you have assessed your finances and organizational capabilities. The total cost of preparing your own cover letter and sending it out to a list you have compiled will certainly be less than hiring a service to do mailings for you. The question to be dealt with is *will you actually do it?* Money spent to get your resumes out in an orderly, timely fashion is money well-spent, money that is working for your career. Saving money is nice, even commendable, but you are not accomplishing anything by saving that money if your picture/resumes are sitting at home on a shelf.

Getting the Right Picture

by Toni Reinhold

One of the most effective marketing tools an actor can use is a headshot. Generally accompanied by a resume, a headshot is your proxy at almost all initial meetings with agents, producers, casting directors, and other key industry professionals.

No one closes the door on a headshot, puts it on hold for half an hour, fails to return its phone calls, or tells it to go away. A headshot sent by mail usually reaches its target swiftly and at that point either fulfills its mission—which is to create so much interest that you are asked to appear in the flesh—or fails so miserably that the only file it reaches is the circular one under someone's desk.

A headshot is one of the few things over which an actor has so much control. You decide when to have it taken and by whom, how much you are willing to pay for it, if the quality is acceptable, how soon you need it, what image you wish to project through it, the kind of work you want to attract with it, and to whom it will be sent.

Having a headshot done is one of the first things you should do to get your career rolling. Because a headshot must deliver a very personal message about you, you must choose a photographer who is right for you—someone who can best capture your individual message on film in the most effective way.

Choosing the right photographer is not something you can do with a random phone call. Many photographers offer headshot services and are qualified to take attractive, usable photos. Most professionals will agree that good chemistry must exist between actor and photographer and that the quality of the photographer's work must be A-1. However, more than personality and art enter into this picture. Other factors must be considered. Prices and services included in photographers' fees vary greatly and must be weighed when you make your decision. You should also have an idea of the image you want to present in your headshots and this must be communicated to photographers. You need someone who can relate to you and what you are trying to achieve at this stage of your career.

Many photographers understand the needs of performers and are willing to do what is necessary to produce exciting, effective headshots. There are those, however, who offer little more than a few rolls of exposed film. As New York-based photographer Bruce Cahn has noted, "There is a growing tendency for photographers to give the actor exposed rolls of film rather than pictures. This is unfairly taking advantage of the performer. Lab procedures and development times vary so widely that to get a quality image this way, you have to be lucky. And if the picture is sloppily done, every party involved gets to lay the blame elsewhere."

Photographer Ron Berlin distributes printed lists to his prospective New York City customers with information about headshots, fees, and services, along with do's and don'ts that contribute to the success or failure of a photo shoot. Berlin says he encourages potential clients to read his list and to follow up by asking questions. "You must ask questions of every photographer you interview," he says. "The selection process should not only be fun, but part of educating yourself as an actor. I spend 40 minutes with potential clients when they first come into my studio because there are things they need to talk about, such as posing techniques and lighting. There are subtle differences among pictures that contribute to the overall good appearance of a photograph. You want to have as many of those differences working in your favor as possible. The whole headshot event is designed to produce an advertising photograph and the person in the picture is the product being promoted. Once you see the project that way, the question becomes, What am I advertising? What am I promoting? Just take it from there."

Most photographers feel that it is important to achieve a good rapport with a client. "When actors are being photographed for a headshot, they are letting their hair down and unmasking themselves, or at the very least presenting a different set of masks. They should feel comfortable about doing that," Ron Berlin stresses. "I tell my clients that I can fake almost anything in a photo except a sense of comfort. Photographers shoot in different styles, but I don't think any of us can fake someone looking relaxed and forthright."

THE PORTFOLIO—THE PHOTOGRAPHER'S PRIDE AND JOY

You should ask to see the portfolio of each photographer you interview because it reveals the quality of a person's work. "Seeing portfolios is important," says photographer Art Murphy, who works in New York and Philadelphia. "My portfolio, for example, shows the success I've had with other actors and gives a client something to talk about while deciding whether or not we can work together."

New York-based photographer Nick Granito says variety is important in a portfolio. "Is the photographer equally good with men and women?" asks Granito. "Are you getting a commercial and theatrical shot in one session? Commercial shots are brighter, whereas those used for opera or stage are more dramatically lit. Is the photographer able to use lighting to show contouring on the face? Many photographers use one type of flat bright lighting which does not show 'layers' of personality. Agents want to see as many facets of the actor's personality as possible. Does the photographer employ a variety of angles to complement all faces? We all have a better side. Is the photographer equally adept with older and younger types?"

"If properly lit," Granito continues, "the print should show details of the face, rather than washing them out. Are you able to see highlights in the hair? Can you distinguish a blonde from a redhead? Is the retouching moderate or is it plastic surgery? Do the eyes say something or are they vacant? Is the smile warm, engaging, and energetic as opposed to tense, posed or tentative? Do the pictures look like the person in real life? High-fashion glamour shots with makeup and hair styles not worn on a daily basis are useless if you can't generate that look with an hour's notice."

THE PHOTOGRAPHIC IMAGE

We each have a certain image of ourselves which may or may not coincide with the one we actually project. To be effective, your headshot should reflect the way you look to others. It is important, therefore, to have a realistic idea of the image you want to project before interviewing photographers.

"Not everyone should go for a glamour shot," says New York photographer Ralph

Lewin, "but everyone wants to look so much better in their photos than they do in real life. You should go for a headshot that reflects what you are. Are you a character type? You should know this. I like to discuss what clients want and know what kind of work they are going after. Many people want to look glamorous in their photos, then they go out for glamour parts and don't get them because they don't look like the person in the photo," says Lewin. "I discuss image and type with clients and tell them if I think they would be better off going for something else. When a photographer has been doing this work for a long time, they develop a good idea of things like this."

Realism also scores high with casting directors and agents, many of whom are aware of how much work goes into finding the right photographer and getting a good headshot.

"Unless you are well-schooled in this business, picking a photographer is a tough choice for an actor or actress," says Vicky Vittes, head of the commercial print department at the Carson Adler Agency in New York City. "I feel one of the reasons people have agents is so the agents can recommend photographers. But it's kind of a Catch-22. You can't get in to see an agent unless you have a good picture, but it's hard to get a good picture if you don't have someone recommending the right photographers. I feel that as an agent one of my functions is to look at a person, consider their personality, and then recommend a photographer."

Vittes offers these suggestions to help you narrow down the market. "The most important thing about a headshot is that it should look like you. Don't get a 'signature' picture—a headshot about the photographer's style and not a headshot about what you really look like. If you are a character type, don't get a glitzy, glamorous headshot that is airbrushed to extremes, washed out, and doesn't look anything like you. I also look for clarity in the photo, clean lines, good backlighting, and good contrast. And I want to see some life, something going on behind the eyes. I don't like dead, boring smiling shots."

Jerry Saviola, casting director at Grey Advertising in New York City, says he and his colleagues are also looking for the "real thing." "I look for a headshot that is accurate and honest—and all I mean by honest is that it isn't too artificially posed," he notes. "Sometimes what is attractive is just an expression on the face. It's very important that the picture look like the person. That sounds like not a lot to ask for, but we get pictures that look nothing like the person."

PHOTOGRAPHERS SURVEY

The 27 questions below are from a survey of 36 photographers in the New York City area, conducted by *Back Stage*. The answers to the questions help provide an overview of the range of prices, contents of headshot packages, costs and related services that are generally available. These questions also supply you with a ready-made checklist to be used when you begin your search for a photographer.

How much do you charge for a headshot photo session?
Prices were from $150 to $300 on the average though some photographers quoted a bottom and a top figure. The bottom/top figures ranged from $50 to $120 to $350 to $655. One photo studio offers a $65 package that included 72 color shots, chrome transparencies, internegs, and an 8×10 color enlargement. At least one photographer charges $25 more for women's headshots, while another charges $300 for single style photos and $350 for two styles of photos, such as commercial and theatrical.

Many photographers base their prices on the number of rolls of film included in the shoot and then add extra charges for additional rolls of film. These charges vary from $5 to $50 per roll. Some photographers said they will shoot extra film at no additional charge if it is warranted. Tax may or may not be included in the price.

How much time do you allocate for each session?
This depends on a variety of factors, including how many rolls of film are shot, how many changes of clothing are allowed, and how much time is put into lighting. Answers varied from one to three hours for 72 shots, with a typical session lasting about two hours. While some photographers stated that a session could last as little as 45 minutes, most said they would give as much time as necessary. There are photographers who book only two shoots a day so clients have time to comfortably work their way through a session. Some photographers take Polaroid photos before each pose to check lighting, hair, and makeup, and this can add on time.

How many shots are included?
A typical photo session can include anywhere from 72 to 180 shots. Sometimes the number depends on how many shots a client wants. The number of shots may also vary according to the size of film used.

The term *format* refers to the size of film. There is 35mm format and 120 format, which is the next size up from 35mm. Film in 120 format comes with several numbers of exposures per roll, such as 8, 10, 12 or 16. This format offers fewer shots per roll than 35mm, and sometimes as few as 40 shots in a session are taken on this size film. This is an important distinction to make, since the price of a session may be greatly increased if a client wants 72 frames shot on 120-size film. Because of the difference in clarity offered by this size film (many photographers feel that larger format film results in better quality pictures), some photographers suggest clients have photos taken on both 35mm and 120 format film during the same session. When photographers start talking rolls of film, you should be asking the number of shots per roll.

Does the session include negatives and prints in one price? Do you give negatives to your clients?
About half the photographers who answered said negs are included. One photographer said each sitting includes 72 poses no matter what size film a client chooses. Almost all photographers said blowups are included in their fees. Those photographers who keep the negatives say it is their way of controlling the quality of reproductions. Some say it is also a way to bring clients back when they want prints from a particular shoot.

If negatives are not included, how much do you charge a client to purchase them?
Many photographers said they will not sell negatives. Photographers who said they would sell negatives separately to their clients cited these prices: $30 per roll; $30 to $80 per shoot; $25 for headshot negatives or more if the shoot is more complex. Some photographers double their fees when negatives are included. For example, a $175 photo session would be increased to $350 if the negatives were included.

Do you have a portfolio an actor can see?
All photographers answered yes to this question. Several noted that they also have samples of reproductions from sittings and composites, Polaroids, "before" and

"after" retouched photos, original and reproduced 8 × 10s, postcards, and contact sheets.

Are hair and makeup included in your fee?

Most photographers said no, but there are those who include makeup in their fee. Several said they assist in makeup and hair styling. Some photographers say that special makeup techniques are needed for black and white photos. While not all photographers agreed with this, many said they do advise clients to have makeup professionally applied for the shoot. Most photographers agreed that men should not use makeup for a photo session, and advise clients to wear their hair as it is normally worn so photos will look realistic.

If hair and makeup are not included, do you provide these services for an additional fee? How much? If not, do you recommend a hairdresser/ makeup artist?

The majority of photographers said they will recommend someone. Flat fees cited for hair and makeup ranged from $40 to $100, with an average price of $70. Fees for makeup ranged from $25 to $65, with an average price of $40. Flat fees for hair ranged from $45 to $50. Some photographers have a hairstylist/makeup artist on staff who works with clients for an additional fee.

Do you airbrush? Retouch? How much does this cost?

Airbrushing is used to soften or correct large areas of a photo. Retouching is generally used for smaller areas, such as dark circles under eyes. Most photographers only offer retouching. Those who do not perform either of these services usually refer clients to labs or individuals who specialize in such work. Some photographers report that complete retouching is included in their headshot fees but most say there is an additional airbrushing/retouching charge ranging from an hourly rate of $25 to $50 to a flat rate of $35 per headshot. Several respondents said their fee includes a minimal touchup, but some photographers said you can get a "full retouch" for as little as $10.

What should a man or woman bring to a photo session to be fully prepared?

Almost all photographers who were queried said they discuss this with clients prior to a session. Although answers varied, many cited these things: an average of four changes of clothing with an emphasis on shirts, tops, and jackets; records or tapes that will help you relax; makeup (including a base for women); hair brush and accessories; props as discussed including glasses, hats, hair clips; clean face, clean hair, and a good haircut; understated jewelry including an assortment of earrings; a positive attitude; energy; a sense of humor; curling iron; clean-shaven men should shave closely beforehand and bring shaving gear; self-confidence and a favorite picture of yourself. Photographers warn against clothing that detracts from the face, and white or black garments. Many suggested pastel or rich colors.

"Having your hair cut before a shoot is the worst thing you can do," says photographer Marie Ruggiero. "The hair never looks right. It always looks best a week to 10 days after a cut. And actors and actresses make a mistake by coming in with a fixed idea of the pose they want. They pose for hours figuring it out. If you want natural pictures, it's the worst thing to do. It's up to the photographer to catch that special pose."

How soon after the photo session do you provide proofs?
These are contact sheets from which photos are selected for enlargement. Delivery time to the client varies from one day to a week.

Do you make prints for your clients or must they have them made by an outside vendor? Do you recommend someone?
Most of the photographers in the survey said they make their own enlargements. Some of them responded that they would recommend a lab for volume reproductions.

If you make prints, how soon after proofs are reviewed will a client have them?
Answers ranged from one day to two weeks, and in one instance as little as one and a half hours. Several photographers offer rush service, but they usually charge extra for this.

Do you do location shoots, studio shoots, or both?
Many photographers do both, although one-fourth of those interviewed said they do only studio work.

Do you charge extra for location shoots?
Most photographers charge extra for location shoots. Additional charges ranged from traveling expenses to a general surcharge of $75. Extra costs could run as high as 20 percent of the session fee, or could consist of a $50 travel fee. Some photographers base extra charges upon the whereabouts of the location or the time involved.

Do you provide studio sets for composites?
The majority of the photographers responded yes to this question, although some offer only limited props and sets. There can be an extra charge for the use of sets, but this is not usual.

How far in advance must a photo session be booked?
Responses varied from two days to three weeks. Some photographers did not specify a time limit, while others stated that they would work with emergencies and rush bookings up to the day of the session.

Do you require a deposit at the time the session is booked? How much?
Responses were fairly evenly divided, with deposit requirements ranging from $50 to 50 percent of the photo session price. Deposits may also be demanded for weekend, evening, or holiday shoots.

How far in advance of a session can a person cancel? Do you charge a cancellation fee?
Answers varied from the day of the session to three days' notice; most photographers said they would appreciate a minimum of one day's notice. The majority of photographers said they do not charge a cancellation fee.

Do you refund the deposit or reshoot if a person is unhappy with the results of the shoot?
Although a few photographers did not specify a policy regarding this, most said they would reshoot. Some charge a fee for this, some do not. Generally, photographers are not willing to issue a refund, but it is rare to encounter one who will neither reshoot nor issue a refund. Some photographers replied that they would only con-

sider a reshoot if a client's unhappiness is caused by technical problems or if they had made mistakes.

How many original shots and prints of each are included in your photo session fee?
Answers varied greatly on this question although a good percentage of photographers surveyed set a standard that includes two 8×10 prints—one each of two poses. Some photographers do not include any prints in their price although this is not usual. Others said the number of enlargements included varied with the number of rolls of film shot.

How much do you charge for each additional original shot a person wants printed and how many prints are included for that charge?
Prices range from $6 to $45 and all were for single enlargements. Photographers who charge $30 to $45 per enlargement stated that prices include retouching.

Do you provide volume reproductions? How much do you charge for 50? 100? 500?
Most photographers said they do not provide volume prints. Among those who do, these prices were cited: $20 to $35 per 50, $34 to $55 per 100, $150 to $230 per 500; $38 per 25, $50 per 50, $62 per 100 with a borderless 8×10 negative; $114.50 per 500 plus name on photo free; $95 per 100, $150 per 100 color prints.

Do you print postcards? How much do you charge for 50? 100? 500?
Most photographers were not equipped to do postcards. Those who were equipped quoted the following prices: $27 per 100, $110 per 500; $72 per 200 with negative; $64.50 for 1000, and for color work as much as $150 per 100.

Do you also photograph children? Are your fees different for these sessions? What are they?
Almost all respondents said yes to this question and more than half of these charge the same for children as they do for adults. Most of those whose prices differ charge less for photographing children. Prices range from $65 to $250, and some photographers have a sliding scale based on a child's age. Generally, children's packages vary as widely as adults.

Do you offer clients a discount if they return for updated photos? How much?
Close to half the photographers surveyed do not offer such a discount. When it is given it ranges from $25 off to 10 to 25 percent off the session fee to charging an "old fee" rather than an updated one.

How often should headshots be updated?
All photographers agreed that children's photos should be updated annually. There was little agreement on how often adults should have new photos taken, although on the average photographers thought it should be done every two years. The one point on which they all agreed is that if your look changes drastically, photos should be updated as soon as possible.

Once you've selected a photographer, there are a few other considerations that will help to ensure a good headshot. Do not cut corners just to keep your costs down.

Ms. Vittes offers this advice: "Sometimes when women are having their headshots taken for the first time, especially if they are new in the business, they want to save a little money and think they will take the easy route and do their own hair and make-up. That's a big no-no. Hire a stylist. I don't know of any commercial photographer who doesn't work with a stylist on the set or have somebody they recommend."

Trends also affect the way your headshot should look. Vittes notes, for example, that from the '60s to the late '70s and early '80s, glossies were "in." "Now," she points out, "a matte finish is preferred. I think it looks cleaner and has a more tangible texture. But as far as the look of an actor goes, that depends on who the actor is and on his or her type."

Vittes recommends a cautious approach in the search for a photographer. "Just remember to be very selective," she says. "It's a buyers' market and you can choose whom you want. You have the right to go to every photographer you think you might be interested in. You have the right to look at their books. You have the right to say, 'I want to think about it.' You don't have to make a decision on the spot and you should not feel pressured into making a decision right away. Take your time and make sure you are making the right choice. Don't go to somebody who has been recommended by other actors if you don't feel comfortable with them. If you don't feel comfortable with the photographer you are not going to get a good session. The most important thing is to get the best shot you can."

Don't overlook decisions that are related to your headshots either, such as having postcards printed. Vittes suggests calling agents and asking if they want to receive postcards, because some, like her, do not. "I think postcards serve a purpose for people who cast soap extras, for example, to remind them that you are around," says Vittes. "I don't like postcards. If I'm going to work with you, I'm going to work with you. I don't need to be reminded that you're around. There are other agents who don't like them either. A casting agency here was receiving postcards every week from an actor. He was never called by the agency—a good indication of whether or not your cards are working—but he kept sending postcards. The agency saved all the cards for a year, and then called the actor and said, 'Your postcards are ready, You can pick them up now.' You have to be able to take a clue! It's perfectly acceptable to call an agency and ask if you should send periodic postcards."

These guidelines should help you to locate the best photographers in town and then narrow down the possibilities to the one who is right for you. Choosing a photographer can be time consuming because of the many factors which should enter into your decision. You will discover, however, that it is time well spent on your career when the result of your photo shoot is an effective, attractive headshot that should help you get work.

Temporary Services

by Andrea Wolper

Let's face it: nobody becomes a performer because they long to type and file; however, many performing artists work as temporary office workers while pursuing theatrical careers; it is an ideal way to keep bills from accumulating into mountains of unpaid debts between engagements. In fact, working temp can be as near to perfect a solution to the problem of remaining solvent while chasing artistic dreams as you're likely to find. If you know how to type, or take dictation, or use a computer or some other type of office equipment, you can put these skills to good use as a temporary worker. The financial stability gained working as a "temp" can go a long way toward nurturing the spirit of the struggling actor who is out there making the rounds, or standing in an audition line.

Perhaps the best reason for relying on temporary office employment is the flexible time schedule that it offers. For performing arts people, this is an invaluable commodity. Got an audition on Monday, Commercial class on Wednesday? Okay, work Tuesday, Thursday, and Friday. Rehearsing a show during the day? Fine—you can make some extra money doing word processing at night or on weekends. Touring for a few weeks, a couple of months, or more? No problem—you can go back to work as soon as you're ready. Need some extra money for new headshots? Work full-time this month and ease up a little the next.

As a temporary employee you work when you want to work, and if you keep your skills up-to-date you shouldn't have a problem getting assignments. Just remember that when you do accept a job, whether it is for one day, one week, or one month, you will be expected to uphold your commitment to complete that assignment.

Along with reasonable-to-excellent hourly wages for skilled workers, quite a few temp services offer a number of bonuses and benefits including insurance packages, child-care reimbursement, and paid vacations and holidays. But don't start packing just yet—if you're not working on a nearly full-time basis, you probably won't qualify for these extras.

If, on the other hand, you're planning to work pretty steadily (three or more days a week, every week), be sure to sign up with a service that offers the benefits you need. There are services that offer referral bonuses, free training to upgrade skills, paid vacations and holidays. Some offer medical and/or dental insurance plans, life insurance, even profit-sharing and credit unions. Whenever you interview at a temporary service, ask about benefits and bonuses. Find out exactly how many hours you'll have to log to become eligible, and how to take advantage of what's offered once you do.

Even if you don't plan to work often enough to take advantage of the variety of bonuses and benefits, chances are you'll find plenty of other advantages to working as a temp. You may simply enjoy the freedom of not being tied to a regular schedule, of remaining detached from corporation politics, or you may find it stimulating to see new walls and new faces when you feel it's time to move on.

To get yourself started, choose the two or three or four services that seem to be right for you. Talk to friends and fellow artists who've done temp work and ask them to recommend good services. Once you've made your choices, telephone those companies and find out when they interview applicants. Some will give you an appointment; many have specified open hours. Next, put on your best audition or interview outfit; you're going to be playing the role of office worker or trade show representative for the time being, so dress the part. You'll want to make the best impression you can on the folks who are going to be thinking of you for jobs.

If you have a job resume, take it with you to the interview, even though you'll probably be asked to fill out an application. Be prepared to be interviewed and to supply checkable references. (Some services check references, some don't.) If you go to the service early in the day, you just might be offered work then and there. You'll probably be tested for any skills you claim to have, such as typing, shorthand, or word processing. Even if you're only qualified to work as a clerk, you may be tested for math and alphabetization ability. Don't be anxious about the tests. Although expectations differ from service to service, they will try to place you if you have any aptitude at all for the requirements of a particular job.

When you register for work be sure to find out exactly what is required of you regarding general procedure. Are you expected to phone that service more than once a day? If you don't understand the procedure you could lose out on jobs.

WORDS ON WORD PROCESSING

To learn word processing or not to learn—that is the question. And a good reason for learning word processing is that insofar as temporary office employment is concerned, word processing is where the money is. Anyone who can type reasonably well can learn word processing. The most convenient way to learn is to qualify for the free training that some temporary services offer, or to be lucky enough to be trained at an office where you are working. But if you're considering paying for training, don't expect to earn top dollars right away. It may take a while to acquire the experience that will earn you a spot as a "regular" with a temp service. "Most clients prefer people with work experience," according to Richard Ackerman of Eastern Office Temps, "but things are changing now. It's true there are some machines on which prior experience is necessary. In other cases, however, if our employees have good training or experience on one software, we may be able to send them out to work on others." Because a working knowledge of one type of computer doesn't translate to that of another in the way typing on a Silver-Reed means you can just as easily use a Brother or an Olivetti, some explanation of the unfamiliar machinery is always necessary. If you haven't learned word processing on one of the more popular machines, you may be out of luck. Some temp services, like FreelancersLegal in New York City, have a training room stocked with various types of software. At this company, employees who have solid experience with one computer can train themselves to use another at a charge of only $5 an hour.

To a typist, breaking word processing might seem as difficult as getting a union card—it can look darn near impossible. But have faith, new word processing operators enter the job market every day and if you're determined, you can too.

Whether you're a word processing operator, a messenger, proofreader, paralegal professional, caterer-waiter, telemarketer, stenographer, or the best little product demonstrator that ever lived, there's a temporary job out there that has your name on it. So what if you can't type—you can pick up a phone and take a message, can't you? So you haven't the faintest idea what CRT means and you never heard of key punch; that's okay—maybe you can be a fragrance model, a customer service representative, a researcher, product demonstrator, or inventory clerk. Some temporary services even send out make-up artists, specialty acts, and industrial workers. At the very least, with all that experience you've had sending out pictures and resumes, you're certainly qualified to stuff envelopes! The bottom line is that if you're reliable, responsible, can dress yourself neatly, and are personable and reasonably articulate, you should be able to find a temp service that will be able to place you.

Telephone Answering Services

by Toni Reinhold

There are many advantages to hiring a telephone answering service. The most obvious one, of course, is that calls are taken for you when you are not at home. Additionally, there is the personal interaction that occurs between an answering service and your callers. Many agents and casting directors prefer to leave a message with a service rather than on an answering machine tape. Also, you can give out the answering service number instead of your home number when it is prudent to do so. Then there are such benefits as wake-up calls, and the secretarial-type calls a service can make for you. For example, if you are too busy to make a certain call, say to cancel a doctor's appointment, an answering service can do it for you. But all such advantages are of little value if your service is not a reliable one.

When you call for information about an answering service, ask some basic questions about services and costs. You can get a "feel" for what the service is like over the phone. If the people you talk to are evasive about the services they offer, be wary about using the company. You are looking for people who are communicative and responsive, who give you a sense that their company is well-organized, responsible, and well-run. If the operators take forever to pick up the phone and then put you on hold for a long time, you had better look elsewhere for your service.

Find out if the service you are interested in is open 24 hours a day, seven days a week, including holidays. Also, call the Better Business Bureau and ask if any complaints have been lodged against this service. If possible, visit the service to see what kind of an operation it is. Is it operating in someone's kitchen with two phones or is it located in a legitimate office with a full staff? Make sure the service is theatrically oriented. You need an answering service that is cognizant of the realities of the entertainment industry and that understands the importance of a call from an agent, director, or producer. Finally, ascertain that *your* service uses live operators around the clock, and not an answering machine after a certain hour.

AN ANSWERING SERVICE SURVEY

Since phone calls and correct messages are so vital to performers, *Back Stage* surveyed 14 New York theatrical answering services to find out what kind of services are typically offered, and how much they cost. These companies have been in business from five to 36 years. Here is a summary of the questions asked in the survey.

Do you offer a 24-hour service?
Only two of the 14 services did not. They operate Monday through Friday from 10 A.M. to 6 P.M.

Is your service open seven days a week?
Most said yes, but one service noted that it is closed on Thanksgiving, Christmas and New Year's Day.

Do you offer call forwarding?
All but one company offers this service.

What is the fee for using your number? a client's number?
Fees for using the service number ranged from $6 a month for an eight-hour service (10 A.M. to 6 P.M.), to $25 a month for a 24-hour service. Fees for picking up on a client's number (direct pick-up) ranged from $30 per month for eight-hour service to $85 per month for 24-hour service.

Do clients use your number, their own or both?
Eight of the services said that clients may use the service number or their own. The remaining six services offer only the use of their own number.

Do you require a deposit?
Nine of the 14 services require a deposit of one to two months.

What is the initial cash outlay?
Initial cost can run as high as $50 when the deposit is included.

Do you ask clients to sign a contract?
All said no.

Do you offer mail services? If so, is there an extra charge for this service?
All but one of the services offer mail pick-up and forwarding. Fees ranged from an additional $2 per month to $10 per month.

Do you have weekly, monthly, or yearly rates?
Three of the services polled offer only monthly rates. The rest offer monthly and yearly rates. Some services offer special rates. For example, if you pay for 11 months, you get the 12th month free or by paying a year in advance, you receive two free months of service. Discounted quarterly, and semiannual rates are also offered.

Do you offer any free months to your clients?
Six respondents said no. Some of the free monthly offerings were: two free months when a client joins a service through an advertisement; one free month to a client who recommends a new client; one free month for paying a year in advance; one free month for making a quarterly payment at the time you sign up and a free month every semi-annual payment.

Do you make wake-up calls? Is there an extra fee for this service?
All but one service said they make wake-up calls. Fees ranged from 25 cents to 50 cents per call.

What are the advantages of subscribing to a telephone answering service instead of having a home answering machine?
The following advantages were cited: no hang-ups, personalized live phone voice, no machine breakdowns, screening of calls, security of not circulating your private number, constant tracing, out-of-town coverage, and wake-up calls.

Do you offer limited or unlimited calls? If calls are limited, what are the conditions?

Some services offer limited and unlimited calls depending upon the type of service to which customers subscribe. For example, one service limits call-forwarding to 100 calls a month, but calls coming in on the service's number are unlimited. One service offers unlimited calls but charges extra for long personal messages. Another service offers unlimited calls to freelance professional customers and another offers unlimited calls "within reason." Still another service offers 65 messages a month free and charges 25 cents for each additional message.

Do you offer call tracing? If so, is there an extra fee for this?

All of the services offer call tracing (locating a client during the day to give them important messages). Prices ranged from free to 25 to 40 cents per call.

Do you offer on-tour coverage?

Almost all replied yes. Some services have a toll-free number on which clients may call when they are out of town. One service charges a fee for use of this number. Some services will also call their clients, person-to-person collect.

Do you offer beeping?
If so, is there an additional charge for this service?

All but two services will beep their clients. There may be an additional fee for this service, ranging from 30 to 50 cents per beep.

Do you have conference room or office space available?

Only five services responded yes to this question, but they did not stipulate fees.

New York's Performing Arts Book Stores

by Victor Gluck

New York is a city that has everything. It should come as no surprise that if you can't find a book in this city it probably can't be found anywhere. In New York's performing arts book stores you can locate a score for a Kurt Weill musical, the labanotation for a ballet by Balanchine, the collected plays of Eugene O'Neill, and Bette Davis's first autobiography. In addition, you can find *Playbills*, souvenir programs, plays on record, original drawings for set designs, manuscript copies of unpublished plays, first editions, foreign imports, and theater, film, and dance annuals.

Various book stores have larger collections of special categories or a staff member who is a respected authority on a particular subject. Applause Theater Books can certainly boast the largest selection of modern British plays. However, if you're looking for an acting edition of a script, your best bet might be to go immediately to Samuel French, Inc. or the Dramatists' Play Service, which boast that they have their complete in-print catalogues available. The archives of such establishments are not to be forgotten either. Some used book stores, such as the Gotham Book Mart, have shelves devoted to important authors such as Tennessee Williams, Shaw, and Shakespeare. Targeting your need to the right book store is an art in itself.

Whether as a service to their customers or as a publicity idea, many stores offer interesting and unusual activities. Book signing parties, readings by authors of their latest books, demonstrations, classes, and play readings are some of the possible offerings. In addition, many book stores have mailing lists of free catalogues, publications, or sale items.

Whatever your interest as a performer, you should be able to track down the information you need somewhere in the vast array of New York's performing arts book shops.

New York's Performing Arts Book Stores

DANCE

THE BALLET SHOP
1887 Broadway
New York, NY 10023
(212) 581-7990

CAPEZIO DANCE/
THEATRE SHOP
755 Seventh Ave., 2nd fl.
New York, NY 10019
(212) 245-2130

CAPEZIO EAST
136 E. 61st St.
New York, NY 10021
(212) 758-8833

CAPEZIO AT STEPS
2121 Broadway
New York, NY 10023
(212) 799-7774

DANCE NOTATION
BUREAU BOOKSTORE
Princeton Book Company
P.O. Box 109
Princeton, NJ 08540
(609) 737-8177

TAFFY'S OF NEW YORK,
INC.
1776 Broadway, 2nd fl.
New York, NY 10019
(212) 586-5140

FILM

APPLAUSE CINEMA
BOOKS
100 W. 67th St.
New York, NY 10023
(212) 787-8858

JERRY OHLINGER'S
MOVIE MATERIAL
STORE INC.
242 W. 14th St.
New York, NY 10011
(212) 989-0869

THE SILVER SCREEN
35 E. 28th St.
New York, NY 10016
(212) 679-8130

MUSIC

COLONY RECORD AND
TAPE CENTER
1619 Broadway
New York, NY 10019
(212) 265-2050

LINCOLN SQUARE
MUSIC CO.
1623 Union Port Road
Ste. 109
Bronx, NY 10462
(212) 823-3272

THE MUSIC
EXCHANGE INC.
151 W. 46th St., 10th fl.
New York, NY 10036
(212) 354-5858

MUSIC PEOPLE
720 Seventh Ave.
New York, NY 10036
(212) 869-1155

THE MUSIC STORE AT
CARL FISCHER
62 Cooper Square
New York, NY 10003
(212) 677-0821

THE JOSEPH PATELSON
MUSIC HOUSE
160 W. 56th St.
New York, NY 10019
(212) 582-5840

SCHIRMER MUSIC
61 W. 62nd St.
New York, NY 10023
(212) 541-6236

THEATER

APPLAUSE THEATRE
BOOKS
211 W. 71st St.
New York, NY 10023
(212) 496-7511

THE DRAMA BOOK
SHOP
723 Seventh Ave.
New York, NY
(212) 944-0595

DRAMATISTS PLAY
SERVICE
440 Park Ave. So., 11th fl.
New York, NY 10016
(212) 638-8960

SAMUEL FRENCH INC.
45 W. 25th St., 2nd fl.
New York, NY 10010
(212) 206-8990

SHAKESPEARE AND CO.
BOOKSELLERS
2259 Broadway
New York, NY 10024
(212) 580-7800

RICHARD STODDARD
PERFORMING ARTS
BOOKS
18 E. 16th St., Rm. 202
New York, NY 10003
(212) 645-9576

THEATRE ARTS
BOOK SHOP
405 W. 42nd St.
New York, NY 10036
(212) 564-0402/3

THEATRE
COMMUNICATIONS
GROUP
355 Lexington Ave.
New York, NY 10017
(212) 697-5230

THEATREBOOKS
1600 Broadway, Rm. 312
New York, NY 10019
(212) 757-2834

USED BOOKS

GOTHAM BOOK MART &
GALLERY, INC.
41 W. 47th St.
New York, NY 10036
(212) 719-4448

GRYPHON BOOKSHOPS
(Main Store)
2246 Broadway
New York, NY 10024
(212) 362-0706

GRYPHON RECORD
SHOP
251 W. 72nd St.
New York, NY 10023
(212) 874-1588

STRAND BOOK
STORE INC.
828 Broadway
New York 10003
(212) 473-1452

The Business of Acting

by Don Snell

Show business is a business. Actors, dancers, singers—all are engaged in the *business* of entertainment. That art may also be considered a business is a reality that many performers have difficulty coming to grips with. They feel that what really is important is their art. This may be true. But a little business savvy won't hurt, and may help get *your show* on the road. So take a moment now and then, to give some serious thought to the business side of show business. You may be able to give a boost to your own career.

Show business is a business of name and facial recognition. Recognition is, in fact, one of the most important elements to a successful career. You should establish a professional name as early as possible in your career and stick with it. It is this name that you should register with the trade unions—it is this name that you will want people in the industry to think of when they are searching for talent. And it is important that people associate your name with your face. One way to assure such an association is to get a photograph that looks like you and to use it over and over. Repetition is the key to recognition.

The next order of business is to define your type. In other words, typecast yourself. The easiest way to do this is to look at a *Player's Guide* and look for the *type* that matches you. If you are unsure what type you are, write down all the types listed and then cross off the ones you are not. Try to make an objective appraisal of the *age range* you are right for, too. Performers are cast according to type and age; if you have a clear idea of your type and age range, it will make it easier for you to be categorized and cast.

Now you are ready to tackle the business end of show business. So the first thing to do is to set yourself up as a business. For this purpose, think of yourself not so much as a performing artist, but as someone who provides entertainment services. This will help you "push" or "sell" yourself. Many performers are reluctant to do this, but it is something worth doing. Self-promotion becomes easier when you are thinking in terms of selling a "service," rather than selling "yourself." Next, set up a space for your office. Put all your office "tools" in order. First and foremost of these are your picture and resume—they must, of course, be first-rate. Then you should have a wall calendar, appointment book, Rolodex, file cabinet, file folders, stationery, business cards, telephone, and so on.

Once your office is set up, you are ready to make contact with the industry. But whom do you contact? To find this out, do a market study—talk to working performers, consult directories (these you can find in performing arts bookshops or in the public library in your city) and find out where the work is and who is involved in its development and production. Investigate television, film, theater, radio, commercials, industrials, voice overs—whatever. Then make contact. Apply for the job. Let the powers that be know who you are, what you do, and how to reach you. Approach acquiring an agent in the same way. You only need one agent, but contact 100 agents. Learn to arrange the information and data that you accumulate into a well-organized filing system. If you do so you will discover that the entertainment industry is not as overwhelmingly immense as it appears to be at first glance. In New York City, for example, there are not thousands of television agencies. On the contrary, the figure is closer to 150.

After you have done your market study, set your goals. Every business does this; having goals is like having a crystal ball to look into. Make sure, however, that your goals are realistic and obtainable. Companies assess the market by looking at the sales histories of other companies. You can approach show business in the same way by looking at the performance records of other entertainers. Your goals can be charted in a number of ways: short term, long term, dollars, number of days worked, etc. After you have set your goals, go after them, but keep them flexible and in touch with changing trends in the industry. At the beginning of each week have a "sales meeting" with yourself. Set a goal for the week and strive for it all week long. At the end of each month, monitor your progress with a sales report showing how many auditions you have gone to, how much work you have gotten, and your gross income for the month.

You will have a much better chance of succeeding in show business if you approach it as a business. In the final analysis, of course, success cannot be judged by financial criteria alone, nor by the barometer of fame. Some make it in this business, and some don't, and talent is often enough not the determining factor. What is important is that you use and enjoy your talent and that you give that talent and show business your best shot. With the application of a little business sense, you will be able to create many more opportunities for yourself, and there is greater likelihood that you will succeed.

PART TWO

Training

Shopping for the Right Class

by Fred Silver

Many performers who have had careers in show business came to the realization early on that in order to succeed, they must study hard and become well-schooled in their craft. To have any real chance of success, a performer must be prepared. This means that your specialty, whether it be comedy, drama, dance, music—whatever, must be honed and finely polished. If you are wise you will make certain that if and when that big break does come you will be ready for it. That is why many hopeful performers enroll in acting school. In the entertainment industry, there are all kinds of schools and classes, from accredited to non-accredited, from crash courses in "method" acting to degree courses in theater, from scene study to acting in commercials, from musical theater auditioning to soap opera performing, from lessons taught by charlatans whose main concern is *your* pocketbook, to lessons taught by seasoned professionals who have a very real sense of dedication and responsibility to their students. With so many choices out there, it is not always easy to make a selection. Some of the factors that should be considered in choosing a class are discussed below.

One of the first things to ask is: How large is the class? Also, how often does it meet, and if it is a performance class, will you be given plenty of opportunity to perform?

Large classes are exciting to be in because of the high energy level they generate. Often the reason they are well-populated though, is that they are less expensive. The principal drawback to a large class is that you may not get to perform often. Ideally, a *performance* class should have a maximum of 14 people in it and should last approximately three hours so that everyone has a chance to work.

Does the class provide a safe space? This is a very important question for a performer to ask—safe in this instance meaning psychologically safe. Because performers must feel free to take risks on stage without getting a battered ego. Unfortunately there do exist teachers who delight in humiliating their students. One way to unearth such teachers is to make inquiries among other performers and students in the trade.

One of the best methods of finding out what a teacher is like is to audit a class. Often a fee is charged for auditing, but this is usually applied toward tuition if you decide to take the class. Some teachers, however, do not permit auditing because it threatens the emotional security of those students who are not ready for strangers to see them emotionally naked.

Tuition and class fees vary. Generally the larger the class, the less it will cost. Private teachers sometimes like to be paid in full before each class. Teachers who allow you to stretch payments may also charge you a higher fee.

Schools usually require you to sign a contract that prohibits refunds. Teachers running their own classes will naturally determine their own refund policies. It is always advisable to inquire about refund policies before enrolling in a class.

In summary, a classroom can be an ideal environment for perfecting the skills that you need in order to better yourself as a performer. There you have an opportunity to assimilate what your teacher has to offer and you have a chance to learn from your classmates, both by watching them perform and by performing in front of them.

Acting Schools, Teachers, and Coaches

Below is a listing of stage and commercial acting schools, teachers, and coaches in New York City that were contacted by *Back Stage*. Although the listing is extensive, it is not all-inclusive.

THE ACTING STUDIO INC.
31 W. 21st St.
New York, NY 10010
(212) 206-8608
James Price

THE ACTORS ADVENT LTD.
Esther Brandice, Dir.
212 W. 29th St.
New York, NY 10001
(212) 242-3900

THE ACTORS CORE
At Westbeth
55 Bethune St. (B633)
New York, NY 10014
(212) 633-9560
Nancy Gabor, Janet Merry Doeden

ACTORS IN ADVERTISING
39 W. 19th St.
New York, NY 10011
(212) 645-0030

ACTORS MOVEMENT STUDIO
305 W. 98 St.
New York, NY 10025
(212) 222-5656
Joe Catalano

STELLA ADLER CONSERVATORY OF ACTING
130 W. 56th St.
New York, NY 10019
(212) 246-1195

ELAINE AIKEN
Actors Conservatory, Inc.
750 Eighth Ave., New York, NY
(212) 764-0543

WILLIAM ALDERSON ACTING STUDIO
276 W. 43rd St., 5th fl.
New York, NY 10036
(212) 924-6627

AMARANTH PRODUCTIONS
250 E. 87 St.
New York, NY 10128
(212) 360-7006
Pamela Childs

AMERICAN ACADEMY OF DRAMATIC ARTS
120 Madison Ave.
New York, NY 10016
(212) 686-9244

AMERICAN ENSEMBLE STUDIO THEATRE
Stanley Harrison, Artistic Dir.
Classes held at Minskoff Studios
1515 Broadway, 3rd fl.
New York, NY
(212) 757-6178

THE AMERICAN MIME THEATRE
24 Bond St.
New York, NY 10012
(212) 777-1710

AMERICAN MUSICAL AND DRAMATIC ACADEMY
2109 B'way
New York, NY 10023
(212) 787-5300; 1-800-367-7908

AMERICAN THEATRE OF ACTORS
314 W. 54 St.
New York, NY 10019
(212) 581-3044
James Jennings

MARTIN BARTER
400 W. 40th St.
New York, NY 10036
(212) 541-7600 (S)

JOHN BASIL
(212) 695-5360

JO ANNA BECKSON
Theater 22
54th W. 22 St.
New York, NY 10011
(212) 586-6300

JULIE BOVASSO
c/o Producer's Club Theatre
358 W. 44 St.
New York, NY 10036
(212) 807-8303

JERROLD BRODY
% Producer's Club
358 W. 44 St.
New York, NY 10036
(212) 246-9069

MADELYN J. BURNS SEMINARS
121 W. 27th St.
Suite 503
New York, NY 10001
(212) 627-8880; (212) 245-3332

LEN CALDER
(212) 757-7554

JONATHAN CANTOR
308 W. 30 St.
New York, NY 10001
(212) 594-4638

MICHAEL CHEKHOV STUDIO
14 W. 36th St.
New York, NY 10018
(212) 736-1544

CIRCLE IN THE SQUARE THEATRE
SCHOOL
1633 Broadway
New York, NY 10019
(212) 307-2732

BOB COLLIER'S TV SUCCESS
SEMINARS
1560 Broadway
Suite 509
New York, NY 10036
(212) 719-9636

CONSERVATORY AT CSC
136 East 13 Street
New York, NY 10003
(212) 677-4210

CORNER LOFT STUDIOS
99 University Place
New York, NY 10003
(212) 228-8728
Elaine Gold

THE CREATIVE ACTOR'S WORKSHOP
451 W. 43 St.
New York, NY 10036
(212) 245-1237
Jeffrey Zeiner

DOUBLE IMAGE THEATRE
444 W. 56th St.
New York, NY 10019
(212) 245-2489
Helen Waren Mayer

EN/CORE STAGE COMPANY
326 E. 93rd St., 1B
New York, NY 10128
(212) 410-1906
Kate Harper

ENSEMBLE STUDIO THEATRE
549 W. 52nd St.
New York, NY 10019
(212) 581-9409

WILLIAM ESPER STUDIO
250 Third Ave.
New York, NY 10010
(212) 673-6713

FACES/TONY PANN
251 W. 97 St., 1D
New York, NY 10025
(212) 222-4234

THE FILM ACTING STUDIO
90 Lexington Avenue, Suite 1H
New York, NY 10016
(212) 684-3094
Jeffrey D. Stocker

GENE FRANKEL THEATRE
WORKSHOP INC.
24 Bond St.
New York, NY 10012
(212) 777-1710

GINGER FRIEDMAN
303 E. 83rd St., 15-B
New York, NY 10028
(212) 472-1714

FRED FUSTER
(212) 662-4562

CATHERINE GAFFIGAN
400 W. 43 St.
New York, NY 10036
(212) 594-9871

JULIE GARFIELD
Actors & Directors Lab
412 W. 42nd St.
New York, NY 10036
(212) 581-6439

KATHRYN GATELY AND RICHARD
POOLE
442 W. 42nd St.
New York, NY 10036
(212) 517-1677

FRANK GIRARDEAU
630 Ninth Ave., #910
New York, NY 10036
(212) 279-2174

GILLIEN GOLL
(212) 581-6470

GERRY GOODMAN
318 E. 11th St.
New York, NY 10003
(212) 730-1188

MICHAEL GRAVES
272 W. 77th St., 1-B
New York, NY 10024
(212) 362-0807

MARIA GRECO ASSOCIATES
1261 Broadway
New York, NY 10001
(212) 213-5500

HB STUDIO
Herbert Berghof, Uta Hagen
120 Bank St.
New York, NY 10014
(212) 675-2370

NICO HARTOS
159 W. 53rd St.
New York, NY 10019
(212) 541-8293

PRUDENCE HOLMES
255 W. 108th St.
New York, NY 10025
(212) 864-6525

MICHAEL HOWARD STUDIO
152 W. 25th St.
New York, NY 10001
(212) 645-1525

HUDSON GUILD THEATER
441 W. 26th St.
New York, NY 10001
(212) 760-9836
Geoffrey Sherman, Producing Dir. Steve
Ramay, Assoc. Dir., and head of casting

IZA ITKIN
251 W. 19th St.
New York, NY 10011
(212) 242-5591

CHARLES KAKATSAKIS
202 W. 80th St.
New York, NY 10024
(212) 362-5757

CHARLES KEBBE
38 E. 85th St.
New York, NY 10028
(212) 879-3833

ED KOVENS
780 Greenwich St., 1-P
New York, NY 10014
(212) 929-3125

SARAH LOUISE LAZARUS
210 W. 70th St.
New York, NY 10023
(212) 316-6873

RICHARD LICHTE
(212) 862-7230

RICK LOMBARDO
111 Hicks St., 5-L
Brooklyn, NY 11201
(718) 834-9331

JUDY MAGEE
401 E. 89th St.
New York, NY 10128
(212) 722-5694

MANHATTAN CLASS COMPANY
Nat Horne Theater
442 W. 42nd St.
New York, NY 10036
(212) 239-9033

MANHATTAN PUNCH LINE COMEDY
INSTITUTE
410 W. 42nd St.
New York, NY 10036
(212) 239-0827

VALERIE MANN
(718) 499-6388

ERNIE MARTIN STUDIO THEATER
311 W. 43rd St., 5th fl.
New York, NY 10036
(212) 397-5880

BOB McANDREW WEEKEND
BREAKTHROUGH ACTING
WORKSHOPS
Contact Jonathan Slaff: (212) 924-0496

DOLORES McCULLOUGH
Box 1403
350 Canal St.
New York, NY 10013
(212) 473-8651

MARGO MCKEE'S SOUNDSTAGE
224 W. 49th St.
New York, NY 10019
(212) 747-5436

EDWARD MOOR
(212) 475-3311

SONIA MOORE STUDIO OF THE
THEATRE
485 Park Ave.
New York, NY 10022
(212) 755-5120

MICHAEL MORIARTY
(212) 581-0297

GEORGE MORRISON
220 W. 10th St.
New York, NY 10014
(212) 242-7706

DOUG MOSTON
Drama Project, Box M
151 1st Ave.
New York, NY 10003
(212) 674-1166

NATIONAL SHAKESPEARE
CONSERVATORY
591 B'way
New York, NY 10012
(212) 219-9874; 1-800-472-6667

ANTHONY NAYLOR
Joe Gardner, Bus. Mgr.
310 W. 47th St., #3D
New York, NY 10036
(212) 581-0919

NEIGHBORHOOD PLAYHOUSE
340 E. 54 St.
New York, NY 10022
(212) 688-3770

RUTH NERKEN
(212) 362-5277

NEW CONSERVATORY THEATRE
WORKSHOP
334 Bowery
New York, NY 10012
(212) 777-1855

PANARO WORKSHOP THEATRE CO.
c/o Panaro Production
60 E. 42nd St., Suite 1158
New York, NY 10165

LINDA PERHACH
221 W. 14th St.
New York, NY 10011
(212) 382-3535

TODD PETERS
345 W. 85th St., #27
New York, NY 10024
(212) 873-5836

ELAINE PETRICOFF
80 Perry St.
New York, NY 10014
(212) 463-8121

PLAYWRIGHTS HORIZONS
416 W. 42nd St.
New York, NY 10036
(212) 564-1235

JACK POGGI
880 W. 181 St.
New York, NY 10033
(212) 928-6882/(212) 382-3535

DANIEL POLLACK
890 West End Ave.
New York, NY 10025
(212) 663-8143

RAPP THEATRE COMPANY
220 E. 4th St.
New York, NY 10009
(212) 995-2245; 529-5921

ROBERT RAVAN
For audition/appointment call:
(212) 382-3344

REED & MELSKY
928 Broadway
New York, NY 10010
(212) 505-5000

REED SWEENEY REED
1780 Broadway
Suite 901
New York, NY 10019
(212) 265-8541

RIVERSIDE SHAKESPEARE COMPANY
165 W. 86th St.
New York, NY 10024
(212) 877-6810

JOHN RODDICK
John Houseman Theater
450 W. 42nd St.
New York, NY 10036
(212) 757-6300(S)

DYLAN ROSS
408 W. 48 St.
New York, NY 10036
(212) 757-0716

ROUNDABOUT THEATRE
CONSERVATORY & ENSEMBLE CO.
100 E. 17 St
New York, NY 10003
(212) 420-1360

T. SCHREIBER STUDIO
83 E. 4th St.
New York, NY 10003
(212) 420-1249

MICHAEL SCHULMAN THEATRE
WORKSHOP
94 St. Marks Place
New York, NY 10003
(212) 777-3055

RAPHAEL KELLY SHAKESPEARE
STUDIO
168 E. 89 St.
New York, NY 10128
(212) 289-1392, 840-1234 (S)

BARRY SHAPIRO
% Herman Lipson Cushing
24 W. 25th St.
New York, NY 10010
(212) 807-7706

SANDE SHURIN ACTING STUDIO NY
335 W. 38 St.
New York, NY 10018
(212) 563-2298

ROGER HENDRICKS SIMON STUDIO
(212) JU6-6300

JONATHAN SLAFF
Wynn Handman Studio
Carnegie Hall
887 7th Av., Rm. 808
New York, NY 10019
(212) 924-0496

SUSAN SLAVIN ACTORS & SINGERS
ACADEMY
Carnegie Hall
154 W. 57th St., #912
New York, NY 10019
(212) 582-0321

MELODIE SOMERS
118 E. 28th St.
Suite 304
New York, NY 10016
(212) 481-6490

JOANNA C. SPILLER
8 W. 75 St.
New York, NY 10023
(212) 874-5870

ALICE SPIVAK
"Three of Us" Studios
39 W. 19 St.
New York, NY 10011
(212) 924-0561

JOHN STRASBERG, SUSAN GRACE
COHEN, DAVID BLACK & DAVID
BERRY
Upper West Side locations.
(212) 678-8515

THE LEE STRASBERG THEATRE
INSTITUTE
115 E. 15 St.
New York, NY 10003
(212) 533-5500

THEATRE IN ACTION
46 Walker St.
New York, NY 10013
(212) 431-1317

VIDEO ASSOCIATES
311 W. 43rd St.
Suite 601
New York, NY 10036
(212) 397-0018

JACK WALTZER
5 Minetta St.
New York, NY 10012
(212) 473-7056; 840-1234

STUART WARMFLASH
160 W. 71st St.
New York, NY 10023
(212) 787-1945/541-7600

WEIST-BARRON ACTING FOR
TELEVISION
35 W. 45th St.
New York, NY 10036
(212) 840-7025

JOAN WHITE/NEW YORK THEATRE
SCHOOL, LTD.
153 W. 76 St.
New York, NY 10023
(212) 787-1575

FLORENCE WINSTON
(212) 541-7600

WALT WITCOVER
40 W. 22nd St.
New York, NY 10011
(212) 691-4367

MARK ZELLER
236 W. 78th St.
New York, NY 10024
(212) 362-1736

DANA ZELLER-ALEXIS
236 W. 78th St.
New York, NY 10024
(212) 724-4862

GREG ZITTEL
123 Fourth Ave.
New York, NY 10003
(212) 219-2650

Choosing a College Theater Program

by Jill Charles

A choice faced by many theater students about to enroll in college is whether to work toward a Bachelor of Arts or a Bachelor of Fine Arts degree. Equally important is the decision about what kind of school will best provide the skills demanded by the entertainment industry. What are the advantages to enrollment in a private liberal arts school with a small theater department as opposed to matriculation at a state university with a large theater department? And which of these is right for you?

THE BA VERSUS THE BFA DEGREE

The Bachelor of Arts degree is a broad-based, liberal arts program offering courses in all subjects, but with a major in a particular discipline—in this case, theater. The Bachelor of Fine Arts degree, on the other hand, is a more specialized program offering courses in fewer subjects and a major in a particular area of a discipline, for instance, acting, design, directing, and so on. Generally, you have to go through a selection process, such as an audition or an interview, to get into the BFA program, even if you have already been accepted into the university; also, you may be subjected to periodic reviews of your work in which you must meet a certain standard to remain in the program.

One great advantage to the BA degree is the variety of subjects and ideas offered. Studying a broad range of subjects and different points of view and philosophies can lead you to a deeper understanding of life, literature, drama, and a better-informed approach to a wide variety of theatrical roles. The BFA program, focusing more specifically on theater as it does, is geared more toward helping students acquire professional skills than to the development of a humanistic world view. Even so, a good BFA program will ensure that its students are challenged to think, are well-read, and cognizant of the wider points of view that can be found in the study of the humanities. Obviously, when you graduate and go out into the real world, you're going to need to know more than just theater.

DEPARTMENT SIZE

When you begin to investigate various colleges and universities, you can easily determine the size of a theater department from the school's catalogue. The number of faculty listed may be as few as three in a small college, and as many as 20 or more in a large university. The question to consider is: What is the optimum size of a theater department? Generally, a department that offers a BFA program will be larger than one offering only a BA degree. Even so, for a small BA program, you should be wary if less than five members are on the faculty. A faculty of five is probably the minimum required for a good, solid program; fewer than five means that the courses offered will be limited, and the scope of the department may be narrow. In some cases, where there is lots of input from other departments (like English, Dance or Music), a faculty of four could suffice, but with five on the faculty you can be assured of more than one viewpoint in most areas of study. For example, two of the five are more than likely acting/directing people, so this will guarantee some diversity in approach to acting techniques.

FACULTY AND CURRICULUM

When choosing a college, there are, of course, many factors to consider other than what courses to take, or what size school to go to. For example, it is also important to look at the qualifications of the faculty. The catalogue will list their degrees, but that won't tell the whole story. How many on the faculty have been or still are working professionals? This factor will tell a great deal about a department: a more academically-oriented department will hire MA's and PhD's with the expectation that such a faculty will publish articles, write books, and will be more effective in helping students realize academic goals; a more professionally-oriented department will hire MFA's, and people without higher degrees who have extensive experience as directors or designers with the expectation that such a faculty will continue to work professionally while associated with the college, and will help guide students toward professional careers. The attitude a department takes toward its faculty reflects the attitude it will take toward its students and its philosophy in general. Thus, if you are working toward a degree in theater history or dramatic criticism, find a school with a long list of PhD's on the faculty. *But*, if your main concern is performing or design, or if your goal is to work in the profession as soon as you get out of school, then one of your major considerations should be the amount of practical, professional experience your teachers can bring to the subjects they are teaching.

Many colleges and universities integrate working professionals into their programs by hiring them to teach one or two courses a semester—often top-notch people who are too active to take on heavy teaching loads. A working professional can be invaluable to a college program. The director, designer or actor who can illustrate a theory with real-life, on-stage examples or anecdotes from a recent live production can bring theater to life in a classroom. Teachers who are active in the industry also provide students with connections that will be helpful in their careers.

COURSE EVALUATION

A typical BA program in general theater should offer a pretty thorough grounding in all liberal arts subjects. One of the first courses you will be required to take will be "Theater 101," which is a general introduction to theater studies. Required courses and electives in theater history and dramatic literature will also be listed; some of the latter courses will probably be offered through the English Department.

A good theater department should offer a variety of courses that teach actual theater skills. Obviously, you will find such a variety in the larger colleges, but even a theater department in a small school should offer more than simply "Acting." Those acting courses that are offered should go beyond the two-semester introductory level, should also cover areas like mime and improvisation, and should offer electives on a more advanced level. There should also be courses in the basics of voice and movement technique. In theater departments in large colleges you will probably be given the option of taking specialized advanced courses like stage combat, commedia del l'arte, period style, non-naturalistic acting, and so on; in BFA programs, such courses are not just electives, but are a part of the degree curriculum.

You will also be required to take a stagecraft or scenography course, including a lab period in the scene shop, where you will work on sets. The BA theater major should also include basic design courses (scenic, costume, and lighting), and a course in directing. Electives in stage management, arts management and the like should fill out this program. Most departments make an effort to cover special needs of their programs with independent study, advanced seminar, or various catch-all courses that students can tailor to their own needs.

FACILITIES AND PRODUCTIONS

College theaters have some of the best facilities in the country. It is important to remember, however, that the quality of your experience is going to depend more on the faculty and student body than on the facilities. Knowledge of state-of-the-art facilities may be insufficient if you have not learned how to work with more primitive equipment. Production students who are accustomed to pneumatic tools, a welding shop, a computerized lighting board and a stage full of traps and turntables may be at a total loss when they hit their first Off-Off-Broadway or shoestring summer stock experience. While there is certainly an advantage in the marketplace to being fully aware of and able to work with modern theater technology, there is also much to be said for developing skills that can work miracles with more ingenuity than money.

Look closely at the list of mainstage productions at the college you are interested in. Over the last three or four years has this college presented programs that achieve a balance among contemporary, classical, American, and European theater productions? What about African, Japanese, or Chinese theater? If you see nothing but Shakespeare, Brecht and Chekhov, where will your exposure to current American playwrights or contemporary drama come from? Is there a studio series for more current work? Has this school ever done a musical? Be on the lookout that there does not exist a discrepancy between the type of work you will be doing in college and the type of work you want to do when you leave school. Theater history and dramatic literature courses should cover all areas, and theatrical productions should expose you to all styles.

One indication of whether a school offers a well-rounded program may be the student-generated shows. Find out if there is a student drama organization separate from the department, and if so, investigate the relationship between the two. Does the department support, with money and/or enthusiasm, the student group? Or are the two at odds, and seen as mutually threatening? Sometimes a student group can be born out of genuine frustration with a department's refusal to deal with contemporary or experimental works; of course, such a venture may merely be the product of frustrated students who weren't cast in a departmental show. In a healthy department, there will be a crossover between student- and faculty-generated projects, with each group respecting and supporting the other's work.

Some programs are connected to a professional theater company, which shares the college facilities. This may be a summer company or a regional theater which produces a full season of plays, as does the Huntington Theater Company at Boston University, or the Syracuse Stage at Syracuse University. The benefits of such a connection are obvious—students have a chance to work directly with professionals. The opportunity to observe or take part in a professional company in full swing can give students a very definite advantage when they go out into the theater world later on. Of course, the connection between school and professional company must consist of a real and not just a perceived relationship. Does, in fact, a real interaction exist, or is the professional company a totally separate entity? Even if the latter instance is true, the situation isn't necessarily all bad—you still have the presence of live regional theater right at home; nevertheless, make sure your expectations are going to be met. Again, the two institutions, school and theater company, should be mutually supportive of each other's activities, not jealously protective of their own interests.

AFTER GRADUATION

The choices commonly open to students after graduation are those of going on to graduate-study programs or going out into the business/professional world. BA students are the more likely candidates for graduate study, because they have not necessarily prepared or trained themselves to enter directly into the theater profession. The unwritten contract with a BA student is that the college will provide a well-rounded education in all areas of theater and that the student will acquire a firm foundation for further study in specific areas. BA students who decide to pursue a professional career will probably require additional study at the graduate level, at a conservatory or in private study. Since it is necessary to either audition or present a portfolio to get into a graduate program, it should be part of the unwritten agreement between students and school that audition skills and preparation of portfolios are taught, and that counseling in post-graduate schooling is provided.

The unwritten contract between a college and a BFA student *does* promise that these students will be ready to work upon leaving. Some quotes from school ads are pretty clear about this unstated agreement: "Our Graduates Work . . ."; "Connect with the profession"; "Professional Training for the Actor," and so on. The term "Professional Theater Training Program" has been attached to many BFA as well as graduate programs, and if that is what is claimed and that is what you're buying, then make sure you get it. You should expect a minimum of one full semester course dealing with auditioning, putting together a picture and resume, and learning to approach the *business* of acting. If you're a designer, an equal amount of class time should be devoted to putting together a portfolio, learning about union exams, and so forth. If such a course is not listed, inquire if there are guest seminars, or workshops, that will cover this ground. Enlightened schools, however, will go much farther toward preparing you for the professional world. A school that is connected with a professional theater may enable you to graduate not only with a degree, but with reputable professional credits on your resume. (You may also get a start toward your Equity card, although this is by no means crucial.)

CHECKING OUT THE ALUMNI

The kinds of persons who have graduated from a school can tell you a great deal about that institution. For instance, you may ask: How many recent graduates are now working professionals? Does an alumni "network" exist in a major theater center like New York or Chicago? Have any small alumni theater companies been formed that can offer a showcase for graduates? An alumni network can form the basis for some of your first (and best) contacts in the profession. Yale, Juilliard, Carnegie Mellon, and The Theater School (formerly the Goodman), are all prime examples of institutions that have developed national theater networks that can be invaluable for graduates. Smaller colleges can and should offer a similar commitment that will last beyond graduation day.

A college or university's overall philosophy can be stated at great length in promotional material, but its real values are going to be obvious in every aspect of the department's activities. What you sense is what you are going to get. A school that creates a milieu where students and faculty can be open and curious also has provided an environment where you can nurture and develop your own creativity. When you evaluate the school where you will be spending four crucial years of your life, look for signs of people working hard in an atmosphere of productivity, self-imposed discipline as a means of achieving quality work, and mutual respect among students, teachers, peers, and colleagues.

Student Checklist

Ask the department:
- ☐ Who on the faculty is currently working professionally?

- ☐ Do you bring in guest directors and designers?

- ☐ Do you run a summer theater, or encourage students to work at other summer theaters?

- ☐ Do you give credit for summer theater work, or for internships with professional theaters during the school year?

- ☐ How many productions per semester would I be involved in?

- ☐ Are there any restrictions to freshman participation in productions?

- ☐ Are there any restrictions in the departmental casting policy?

- ☐ Are there opportunities in the department for students to direct, design, or write plays?

- ☐ Does the department encourage students to do projects on their own?

- ☐ Are any student productions budgeted by the department?

- ☐ Are graduates prepared to enter the profession?

- ☐ Does an alumni network exist?

- ☐ What are recent graduates doing now? Which grad schools did they get into? How many are currently working in the profession?

Ask the current students:
- ☐ Is the casting policy fair?

- ☐ Have you been taught how to audition?

- ☐ Do you feel that you've been prepared to get work once you graduate?

- ☐ Which areas do you feel are the strengths of the department? The weaknesses?

- ☐ Are the faculty members accessible to students?

- ☐ Did you get to know the guest artists who were brought in?

- ☐ How many productions have you worked on since you entered the program?

- ☐ If you were looking for colleges now, would you choose to come here again?

Ask the graduates:
- ☐ Are there any areas taught at this school in which you feel you now have to make up for a lack of training?

- ☐ Did you apply to any grad schools? Did you get accepted?

- ☐ Were you well prepared to start your career by the time you graduated?

- ☐ Has it been any advantage to your career that you're an alumni of this particular school?

Then ask yourself:
- ☐ Is this the program that will take me where I want to go in four years time?

- ☐ Can I see myself working well in this environment?

- ☐ Do I sense positive energy and enthusiasm in these people?

Studying Dance in New York

by Phyllis Goldman

New York City is a place where dancers may study, learn to perform with finesse and confidence, and find work. There are schools devoted exclusively to ballet and also commercial studios where classes in all kinds of dance are offered. Awaiting students who attain the high degree of proficiency required are the stages of City Center, Lincoln Center, Broadway, the Joyce Theater and countless other performing venues where dancers may practice their profession.

Some dance schools, notably the schools associated with major ballet companies, are very difficult to get into. The School of American Ballet, which was founded by George Balanchine, and the newly formed American Ballet Theater School, for example, select students by audition only. These students are trained in an atmosphere of seclusion and in a curriculum that will eventually produce professional ballet dancers, and in all likelihood, jobs. There are, however, many other options for study, as is self-evident from the list that follows. Also, with the rapid growth of regional ballet, there are more opportunities for study outside of New York City than ever before; this includes study with schools that are associated with major ballet companies—the San Francisco Ballet School and the Pennsylvania Ballet School are two cases in point. As David Howard, who teaches dance in New York City describes it, "There is less need for young people to come to New York City for their professional training. Major companies outside of New York City offer good training and the opportunity to stay near home and family." Whatever the choice of school or of location, it is certain that dancers stay in ballet as a career out of an amalgam of grit, determination, commitment, and resolve. "Ballet is a most intensive career choice," says Alexander Filipov, a teacher in the scholarship program at the American Ballet Theater School.

Broadway shows also demand a solid ballet technique—first and foremost. In fact, you won't be able to pass an audition without it. Of course, you must also be proficient in jazz combination, waltz, or soft shoe—whatever the script dictates. Because of the varied demands of professional theater, privately-owned studios must offer a full program of classes in order to compete. The variety of dance styles offered for study in New York City is mind-boggling. From funky to flamenco; from aerobics to pointe work; Afro-Cuban, mime, theater or jazz dance, tap, belly dance, video dance—it is all to be found in the New York dance studios. Additionally, many studios never close—commercial studios offer classes every hour on the hour, so that Broadway dancers can keep in shape despite a grueling eight-times-a-week show schedule.

Studio directors are eager to make their facilities comfortable. It is also important that a studio be located in a safe, accessible area. Not only should the neighborhood be safe, but also the facilities within the school. Clean dressing rooms, heat, light and security are things to look for and to expect when making a choice of which studio to attend. Be sure to inspect the floor. It should be covered with sponge-like material to absorb the impact of jumping. Look for music or some adequate accompaniment as opposed to a teacher who counts while filing her nails.

In the lofts that once spawned the great innovators of modern dance, such as Martha Graham, Doris Humphrey, Jose Limon and Katharine Dunham, second generation teachers and performers now carry on the same innovative tradition. Many young companies and choreographers have evolved from these sources and today fill the theater spaces with their own eclectic creativity. With such a tradition to draw from, you should be able to find a school or class that will help you fulfill your artistic goals. The diversity of classes offered at the present time is unparalleled in the history of American dance.

Dance Schools and Studios

THE ALVIN AILEY
AMERICAN DANCE
CENTER
(Denise Jefferson, director)
1515 Broadway
New York, NY 10036
(212) 997-1980

ALPHA OMEGA DANCE
STUDIOS
(Andy Torres, director)
9 Second Ave.
New York, NY 10003
(212) 673-7880 or 673-7881

THE AMERICAN DANCE
MACHINE
(Nenette Charisse, chief
instructor)
588 Ninth Ave.
New York, NY 10036
(212) 582-8400

MARY ANTHONY
STUDIO
Mary Anthony Dance
Theatre-Phoenix
736 Broadway
New York, NY 10003
(212) 674-8191

APPLEBY STUDIO
(Russ Bralley, manager)
579 Broadway
New York, NY 10012
(212) 431-8489

ASIAN-AMERICAN
DANCE THEATRE
ASIAN-AMERICAN ARTS
CENTER
(Eleanor S. Yung, artistic
dir.)
26 Bowery
New York, NY 10013
(212) 233-2154 or 233-8660

BALASARASWATI
INSTITUTE OF INDIAN
MUSIC
(Lakshmi, artistic director)
P.O. Box 227
Prince Station
New York, NY 10012
(212) 627-1076

BALLET ACADEMY EAST
340 E. 79th St.
New York, NY 10021
(212) 861-5204

BALLET BASICS AND
JAZZ ARTS BY RITA
COLBY
(Rita Colby)
2121 Broadway, Room 201
New York, NY 10023
(212) 245-3605

BALLET HISPANICO
SCHOOL OF DANCE
167 W. 89th St.
New York, NY 10024
(212) 362-6710

BALLET SCHOOL N.Y.
30 E. 31st St.
New York, NY 10016
(212) 679-0401

BLUE DOOR STUDIO
(Grethe Holby, director)
463 Broome St.
New York, NY 10013
(212) 431-8102

BROADWAY DANCE
CENTER
(Jenny Logas, manager)
1733 Broadway
New York, NY 10019
(212) 582-9304

TRISHA BROWN
COMPANY STUDIO
(Laurie MacFarlane,
company administrator)
225 Lafayette St.
Suite 807
New York, NY 10012
(212) 334-9374

CALDERON
PRODUCTION STUDIO
(Des Calderon, director)
1628 Broadway
New York, NY 10003
(212) 246-0469

THE CENTER
Susana and Satoru Oishi
Hayman-Chaffey
53 Gansevoort St.
New York, NY 10014
(212) 255-7455

CHOREOGRAPHERS
THEATRE
225 Lafayette St.
New York, NY 10012
(212) 925-3721

CLARK CENTER
(Jerry R. Cole, managing
dir.)
254 W. 47 St.
New York, NY 10036
(212) 246-4818

ELINOR COLEMAN
EXERCISE AND DANCE
STUDIO AND DANSE
MIRAGE THEATRE
153 Mercer St., 2nd fl.
New York, NY 10012
(212) 226-5767

CONSORT DANCE
ENSEMBLE, INC.
(Myra Hushansky, director)
303 Park Ave. So., #318
New York, NY 10010
(212) 677-8075

AILEEN CROW SCHOOL
OF ALEXANDER
TECHNIQUE
P.O. Box 1273
Ansonia Station
New York, NY 10023
(212) 787-3883

MERCE CUNNINGHAM
STUDIO
(Alice Helpern, studio
administrator)
55 Bethune St.
New York, NY 10014
Mailing Address: 463 West
St.
New York, NY 10014
(212) 691-9751

RUTH CURRIER DANCE
STUDIO
425 Broome St.
New York, NY 10013
(212) 966-7521

DANCE: JUNE LEWIS
AND COMPANY
(June Lewis, artistic dir.)
48 W. 21 St.
New York, NY 10010
(212) 741-3044

DANCE CONCEPTS
STUDIO
(Edvige Val, Marvin
Gordon, directors)
231 W. 54 St.
New York, NY 10019
(212) 757-1941

DANCE SPACE, INC.
622 Broadway, 6th fl.
New York, NY 10012
(212) 777-8067

DANCE THEATER
WORKSHOP
(Laurie Uprichard, managing
dir.)
219 W. 19 St.
New York, NY 10011
(212) 691-6500

DANCE THEATRE OF
HARLEM
(Arthur Mitchell, exec. dir.,
Ruby H. Herd, dir. of
administration)
466 W. 152nd St.
New York, NY 10031
(212) 690-2800

THE FELD BALLET
THE NEW BALLET
SCHOOL
Katherine Moore,
administrator, New Ballet
School)
890 Broadway, 8th fl.
New York, NY 10003
(212) 777-7710

JERRI GARNER
124 W. Houston St.
New York, NY 10012
(212) 254-3951

GELABERT STUDIOS
(Raoul Gelabert, director)
255-57 W. 86th St.
New York, NY 10024
(212) 874-7188

MARTHA GRAHAM
SCHOOL OF
CONTEMPORARY
DANCE
(Diane Gray, director)
316 E. 63rd St.
New York, NY 10021
(212) 838-5886

ERICK HAWKINS
SCHOOL OF DANCE
(Erick Hawkins, artistic dir.)
38 E. 19th St., 8th fl.
New York, NY 10003
(212) 777-7355

THE HEBREW ARTS
SCHOOL
Abraham Goodman House
129 W. 67th St.
New York, NY 10023
(212) 362-8060

NAT HORNE MUSICAL
THEATRE
(Nat Horne, artistic dir.)
440 W. 42nd St.
New York, NY 10036
(212) 736-7128

DAVID HOWARD DANCE
CENTER
(David Howard, director)
211 W. 61st St.
New York, NY 10023
(212) 757-9877

JOFFREY BALLET
SCHOOL (AMERICAN
BALLET CENTER)
(Gerald Arpino, director;
Edith D'Addario, exec. dir.)
434 Ave. of the Americas
New York, NY 10011
(212) 254-8520

KATHERINE KINGSLEY
DANCE CENTER
244–250 W. 54 St., 4th fl.
New York, NY 10019
(212) 307-6909

SUSAN KLEIN SCHOOL
OF DANCE
(Susan Klein & Barbara
Mahler, directors)
48 Beach Street, 4th fl.
New York, NY 10013
(212) 226-6510

LEZLY DANCE AND
SKATE SCHOOL
(Lezly Ziering, director)
622-626 Broadway
New York, NY 10012
(212) 777-3232

LUIGI'S JAZZ CENTER
211 W. 61st St., 5th fl.
New York, NY 10023
(212) 247-1995

THE MANHATTAN
BALLET SCHOOL
(Elfriede Merman, *nee* von
Buffe Grapputo, director)
1556 Third Ave.
New York, NY 10128
(212) 369-3369

MOROCCO ACADEMY OF
MIDEASTERN DANCE
151 W. 28th St., No. 2E
New York, NY 10001
(212) 736-1424

MULTIGRAVITATIONAL
GROUP/
MULTIGRAVITATIONAL
AERODANCE GROUP
c/o Salz
234 E. 23rd St.
New York, NY 10010
(212) 696-5274

NEUBERT BALLET
INSTITUTE
(Christine Neubert,
director)
Carnegie Hall Studio
No. 819
881 7th Ave.
New York, NY 10019
(212) 246-3166

NEW DANCE GROUP
STUDIO
254 W. 47th St.
New York, NY 10036
(212) 719-2733

NEW YORK ACADEMY
OF BALLET & DANCE
ARTS
231 E. 51st St.
New York, NY 10022
(212) 838-0822

NEW YORK
CONSERVATORY OF
DANCE
30 E. 31st St.
New York, NY 10016
(212) 581-1908

NIKOLAIS/LOUIS DANCE
LAB
(Rick Biles, director)
33 E. 18th St.
New York, NY 10003
(212) 777-1120

92ND STREET YMHA
DANCE CENTER
(Ilona Copen, director;
Laura Masone, asst.
director)
1395 Lexington Ave.
New York, NY 10128
(212) 427-6000, ext. 169

MAY O'DONNEL
MODERN DANCE
CENTER
(Ray Green, exec. director)
263 E. 7th St.
New York, NY 10009
(212) 777-0744

PERIDANCE CENTER
(Igal Perry, artistic director)
33 E. 18th St.
New York, NY 10003
(212) 505-0886

ROD RODGERS DANCE
CO. STUDIOS
(Rod Rodgers, founder/
director)
62 E. 4th St.
New York, NY 10003
(212) 674-9066

SCHOOL FOR CREATIVE
MOVEMENT
(Jack Wiener, director)
20 W. 20th St., 5th fl.
New York, NY 10011
(212) 929-0929

SCHOOL OF AMERICAN
BALLET
144 W. 66th St.
New York, NY 10023
(212) 877-0600

STEPPING OUT
BALLROOM DANCE
STUDIO
(Diane Lachtrupp, Paul
Pellicoro, co-owners)
1845 Broadway
New York, NY 10023
(212) 245-5200

STEPS CONTEMPORARY
AND CLASSICAL DANCE
STUDIOS
(Carol Paumgarten and
Patrice Soriero, directors)
1845 Broadway, 4th fl.
New York, NY 10023
(212) 582-7929
2121 Broadway, 3rd fl.
New York, NY 10023
(212) 874-2410

PAUL TAYLOR SCHOOL
552 Broadway, 2nd fl.
New York, NY 10012
(212) 966-6959

THEATRE DANCE
(Lisa Danias, director)
1697 Broadway, 2nd fl.
New York, NY 10019
(212) 247-3755

31/21 STUDIO
(Marjorie Mussman
Hancock, Jonathan Hancock,
directors)
31 W. 21st St., 11th fl.
New York, NY 10010
(212) 989-4814

THE VITAL ARTS
CENTER
(Eleo Pomare, artistic
director)
33 E. 18th St., 3rd fl.
New York, NY 10003
(212) 475-1065/1297

WEST SIDE DANCE
PROJECT
(John DeBlass, Maria
Zannieri, co-directors)
220 W. 80th St.
New York, NY 10024
(212) 580-0915

NINA YOUSHKEVITCH
BALLET WORKSHOP
27 W. 72nd St.
New York, NY 10023
(212) 873-0455

YWCA DANCE
DEPARTMENT
(Lettie Abdelaziz,
coordinator)
610 Lexington Ave.
New York, NY 10022
(212) 735-9755

Finding the Right Singing Teacher

by Fred Silver

To perform in a musical today requires that performers be able to sing better than their counterparts of 20 or 30 years ago. Just listen to cast albums of Broadway musicals of that era and compare the vocal performances with those of more recent vintage. There was a time when dancers in a Broadway show were rarely required to be able to sing; that's what the chorus was for.

Today all that has changed. As the result of tighter budgets only a limited number of chorus personnel are hired and they have to do triple duty. Not only do they have to be able to dance or move; they have to be able to sing and act. Today's chorus people would have been yesteryear's stars. Therefore, to stand any chance of being hired for a musical today, an actor or a dancer must not only be able to sing, but must be able to sing well. To achieve this, many actors seek the services of a singing teacher.

Singing teachers come from varied backgrounds. Some are conservatory-trained and sang opera or lieder before turning to teaching as an occupation. Some were not only classically trained, but had careers in the musical theater and have performed in Broadway shows. This is important because teachers' backgrounds play an important part in how they train their students. Teachers with an operatic background may tend to stress voice placement and *tessitura* better suited to the more classical repertoire, and their teaching of vocal technique may emphasize tone and size at the expense of good diction and ease of singing. Teachers who have had experience acting and who have performed in musical shows tend to be more realistic about the rigors of singing on stage. Giving eight performances a week requires a vocal technique that prevents strain and helps the voice to endure the rigorous demands of today's musical.

How then do you select a singing teacher? Here are some answers to commonly asked questions that should prove useful in helping you find the singing teacher that is right for you.

How long should the duration of the lesson be?

Thirty minutes is the maximum length of time for a beginner and that one lesson per week is the minimum amount of time you will need. After all, a voice lesson is a vocal workout that is as vigorous, in its own way, as any workout in a gym. By the end of a half-hour there may be some vocal fatigue, but there should not be pain. If there is any pain, burning, or hoarseness something is very wrong and you are studying with the wrong singing teacher. The end of a good lesson is accompanied by a happy sense of release of tension and relaxation.

Should I study with a teacher of the same gender?

It doesn't really matter. A good singing teacher is able to communicate sound vocal techniques and the theory behind them no matter what gender you are. Sometimes, if the student is very new to singing and very self-conscious, it may be wise to select a teacher of the same sex if it makes the student feel more comfortable.

How long should it take to develop my voice so that I can be ready to audition and perform?

It depends on several things. How often you have lessons, how frequently you practice your vocal exercises, how quick you are in absorbing and putting into practice the new techniques you are learning. It could take anywhere from a minimum of six months to several years before you reach the level of development you need. Voice building is very much like body building. You are developing muscular control through frequency of repetition and resistance.

What can I expect to happen during a lesson?

Your singing teacher will put you through a series of *vocalises* (vocal exercises) that exercise and navigate all ranges of your voice in a way that keeps tension to a minimum and results in a free and honest sound in all vocal registers. The voice teacher will teach you how to stand as well as how to breathe. You will also be learning where to place your tongue so it doesn't get in the way as well as learning how to relax your jaw and facial muscles. Ideally, you will learn through positive reinforcement how to produce the largest and most focused sound you can.

How, and where do I find a good voice teacher?

Ask everyone you know who sings well who they've studied with. Often they will have found someone they wanted to stay with after trying out others they didn't like. You can gain from their experience. There are also organizations like NYSTA (New York Singing Teachers Association) and NATS (National Association of Teachers of Singing). Contact them, or your own state organization, for their list of teachers. Also, look in *Back Stage* and other trade magazines and publications in which many singing teachers place ads. Don't be afraid to audition a singing teacher.

What questions should I ask a singing teacher in deciding whether they're the right one for me?

The first question could be: How much are the lessons going to cost? A realistic fee would start between $25 and $40 for a half-hour lesson from a good teacher. Obviously you can't pay more than you can afford. One well-known voice teacher in Los Angeles now gets $250 per hour. Of course, these prices are geared to stars, who can afford such a price. But such prices need not concern you for now. You can certainly find a teacher who will work wonderfully for you at a price you can afford.

Next, ask about the students whom the teacher has trained. It would especially be noteworthy to know how many of his or her students have sung, or are singing in Broadway or Off-Broadway shows.

Try to find out what the singing teacher wants to do for you and make it clear that you are primarily interested in singing the repertoire of the musical theater. Mozart arias may be challenging to sing at lessons but will hardly be suitable when auditioning for a musical.

And finally, make certain that you are getting a voice teacher and not a vocal coach. The voice teacher trains you to develop your vocal instrument while the vocal coach helps you select material and teaches you to sing it. Study with a voice teacher first. Later, when your voice is ready, you may begin to look for a vocal coach.

Voice Teachers and Coaches

Vocal Coaches

DAVID AND NANCY
ADAMS
221 W. 82nd St.
Apt. 2D
New York, NY 10024
(212) 595-3324/2886

MME. LENORE
ALESSANDRO
Lenore Alessandro Studio
2109 Broadway
New York, NY 10023
(212) 799-7280

ELIZABETH ARRIGO
175 W. 76th St. 2C
New York, NY 10023
(212) 874-0998

GEORGE AXILTREE
(see Voice Teachers)

JOE BOUSARD
(see Voice Teachers)

LINDA AMIEL BURNS,
DIRECTOR
John Houseman Theater
Ctr.
450 W. 42nd St.
Suite 2E
New York, NY 10036
(212) 564-3455

DEAN BURRIS
252 W. 11th St.
New York, NY 10014
(212) 627-1048

SHIRLEY CALLAWAY
(see Voice Teachers)

LANA CANTRELL
300 E. 71st St.
New York, NY 10021
(212) 249-6046

JANICE CAVALIER
Cavalier Vocal Studio
(see Voice Teachers)

LARRO CHELSI
17 Park Ave.
New York, NY 10016
(212) 689-4596

ANDREW COOKE
318 W. 100th St.
Apt. 4A
New York, NY 10025
(212) 866-8982

CHRISTOPHER DENNY
7 W. 14th St.
Apt. #20R
New York, NY 10011
(212) 929-5198

MARY FEINSINGER
(see Voice Teachers)

BOB GERARDI
Sherman Square Studios
(see Voice Teachers)

ELIZABETH HOWELL
325 Central Park West
New York, NY 10025
(212) 864-6472

JEFFREY KLITZ
300 E. 40th St.
New York, NY 10016
(212) 867-1799

ESTON KRIEGER
Eston Krieger Studio
(see Voice Teachers)

RONA LESLIE
(see Voice Teachers)

SHELLEN LUBIN
509 W. 110th St.
Apt. 11B
New York, NY 10025
(212) 864-2380

ROBERT MARKS
850 Seventh Ave.
Suite 804
New York, NY 10019
(212) 664-1654

MICHAEL McASSEY
150 W. 47th St.
Apt. 5A
New York, NY 10036
(212) 354-8468

ALVA NELSON
202 W. 138th St., #3
New York, NY 10030
(212) 690-2407

RON PANVINI
(see Voice Teachers)

HAL SCHAEFER
101 Greene St.
New York, NY 10012
(212) 941-9753

TOM SHEPARD
(see Voice Teachers)

FRED SILVER
Fred Silver Studio
173 W. 78th St.
New York, NY 10024
(212) 724-3813

MARY SMALL
165 W. 66th St.
New York, NY 10023
(212) 580-3339

ELLY STONE
251 W. 92nd St.
New York, NY 10025
(212) 874-7871

GRACE TESTANI
(See Sight-Singing Teachers)

THOMAS WHITNEY
780 Riverside Dr.
New York, NY 10032
(212) 926-2491

ARABELLA YOUNG
Ansonia Hotel
73rd St. & Broadway
New York, NY 10023
(212) 354-1422

Voice Teachers

DAVID AND NANCY
ADAMS
(See Vocal Coaches)

EDWARD ALBANO
Albano Voice Institute
152 W. 72nd St.
New York, NY 10023
(212) 362-2331

LOWELL ALECSON
411 W. 44th St.
New York, NY 10036
(212) 246-4889

MME. LENORE
ALESSANDRO
Lenore Alessandro Studio
(see Vocal Coaches)

ELIZABETH ARRIGO
Elizabeth Arrigo Studio
175 W. 76th St.
Apt. 2C
New York, NY 10023
(212) 874-0998

GEORGE AXILTREE
222 W. 15th St.
Apt. 8C
New York, NY 10011
(212) 255-2565
HB Studio: (212) 675-2370

JOE BOUSARD
990 Sixth Ave., at 37th St.
Apt. 8A
New York, NY 10018
(212) 594-2249

LINDA AMIEL BURNS
The Singing Experience®
(see Vocal Coaches)

SHIRLEY CALLAWAY
59 W. 76th St.
Apt. 5F
New York, NY 10023
(212) 496-2476

JANICE CAVALIER
Cavalier Vocal Studio
161 W. 54th St.
Apt. 1102
New York, NY 10019
(212) 265-5316

LARRO CHELSI
(see Vocal Coaches)

DAVID SORIN COLLYER
50 W. 67th St.
New York, NY 10023
(212) 362-2225

ANTHONY DI LEVA
160 W. 73rd St.
New York, NY 10023
(212) 874-0756

J. ERIC DOUGLAS
777 West End Ave.
New York, NY 10025
(212) 666-1166

SHIRLEE EMMONS
12 W. 96th St.
New York, NY 10025
(212) 222-5154

DR. DAVID FAIRCHILD
Dr. David Fairchild Voice
Studio
166 W. 72nd St.
Apt. 9A
New York, NY 10023
(212) 873-6630
(914) 337-6405

MARY FEINSINGER
99 E. 4th St.
Apt. 5C
New York, NY 10003
Ansonia Hotel
B'way & 73rd St.
Studio 13–131
New York, NY 10023
(212) 674-1194

CARMINE GAGLIARDI
200 W. 70th St.
New York, NY 10023
(212) 799-7325

AMRI GALLI-CAMPI
Galli-Campi Studio
850 Seventh Ave.
Studio 904
New York, NY 10019
(212) 582-7466. (718)
528-3579

BOB GERARDI
Sherman Square Studios
160 W. 73rd St.
New York, NY 10023
(212) 874-6436

NOEL HART
Studio Address:
129 W. 67th St.
New York, NY 10023
(914) 779-3985

RICHARD L. HILTY
150 W. 80th St.
Apt. 4C
New York, NY 10024
(212) 362-5257

ELIZABETH HOWELL
Howell Studio
325 Central Park West
New York, NY 10025
(212) 864-6472

KATHLEEN JENKINS
55 W. 26th St.
New York, NY 10010
(212) 213-6362

JAY KERR
1697 Broadway
Suite 605A
(Ed Sullivan Bldg.)
New York, NY 10019
(212) 582-5118

ESTON KRIEGER
400 W. 119 St.
New York, NY 10027
(212) 663-3248

GENETTE LANE
3950 Blackstone Ave.
Apt. 5C
Riverdale, NY 10471
(212) 549-3567

MARTIN LAWRENCE
260 W. 72nd St.
New York, NY 10023
(212) 787-4614

RONA LESLIE
142 West End Ave.
New York, NY 10023
(212) 724-3082

SHELLEN LUBIN
(see Vocal Coaches)

BARBARA MAIER
365 W. 28th St.
New York, NY 10001
(212) 255-2906

DEE MARTIN
Dee Martin Voice Studios
Ansonia Hotel
73rd & Broadway
New York, NY 10023
(212) 696-2030

GENE McLAUGHLIN
2109 Broadway
New York, NY 10023
(212) 787-4982

CARLO LIFAVI MENOTTI
160 W. 73rd St.
New York, NY 10023
(212) 874-0867

YVONNE NAUM
2109 Broadway
New York, NY 10023
(212) 362-4698

RON PANVINI
Ron Panvini Studio For
Singers
160 W. 73rd St.
New York, NY 10023
(212) 595-4952

JANET PAVEK
Janet Pavek Studio
200 W. 79th St.
New York, NY 10024
(212) 496-0534

HAL SCHAEFER
(see Vocal Coaches)

TOM SHEPARD
484 W. 43rd St.
Apt. 35K
New York, NY 10036
(212) 541-7600 (service)

FRED SILVER
(see Vocal Coaches)

MARY SMALL
(see Vocal Coaches)

ALLYSON STARR
"Singer's Studio"
"The Art of Performing"
101 W. 57th St.
New York, NY 10019
(212) 582-6448

HELEN STEPHENSON
19 W. 69th St.
New York, NY 10023
(212) 496-6337

JOYCE SUSKIND
200 W. 70 St.
Apt. 9M
New York, NY 10023
(212) 362-0135

MARK ZELLER
The Mark Zeller Workshop
236 W. 78 St.
New York, NY 10024
(212) 362-1736

Sight-Singing Teachers

EDWARD ALBANO
(see Voice Teachers)

GEORGE AXILTREE
(see Voice Teachers)

PAUL CAPUTO
1275 E. 48th St.
Brooklyn, NY 11234
(212) 594-3688
(718) 444-7270

MAURICE FINNELL
Maurice Finnell Studios
Hotel Ansonia
2109 Broadway
Studio 977
New York, NY 10023
(212) 722-6215

PARKS HILL
66 Seventh Ave., #3A
New York, NY 10011
(212) 675-2153

HELEN HOBBS JORDAN
119 W. 57th St.
New York, NY 10019
(212) 757-3689

LUBA TCHERESKY
915 West End Ave.
New York, NY 10025
(212) 222-8585

GRACE TESTANI
SOJ Music Studios
246 W. 46th St.
New York, NY 10036
(212) 222-6632
Studio: (212) 869-0226

THOMAS WHITNEY
(see Vocal Coaches)

ARABELLA YOUNG
(see Vocal Coaches)

PART THREE

Finding The Work

AEA, AFTRA, and SAG Agents

by Marje Fields

Talent agencies represent the interests of performing artists in all areas of the entertainment industry. They are the representatives franchised by Actors' Equity (AEA), the Screen Actors Guild (SAG), and the American Federation of TV & Radio Artists (AFTRA) to negotiate contracts for performers. These three trade unions have established a body of regulations that talent agents must abide by. In addition, these representatives are also regulated in New York and California by state laws. These regulations protect the performer in a manner similar to that of other consumer protection legislation. The regulations have been in existence for over 50 years, and prescribe a high standard of business ethics and personal behavior for agents. No other performer's representative—lawyer, personal manager, or publicity agent—is so tightly regulated. Armed with your union's assurance that it has investigated an agency, you can set your mind at ease with regard to an agency's reliability and ethics, and can proceed to concentrate on finding the agency that can best develop your talents.

WHAT AN AGENT DOES
It is the agent's business to seek out talented artists and help them develop their careers. It is the agent who can open doors and lead the performer through them, who can give suggestions that advance a career. The agent advises, urges, listens, lectures, negotiates, soothes, worries, and, finally, applauds.

HOW TO APPROACH AN AGENCY
Once you have determined that an agency handles your particular range of talents, send them an 8 × 10 black and white headshot, on the back of which you have attached your resume. If the agency is interested, one of their agents will phone you to come in and see them. At the initial interview, the agent will try to determine whether there is a possibility that the agency can help you develop your career. Of course, no decision can be reached until the agent has seen your work. If, however, the agency is interested, they will ask you to let them know when that opportunity arises—when you are performing in a showcase, a reading, a non-union rep company, and so forth.

Agents are invited to every showcase and production in town. Many of them see something every evening in order to search out talent. Although there are more actors than agents, and occasionally an agent will seem brusque when turning down your request for an appointment, *they do need you*. An agency's business and reputation is built on the quality of the talent they represent.

HOW TO WORK WITH AN AGENCY

When an agency decides it can work with you (this is a crucial decision because agencies only make money when their clients are employed) the agency will proceed in one of two ways:

Signed Clients: If your talents fall within the range of the agency's expertise, you will be asked to sign one or more of the exclusive management contracts provided by each of the three unions. These contracts establish a legal relationship between you and the agency. It can also be considered as a show of faith in your talents. Whatever work you get that is within the union's jurisdiction during the term of this contract (first contracts can be a year with SAG and AFTRA and no more than 18 months with AEA) is commissionable by the agency.

Freelance: If representatives at an agency wish to become further acquainted with your work, and if, in their estimation, there is not enough demand for your type or talent, they may ask if you will work on a freelance basis with them. If you agree to this arrangement, you must sign an agreement that will guarantee that you will pay commission if you get a part that the agent has submitted you for. Many actors with particular specialties work this way and, in fact, prefer a freelance arrangement, wherein they can be submitted for auditions by more than one agent.

AGENCY FEES

Union-franchised agents can charge you 10 percent of your salary for a job they helped you secure. This 10 percent covers costs of sending you out on auditions, bringing casting directors to see you in showcases, advising you, counseling you, and submitting you for work regionally or nationally.

SUMMARY

Agents work primarily with union actors, but they do advise beginning talent on how best to pursue union credentials. Agents work within strict union guidelines. Agencies either ask you to sign union-devised contracts in which they represent you exclusively or as freelancers. All agreements are legally binding and the agency fee is 10 percent.

AEA, AFTRA, and SAG Agents

NEW YORK CITY AREA AGENTS

The following is a list of AFTRA-, Equity-, and SAG-franchised agents in New York City. Contact the agency departments at the individual unions for specific information: AFTRA, 200 Madison Ave., New York, NY 10016, (212) 532-0800; Actor's Equity Association, 165 W. 46th St., New York, NY 10036, (212) 869-8530; SAG, 1515 Broadway, New York, NY 10036, (212) 944-1030.

A = AFTRA   E = AEA   S = SAG

ABRAMS ARTISTS &
ASSOCIATES, LTD.
420 Madison Ave.
Suite 1400
New York, NY 10017
(212) 935-8980   A–E–S

ACTORS GROUP AGENCY
157 W. 57th St.
Suite 604
New York, NY 10019
(212) 245-2930   A–E–S

BRET ADAMS
448 W. 44th St.
New York, NY 10036
(212) 765-5630   A–E–S

AGENCY FOR THE
PERFORMING ARTS
888 7th Ave.
New York, NY 10106
(212) 582-1500   A–E–S

AGENTS FOR THE ARTS
1650 Broadway
Suite 306
New York, NY 10019
(212) 247-3220   A–E–S

BONNI ALLEN TALENT
250 W. 57th St.
New York, NY 10107
(212) 757-7475   A–E–S

MICHAEL AMATO
AGENCY
1650 Broadway
New York, NY 10019
(212) 247-4456   A–E–S

THE AMBROSE
COMPANY
311 W. 43rd St.
Suite 1401
New York, NY 10036
(212) 586-9110   A–E–S

AMBROSIO/MORTIMER
& ASSOCIATES, INC.
165 W. 46th St.
New York, NY 10036
(212) 719-1677   A–E–S

AMERICAN
INTERNATIONAL
TALENT
303 W. 42nd St.
Suite 608
New York, NY 10036
(212) 245-8888   A–E–S

BEVERLY ANDERSON
1501 Broadway
Suite 2008
New York, NY 10036
(212) 944-7773   A–E–S

ANDREADIS TALENT
AGENCY, INC.
119 W. 57th St.
Suite 711
New York, NY 10019
(212) 315-0303   A–E–S

ARTISTS' AGENCY
230 W. 55th St., #29D
New York, NY 10019
(212) 245-6960   A–E–S

ASSOCIATED BOOKING
1995 Broadway
New York, NY 10023
(212) 874-2400   A–E–S

RICHARD ASTOR
1697 Broadway
New York, NY 10019
(212) 581-1970   A–E–S

BARRY AGENCY
165 W. 46th St.
New York, NY 10036
(212) 869-9310   A–E–S

BAUMAN, HILLER &
ASSOCIATES
250 W. 57th St.
New York, NY 10019
(212) 757-0098   A–E–S

PETER BEILIN
230 Park Ave.
New York, NY 10169
(212) 949-9119   A–S

BETHEL AGENCIES
513 W. 54th St.
Suite 1
New York, NY 10019
(212) 664-0455   A–E–S

J. MICHAEL BLOOM,
LTD.
233 Park Ave. South
New York, NY 10003
(212) 529-5800
(212) 529-6500   A–E–S

BOOKERS, INC.
39 W. 19th St.
New York, NY 10011
(212) 645-9706   S

BOULEVARD TALENT
GROUP
35 E. 21st St., #7E
New York, NY 10010
(212) 473-1900   S

BRESLER, KELLY,
KIPPERMAN AGENCY
111 W. 57th St.
Suite 1409
New York, NY 10019
(212) 265-1980   E–S

DON BUCHWALD &
ASSOCIATES, INC.
10 E. 44th St.
New York, NY 10017
(212) 867-1070;
867-1200   A–E–S

CARSON/ADLER AGENCY
250 W. 57th St., #729
New York, NY 10107
(212) 307-1882;
307-6231   A–E–S

RICHARD CATALDI
AGENCY
180 7th Ave., #1C
New York, NY 10011
(212) 741-7450   A–E–S

CELEBRITY TALENT
INC.
575 Madison Ave., #1006
New York, NY 10022
(212) 605-0515   A–S

COLEMAN-ROSENBERG
210 E. 58th St.
New York, NY 10022
(212) 838-0734   A–E–S

BILL COOPER
ASSOCIATES, INC.
224 W. 49th St.
Suite 411
New York, NY 10019
(212) 307-1100   A–S

CREATIVE I ARTISTS
Five Union Square West
Fifth Fl.
New York, NY 10003
(212) 989-0800   A–S

CUNNINGHAM, ESCOTT,
DIPENE AND
ASSOCIATES
118 E. 25th St.
New York, NY 10010
(212) 477-1666   A–S

JANE DEACY AGENCY
181 Revolutionary Rd.
Scarborough, NY 10510
(914) 941-1414   A–E–S

DESPOINTES-CASEY
ARTISTS
75 Varick St.
Suite 1407
New York, NY 10013
(212) 334-6023   A–S

DIAMOND ARTISTS
119 W. 57th St.
Suite 808
New York, NY
(212) 247-3025   A–E–S

GINGER DICCE TALENT
AGENCY
1650 Broadway, #714
New York, NY 10019
(212) 974-7455   A–E–S

GLORIA DOLAN, LTD.
1339 York Ave.
New York, NY 10021
(212) 696-1850   A

DOUGLAS, GORMAN,
ROTHACKER AND
WILHELM, INC.
1650 Broadway
Suite 806
New York, NY 10019
(212) 757-5500   A–E–S

DAVID DRUMMOND
TALENT
102 W. 75th St.
New York, NY 10023
(212) 877-6753   E–S

DULCINA EISEN
ASSOCIATES
154 E. 61st St.
New York, NY 10021
(212) 355-6617   A–E–S

ENTERTAINMENT
ASSOCIATES, INC.
Lakeview Common
Gibbsboro, NJ 08026
(609) 435-8300   S

FTA TALENT AGENCY,
INC.
401 Park Ave. South
New York, NY 10016
(212) 686-7010   A–S

FACES TALENT AGENCY
567 Third Ave.
New York, NY 10016
(212) 661-1515   S

MARJE FIELDS, INC.
165 W. 46th St.
New York, NY 10036
(212) 764-5740   A–E–S

FLICK E & W TALENT,
INC.
881 Seventh Ave.
New York, NY 10019
(212) 307-1850   S

FORD TALENT GROUP
344 E. 59th St.
New York, NY 10022
(212) 688-8628   A–S

FOSTER-FELL AGENCY
80 Varick St.
New York, NY 10013
(212) 226-4562   E–S

4B TALENTS
UNLIMITED
630 Ninth Ave.
New York, NY 10036
(212) 246-1606   S

FRONTIER BOOKING
INTERNATIONAL, INC.
1776 Broadway
New York, NY 10019
(212) 265-0822   A–E–S

GAGE GROUP, INC.
1650 Broadway
New York, NY 10019
(212) 541-5250   A–E–S

GERSH AGENCY
130 W. 42nd St.
New York, NY 10036
(212) 997-1818   A–E–S

GILCHRIST TALENT
GROUP, INC.
310 Madison Ave.
Suite 1003
New York, NY 10017
(212) 692-9166   A–E–S

HV TALENTS
18 E. 53rd St.
New York, NY 10022
(212) 751-3005   A–S

PEGGY HADLEY
ENTERPRISES
250 W. 57th St.
New York, NY 10107
(212) 246-2166   A–E–S

HARTER/MANNING &
ASSOCIATES
111 E. 22nd St.
New York, NY 10010
(212) 529-4555   A–E–S

MICHAEL HARTIG
AGENCY, LTD.
114 E. 28th St.
New York, NY 10016
(212) 684-0010   A–E–S

HENDERSON-HOGAN
405 W. 44th St.
New York, NY 10036
(212) 765-5190   A–E–S

DIANA HUNT
Royalton Hotel
44 W. 44th St.
New York, NY 10036
(212) 391-4971   A–E–S

IANNONE-DAY AGENCY,
INC.
311 W. 43rd St.
Suite 1405
New York, NY 10036
(212) 957-9550   A–E–S

INTERNATIONAL
CREATIVE
MANAGEMENT
40 W. 57th St.
New York, NY 10019
(212) 556-5600   A–E–S

MARIAN IVRY
1650 Broadway
Suite 906
New York, NY 10019
(212) 586-2760   E

JACOBSON-WILDER &
KESTEN, INC.
419 Park Ave. South
New York, NY 10016
(212) 686-6100   A–S

JAN J. AGENCY
328 E. 61st St.
New York, NY 10021
(212) 759-9775   A–E–S

JOE JORDAN TALENT
AGENCY
156 Fifth Ave.
Suite 711
New York, NY 10010
(212) 463-8455   A–E–S

MARVIN A. JOSEPHSON
555 Madison Ave.
Suite 815
New York, NY 10022
(212) 758-5480   E

JOVANO AGENCY
2320 Main St.
Bridgeport, CT 06606
(203) 336-0597   A–S

KMA ASSOCIATES
211 W. 56th St., 17E
New York, NY 10019
(212) 581-4610   A–S

JERRY KAHN INC.
853 Seventh Ave.
New York, NY 10019
(212) 245-7317   A–E–S

KEARNEY/BISHOP
1697 Broadway
Room 905
New York, NY 10019
(212) 581-6200   S

CHARLES KERIN
ASSOCIATES
25 Central Park West,
   #25Q
New York, NY 10023
(212) 757-8338   A–E–S

ARCHER KING
420 Lexington Ave.
New York, NY 10017
(212) 210-8740   A–E–S

KINGMAN AGENCY, INC.
1501 Broadway, 1808A
New York, NY 10036
(212) 354-6688   A–E–S

ROSEANNE KIRK
161 W. 54th St., #1234
New York, NY 10022
(212) 888-6711   A–E–S

KOLMAR-LUTH
ENTERPRISES
1501 Broadway, #201
New York, NY 10036
(212) 730-9500   A

LUCY KROLL
390 West End Ave.
New York, NY 10024
(212) 877-0627   A–E–S

KRONICK, KELLY &
LAUREN AGENCY
220 Fifth Ave.
New York, NY 10001
(212) 684-5223   A–E–S

L.B.H. ASSOCIATES
1 Lincoln Plaza
New York, NY 10023
(212) 787-2609   A

THE LANTZ OFFICE
888 Seventh Ave.
New York, NY 10106
(212) 586-0200   A–E–S

LIONEL LARNER, LTD.
130 W. 57th St.
New York, NY 10019
(212) 246-3105   A–E–S

DENNIS A LEACH
160 Fifth Ave., #815
New York, NY 10010
(212) 891-3450   A–S

SANFORD LEIGH
AGENCY
440 E. 62nd St.
Suite 1B
New York, NY 10021
(212) 752-4450   A–S

LESTER LEWIS
ASSOCIATES
400 E. 52nd St., #110
New York, NY 10022
(212) 758-2480   A–E–S

L'IMAGE TALENT
GROUP, INC.
35 E. 21st St.
Seventh Floor
New York, NY 10010
(212) 477-2100   S

MMG ENTERPRISES/
MARCIA'S KIDS
250 W. 57th St.
New York, NY 10107
(212) 246-4360   A–E–S

MANNEQUIN MODELS,
INC.
150 E. 58th St., #3500
New York, NY 10155
(212) 755-1456   A–S

MARTINELLI
ATTRACTIONS
888 Eighth Ave.
New York, NY 10036
(212) 586-0963   A–S

MARGE McDERMOTT
216 E. 39th St.
New York, NY 10016
(212) 889-1583   A–S

WILLIAM MORRIS
AGENCY
1350 Sixth Ave.
New York, NY 10019
(212) 586-5100   A–E–S

NEW YORK AGENCY
1650 Broadway, #504
New York, NY 10019
(212) 245-8860   A–E–S

THE NEWS &
ENTERTAINMENT CORP.
221 W. 57th St.
New York, NY 10019
(212) 765-5555   A–E–S

NOBLE TALENT U.S.A.
250 W. 57th St.
Suite 1508
New York, NY 10107
(212) 581-3800   A–E–S

OPPENHEIM-CHRISTIE
13 E. 37th St.
New York, NY 10016
(212) 213-4330   A–E–S

FIFI OSCARD
ASSOCIATES, INC.
19 W. 44th St.
New York, NY 10036
(212) 764-1100   A–E–S

BARNA OSTERTAG
AGENCY
501 Fifth Ave.
New York, NY 10017
(212) 697-6339   A–E–S

PGA, INC.
1650 Broadway
New York, NY 10019
(212) 586-1452   A–E–S

HARRY PACKWOOD
TALENT LTD.
250 W. 57th St.
Suite 1416
New York, NY 10107
(212) 586-8900   A–E–S

DOROTHY PALMER
TALENT AGENCY
235 W. 56th St., #24K
New York, NY 10019
(718) 765-4280   A–E–S

PHOENIX ARTISTS, INC.
250 W. 57th St.
Suite 2530
New York, NY 10107
(212) 956-7070   A–E–S

PREMIER TALENT
AGENCY
3 E. 54th St.
14th Floor
New York, NY 10022
(212) 758-4900   A–S

PROFESSIONAL
ARTISTS, UNLIMITED
513 W. 54th St.
New York, NY 10019
(212) 247-8770   A–E–S

RADIO ACTIVE TALENT,
INC.
476 Elmont Rd.
Elmont, NY 11003
(212) 315-1919   A–S

RASCALS, UNLIMITED
135 E. 65th St
New York, NY 10021
(212) 517-6500   S

NORMAN REICH
AGENCY
65 W. 55th Street
Suite 4-H
New York, NY 10019
(212) 399-2881   S

REVELATION
ENTERTAINMENT CO.,
INC.
601 Halstead Ave.
Mamaroneck, NY 10543
(914) 381-5207   S

WALLACE ROGERS
TALENT
37 E. 28th St.
New York, NY 10016
(212) 889-8233   S

GILLA ROOS LTD.
555 Madison Ave.
New York, NY 10022
(212) 758-5480   A–S

CHARLES V. RYAN
AGENCY
200 W. 57th St.
New York, NY 10019
(212) 245-2225   A–S

SAMES, ROLLNICK
ASSOCIATES
250 W. 57th St.
Suite 703
New York, NY 10107
(212) 315-4434   A–E–S

SANDERS AGENCY LTD.
156 Fifth Ave.
Suite 222
New York, NY 10010
(212) 627-7726   A–E–S

SCHIFFMAN, EKMAN,
MORRISON & MARX,
INC.
156 Fifth Ave.
Suite 523
New York, NY 10010
(212) 627-5700   A–S

WILLIAM SCHILL
AGENCY
250 W. 57th St.
Suite 1429
New York, NY 10107
(212) 315-5919   A–E–S

DICK SCOTT AGENCY
159 W. 53rd Street
New York, NY 10019
(212) 246-6096   E

SCHULLER TALENT/NY
KIDS
276 Fifth Ave.
New York, NY 10001
(212) 532-6005   A–E–S

SELECT ARTISTS
REPRESENTATIVES,
INC.
337 W. 43rd St.
Suite 1-B
New York, NY 10036
(212) 586-4300   A–E–S

MONTY SILVER AGENCY
145 W. 45th St.
Suite 1204
New York, NY 10036
(212) 391-4545   A–E–S

SMITH-FREEDMAN
ASSOCIATES
192 Lexington Ave.
12th Floor
New York, NY 10016
(212) 545-0500   A–E–S

ANTHONY SOGLIO
423 Madison Ave.
New York, NY 10017
(212) 751-1850   A–E

SPOTLITE ENTERPRISES
221 W. 57th St.
Ninth Floor
New York, NY 10019
(212) 586-6750   A–E–S

THE STARKMAN
AGENCY INC.
1501 Broadway
Room 301A
New York, NY 10036
(212) 921-9191   A–E–S

STE REPRESENTATION
888 Seventh Ave.
New York, NY 10019
(212) 246-1030   A–E–S

STEWART ARTISTS
CORP.
215 E. 81st St.
New York, NY 10028
(212) 249-5540   A–S

STRAIN & TENNET
ASSOCS., INC.
1501 Broadway
Suite 1405
New York, NY 10036
(212) 391-0380   A–E–S

STROUD MANAGEMENT
(Daytime soap writers only)
119 W. 57th St.
New York, NY 10019
(212) 315-3111   A–S

TALENT REPS, INC.
20 E. 53rd St.
New York, NY 10022
(212) 752-1835   A–E–S

MICHAEL THOMAS
AGENCY, INC.
305 Madison Ave.
New York, NY 10165
(212) 867-0303   A–E–S

TRANUM, ROBERTSON,
HUGHES, INC.
Two Dag Hammarskjold
Plaza
New York, NY 10017
(212) 371-7500   A–S

TRIAD ARTISTS
888 Seventh Ave.
Suite 1602
New York, NY 10106
(212) 489-8100   A–E–S

GLORIA TROY
34-12 36th St.
Astoria, NY 11106
(718) 392-1290   A–E–S

UNIVERSAL
ATTRACTIONS
218 W. 57th St.
New York, NY 10019
(212) 582-7575   A

UNIVERSAL TALENT
505 Fifth Ave.
10th Floor
New York, NY 10017
(212) 661-3888   S

VAN DER VEER PEOPLE,
INC.
401 E. 57th St.
New York, NY 10022
(212) 688-2880   S

BOB WATERS AGENCY
1501 Broadway
New York, NY 10036
(212) 302-8787   A–E–S

RUTH WEBB
ENTERPRISES
701 Seventh Ave., #9N
New York, NY 10036
(212) 757-6300   S

WILHELMINA ARTISTS
REPRESENTATIVES,
INC.
Nine E. 37th St.
New York, NY 10016
(212) 889-9450   A–E–S

HANNS WOLTERS
10 W. 37th St.
New York, NY 10018
(212) 714-0100   S

PATRICIA WOO AGENCY
156 Fifth Ave.
New York, NY 10011
(212) 989-7171   E

ANN WRIGHT REPS.
136 E. 56th St.
New York, NY 10022
(212) 832-0110   A–E–S

WRITERS & ARTISTS
AGENCY
70 W. 36th St.
Suite 501
New York, NY 10018
(212) 947-8765   A–E–S

BABS ZIMMERMAN
PRODUCTIONS, INC.
305 E. 86th St.
New York, NY 10028
(212) 348-7203   A–E

ZOLI MANAGEMENT,
INC.
146 E. 56th St.
New York, NY 10022
(212) 319-0327   A–E–S

LOS ANGELES AREA AEA AGENTS

The following are Equity franchised agents in the Los Angeles area. The AEA Western Regional Office is located at 6430 Sunset Blvd., Los Angeles, CA 90028; (213) 462-2334.

A TOTAL ACTING
EXPERIENCE
6736 Laurel Canyon
Suite 300
North Hollywood, CA 91606
(818) 765-7244

SALLY AARON ARTISTS
5301 Lauren Canyon Road
Suite 116
North Hollywood, CA 91067
(818) 980-6719

ABRAMS ARTISTS &
ASSOCIATES
9200 Sunset Blvd.
Garden Suite 625
Los Angeles, CA 90069
(213) 859-0625

ABRAMS, RUBALOFF &
LAWRENCE
8075 West Third Street
Suite 303
Los Angeles, CA 90048
(213) 935-1700

THE AGENCY
10351 Santa Monica Blvd.
Suite 211
Los Angeles, CA 90025
(213) 551-3000

AGENCY FOR CREATIVE
TALENT
8500 Melrose Avenue
Suite 210
Los Angeles, CA 90069
(213) 657-5304

AGENCY FOR THE
PERFORMING ARTS
(APA)
9000 Sunset Blvd.
Los Angeles, CA 90069
(213) 273-0744

ALL TALENT AGENCY
2437 East Washington Blvd.
Pasadena, CA 91104
(818) 797-2422

AMBROSIO-MORTIMER
9000 Sunset Blvd.
Suite 900
Los Angeles, CA 90069
(213) 274-4274

FRED AMSEL
6310 San Vicente Blvd.
Suite 407
Los Angeles, CA 90067
(213) 939-1188

THE ARTISTS AGENCY
10000 Santa Monica Blvd.
Suite 305
Los Angeles, CA 90069
(213) 277-7777

ARTISTS FIRST
8230 Beverly Blvd.
Suite 23
Los Angeles, CA 90048
(213) 653-5640

ARTISTS GROUP
1930 Century Park West
Suite 303
Los Angeles, CA 90067
(213) 552-1100

ATKINS & ASSOCIATES
303 S. Crescent Heights
  Blvd.
Los Angeles, CA 90048
(213) 658-1025

BADGLEY, MCQUENNEY
& CONNOR
9229 Sunset Blvd.
Suite 607
Los Angeles, CA 90069
(213) 278-9313

BOBBY BALL AGENCY
6290 Sunset Blvd.
Suite 3045
Los Angeles, CA 90028
(213) 465-7522

RICKEY BARR AGENCY
8350 Santa Monica Blvd.
Suite 206A
Los Angeles, CA 90069
(213) 650-8525

BAUMAN-HILLER &
ASSOCIATES
9220 Sunset Blvd.
Suite 202
Los Angeles, CA 90069
(213) 271-5601

BDP AGENCY
10637 Burbank Blvd.
Burbank, CA 91601
(818) 506-7615

BEAKEL & DEBORO
AGENCY
10637 Burbank Blvd.
N. Hollywood, CA 91601
(818) 506-7615

BELSON & KLASS
AGENCY
144 S. Beverly Dr.
Suite 405
Beverly Hills, CA 90210
(213) 274-9169

MARIAN BERZON
TALENT AGENCY
336 East 17th Street
Costa Mesa, CA 92627
(714) 631-5936

YVETTE BIKOFF
AGENCY, LTD.
9255 Sunset Blvd.
Suite 510
Los Angeles, CA 90069
(213) 278-7490

J. MICHAEL BLOOM &
ASSOCIATES
9200 Sunset Blvd.
Suite 710
Los Angeles, CA 90069
(213) 275-6800

BORNSTEIN BOGART
AGENCY
9100 Sunset Blvd.
Suite 200
Los Angeles, CA 90069
(213) 278-2555

BRESLER KELLY &
ASSOCIATES
15760 Ventura Blvd.
Suite 1730
Encino, CA 91436
(213) 905-1155

ALEX BREWIS
12429 Laurel Terrace Dr.
Studio City, CA 91604
(818) 509-0831

BROOKE DUNN OLIVER
AGENCY
9165 Sunset Blvd.
Suite 202
Los Angeles, CA 90069
(213) 859-1405

CAMDEN ARTISTS
2121 Avenue of the Stars
Suite 410
Los Angeles, CA 90067
(213) 556-2022

THE CARPENTER
COMPANY
1516 West Redwood Street
San Diego, CA 92101
(619) 235-8482

MARY J. CARTER: A
TALENT AGENCY
6525 Sunset Blvd.
Suite 502
Los Angeles, CA 90028
(213) 467-2662

THE CAVALERI AGENCY
6605 Hollywood Blvd.
Suite 220
Hollywood, CA 90028
(213) 461-2940

CENTURY ARTISTS
9744 Wilshire Boulevard
Suite 308
Beverly Hills, CA 90212
(213) 273-4366

CHARTER
MANAGEMENT
9000 Sunset Blvd.
Suite 1112
Hollywood, CA 90069
(213) 278-1690

CNA & ASSOCIATES
8721 Sunset Blvd.
Suite 202
Los Angeles, CA 90069
(213) 657-2063

CONTEMPORARY
ARTISTS
132 Lasky Drive
Beverly Hills, CA 90212
(213) 278-8250

CORALIE JR.
4789 Vineland Avenue
Suite 100
N. Hollywood, CA 91602
(818) 766-9501

ROBERT COSDEN
ENTERPRISES, LTD.
7080 Hollywood Blvd.
Suite 908
Hollywood, CA 90028
(213) 856-9000

THE CRAIG AGENCY
8485 Melrose Place
Suite E
Los Angeles, CA 90069
(213) 655-0236

CREATIVE ARTISTS
1888 Century Park East
Suite 1400
Los Angeles, CA 90067
(213) 277-4545

LIL CUMBER
6515 Sunset Blvd.
Suite 30A
Los Angeles, CA 90028
(213) 469-1919

DADE/ROSEN/SCHULTZ
AGENCY
15010 Ventura Blvd.
Sherman Oaks, CA 91403
(818) 907-9877

DIAMOND ARTISTS
9200 Sunset Blvd.
Suite 909
Los Angeles, CA 90069
(213) 278-8146

EILEEN FARRELL
TALENT AGENCY
10500 Magnolia Blvd.
N. Hollywood, CA 91601
(213) 762-6994

ELLIS ARTISTS AGENCY
119 North San Vicente Blvd.
Beverly Hills, CA 90211
(213) 651-3032

EXCLUSIVE ARTISTS
AGENCY
2501 West Burbank Blvd.
Suite 304
Burbank, CA 91505
(818) 846-0262

WILLIAM FELBER
2126 Cahuenga Blvd.
Hollywood, CA 90068
(213) 466-7629

FILM-THEATRE ACTORS
EXCHANGE
271 Columbus Avenue
Suite 2
San Francisco, CA 94113
(415) 433-3920

THE BARRY FREED
COMPANY
9255 Sunset Blvd.
Suite 603
Los Angeles, CA 90069
(213) 274-6898

KURT FRINGS AGENCY
139 South Beverly Dr.
Beverly Hills, CA 90210
(213) 277-1103

THE GAGE GROUP
9229 Sunset Blvd.
Suite 103
Los Angeles, CA 90069
(213) 859-8777

HELEN GARRETT
TALENT AGENCY
6525 Sunset Blvd.
Suite 205
Hollywood, CA 90028
(213) 871-8707

LAYA GELFF &
ASSOCIATES
16000 Ventura Blvd.
Suite 500
Encino, CA 91436
(818) 906-0925

PHIL GERSH AGENCY
222 North Cannon Drive
Suite 201
Beverly Hills, CA 90210
(213) 274-6611

GEORGIA GILLY
8721 Sunset Blvd.
Suite 103
Los Angeles, CA 90069
(213) 657-5660

HAROLD GOLD &
ASSOCIATES
12725 Ventura Blvd., #E
Studio City, CA 91604
(818) 769-5003

SUE GOLDIN TALENT
AGENCY
6380 Wilshire Blvd.
Suite 1600
Los Angeles, CA 90048
(213) 852-1441

ALLEN GOLDSTEIN &
ASSOCIATES
15010 Ventura Blvd.
Suite 234
Sherman Oaks, CA 91403
(818) 905-7771

JACK GORDEAN
809 North Foothill Road
Beverly Hills, CA 90210
(213) 273-4195

GORES-FIELDS AGENCY
10100 Santa Monica, #700
Los Angeles, CA 90067
(213) 277-4400

MARY GRADY AGENCY
3575 Cahuenga Blvd. West
Suite #320
Hollywood, CA 90068
(213) 851-8872

JOSHUA GRAY &
ASSOCIATES
6736 Laurel Canyon Blvd.,
#306
N. Hollywood, CA 91606
(818) 982-2510

GREENEVINE AGENCY
110 E. 9th St., C-1005
Los Angeles, CA 90079
(213) 622-3016

MITCHELL J.
HAMILBURG
292 S. La Cienega Blvd.
Suite #212
Beverly Hills, CA 90211
(213) 657-1501

HARRIS & GOLDBERG
AGENCY
2121 Avenue of the Stars,
#950
Los Angeles, CA 90067
(213) 553-5200

HENDERSON/HOGAN
AGENCY
247 South Beverly Drive
Beverly Hills, CA 90212
(213) 274-7815

GEORGE B. HUNT
8350 Santa Monica Blvd.
Suite #104
Los Angeles, CA 90069
(213) 654-6600

GEORGE INGERSOLL
6513 Hollywood Blvd.
Suite #217
Los Angeles, CA 90028
(213) 874-6434

INTERNATIONAL
CREATIVE
MANAGEMENT, INC.
8899 Beverly Blvd.
Los Angeles, CA 90048
(213) 550-4000

INTERNATIONAL
TALENT AGENCY
3419 W. Magnolia Blvd.
Burbank, CA 91505
(818) 842-1204

JOSEPH, HELFOND &
RIX INC.
1717 North Highland Avenue
Hollywood, CA 90028
(213) 466-9111

KARG-WEISSENBACH &
ASSOCIATES
329 North Wetherly Drive
Suite 101
Beverly Hills, CA 90211
(213) 205-0435

JOSEPH/KNIGHT
AGENCY
1680 North Vine Street
Suite 726
Hollywood, CA 90028
(213) 465-5474

LEN KAPLAN AGENCY
4717 Laurel Canyon Blvd.
Suite 206
North Hollywood, CA 91607
(818) 980-8811

KELMAN/ARLETTA
7813 Sunset Blvd.
Los Angeles, CA 90046
(213) 851-8822

WILLIAM KERWIN
AGENCY
1605 North Cahuenga Blvd.
Suite #202
Hollywood, CA 90028
(213) 469-5155

THE TYLER KJAR
AGENCY
8961 Sunset Blvd.
Los Angeles, CA 90069
(213) 278-0912

PAUL KOHNER, INC.
9169 Sunset Blvd.
Los Angeles, CA 90069
(213) 550-1060

L.A. ARTISTS TALENT
AGENCY
2566 Overland Ave.
Suite 800
Los Angeles, CA 90064
(213) 202-0254

LANTZ OFFICE
9255 Sunset Blvd.
Suite 505
Los Angeles, CA 90069
(213) 858-1144

MARK LEVIN
ASSOCIATES
208 South Beverly Drive
Suite 4
Beverly Hills, CA 90212
(213) 278-9933

THE LIGHT COMPANY
113 North Robertson Blvd.
Los Angeles, CA 90048
(213) 273-9602

BESSIE LOO
8235 Santa Monica Blvd.
Suite 202
W. Hollywood, CA 90046
(213) 650-1300

LOVELL & ASSOCIATES
1350 North Highland Ave.,
#24
Los Angeles, CA 90028
(213) 462-1672

THE MARTEL AGENCY
7813 Sunset Blvd.
Los Angeles, CA 90046
(213) 874-8131

McCARTT/ORECK/
BARRETT
10390 Santa Monica Blvd.,
#300
Los Angeles, CA 90025
(213) 553-2600

JAMES McHUGH
8150 Beverly Blvd.
Suite 303
Los Angeles, CA 90048
(213) 651-2770

PETER MEYER AGENCY
9220 Sunset Blvd., #303
Los Angeles, CA 90048
(213) 278-4766

THE MINKOFF AGENCY
12001 Ventura Place, #335
Studio City, CA 91604
(818) 760-4501

THE MISHKIN AGENCY
2355 Benedict Cyn.
Beverly Hills, CA 90210
(213) 274-5261

WILLIAM MORRIS
AGENCY
151 El Camino Drive
Beverly Hills, CA 90212
(213) 274-7451

BUD BURTON MOSS
113 N. San Vicente Blvd.
Suite 202
Beverly Hills, CA 90211
(213) 655-1156

H. DAVID MOSS
8019½ Melrose Ave.
Suite 3
Los Angeles, CA 90046
(213) 653-2900

BEN PEARSON
606 Wilshire Blvd.
Suite 614
Santa Monica, CA 90401
(213) 451-8414

PECHET BLANCHARD
BERMAN AGENCY
1925 Century Park East,
#1150
Los Angeles, CA 90067
(213) 556-1971

VICTOR PERILLO
9229 Sunset Blvd.
Los Angeles, CA 90069
(213) 278-0251

PROGRESSIVE ARTISTS
400 South Beverly Drive
Suite 216
Beverly Hills, CA 90212
(213) 553-8561

JACK ROSE
6430 Sunset Blvd.
Suite 1203
Hollywood, CA 90028
(213) 463-7300

THE SANDERS AGENCY
LTD.
721 North LaBrea Avenue
Los Angeles, CA 90038
(213) 938-9113

THE SAVAGE AGENCY
6212 Banner Avenue
Los Angeles, CA 90038
(213) 461-8316

IRV SCHECHTER
9300 Wilshire Blvd.
Suite 410
Beverly Hills, CA 90212
(213) 278-8070

SCHIOWITZ &
ASSOCIATES
7080 Hollywood Blvd.,
#720
Hollywood, CA 90028
(213) 461-0152

DON SCHWARTZ
8749 Sunset Blvd.
Los Angeles, CA 90069
(213) 657-8910

JOHN SEKURA
7469 Melrose Avenue, #30
Los Angeles, CA 90046
(213) 653-5005

SELECTED ARTISTS
AGENCY
13111 Ventura Blvd.
Suite #204
Studio City, CA 91604
(213) 877-0055

DAVID SHAPIRA
15301 Ventura Blvd.
Suite #345
Sherman Oaks, CA 91403
(818) 906-0322

GLENN SHAW
3330 Barham Blvd.
Suite #103
Hollywood, CA 90068
(213) 851-6262

LEW SHERRELL
7060 Hollywood Blvd.
Suite #610
Los Angeles, CA 90028
(213) 461-9955

SHIFFRIN ARTISTS
7466 Beverly Blvd.
Suite #205
Los Angeles, CA 90048
(213) 937-3937

THE SHILOH AGENCY
12023½ Ventura Blvd.
Suite 2
Studio City, CA 91604
(818) 506-8303

SHUMAKER TALENT
AGENCY
6533 Hollywood Blvd.,
#301
Hollywood, CA 90028
(213) 464-0745

SMITH-FREEDMAN &
ASSOCIATES
121 N. San Vicente Blvd.
Beverly Hills, CA 90211
(213) 852-4777

SPOTLITE
ENTERPRISES, LTD.
8665 Wilshire Blvd.
Suite 208
Beverly Hills, CA 90211
(213) 657-8004

STARS, THE AGENCY
777 Davis Street
San Francisco, CA 94111
(415) 421-6272

STE REPRESENTATION
9301 Wilshire Blvd., #312
Beverly Hills, CA 90210
(213) 550-3982

STONE MANNERS
9113 Sunset Blvd.
Los Angeles, CA 90069
(213) 275-9599

WINIFRED STRAND
TALENT AGENCY
9229 Sunset Blvd.
Suite 202
Los Angeles, CA 90069
(213) 278-1561

STRIEMER AND
COMPANY
2040 Avenue of the Stars
4th Floor
Los Angeles, CA 90067
(213) 556-3137

SUTTON/BARTH/
VENNARI
145 S. Fairfax Ave.
Suite 310
Los Angeles, CA 90036
(213) 938-6000

HERB TOBIAS
1901 Avenue of the Stars
Suite 840
Los Angeles, CA 90067
(213) 277-6211

TRIAD ARTISTS, INC.
10100 Santa Monica Blvd.
Los Angeles, CA 90067
(213) 556-2727

20TH CENTURY AGENCY
3800 Barham Blvd.
Suite 303
Los Angeles, CA 90068
(213) 850-5516

VARIETY ARTISTS
INTERNATIONAL
9073 Nemo St.
3rd Floor
Los Angeles, CA 90069
(213) 858-7800

WALLACK &
ASSOCIATES TALENT
1717 North Highland Ave.
Suite 701
Hollywood, CA 90028
(213) 465-8004

ANN WAUGH AGENCY
4731 Laurel Canyon Blvd.,
#5
N. Hollywood, CA 91607
(818) 980-0141

RUTH WEBB
7500 Devista Drive
Los Angeles, CA 90046
(213) 874-1700

MARY ELLEN WHITE,
INC.
151 No. San Vicente Blvd.
Suite 208
Beverly Hills, CA 90211
(213) 653-4731

WILHELMINA ARTISTS
6430 Sunset Boulevard
Suite 701
Los Angeles, CA 90028
(213) 464-8577

NOTA WILLIAMS
TALENT AGENCY
4942 Vineland Avenue
N. Hollywood, CA 91601
(818) 505-9962

WILLIAMSON &
ASSOCIATES
932 North LaBrea Avenue
Los Angeles, CA 90038
(213) 851-1881

CARTER WRIGHT
TALENT
6533 Hollywood Blvd.
Suite 201
Hollywood, CA 90028
(213) 469-0944

WRITERS AND ARTISTS
11726 San Vicente Blvd.
Suite 300
Los Angeles, CA 90049
(213) 820-2240

SCREEN ACTORS GUILD (SAG) BRANCH OFFICES

For a list of SAG agents, contact the branch office that is nearest to you. SAG's national headquarters are located at 7065 Hollywood Boulevard, Hollywood, CA 90028, (213) 465-4600.

5150 N 16th Street, #C-255
Phoenix, AZ 85016
(602) 279-9975

3045 Rosecrans Avenue,
#308
San Diego, CA 94104
(619) 222-3996

100 Bush Street
16th Floor
San Francisco, CA 94104
(415) 391-7510

950 S. Cherry Street, #502
Denver, CO 80222
(303) 757-6226

2299 Douglas Road
Suite West
Miami, FL 33145
(305) 444-7677

1627 Peachtree Street,
N.E., #210
Atlanta, GA 30309
(404) 897-1335

949 Kapiolani Boulevard,
#105
Honolulu, HI 96814
(808) 538-6122

307 N. Michigan Avenue
Chicago, IL 60601
(312) 372-8081

The Highland House
5480 Wisconsin Avenue,
#201
Chevy Chase, MD 20815
(301) 657-2560

11 Beacon Street, #512
Boston, MA 02108
(617) 742-2688

28690 Southfield Road
Lathrup Village, MI 48076
(313) 559-9540

15 S. 9th Street, #400
Minneapolis, MN 55404
(612) 371-9120

906 Olive Street, #1006
St. Louis, MO 63101
(619) 231-8410

1515 Broadway
44th Floor
New York, NY 10036
(212) 944-1030

1367 E. 6th Street, #229
Cleveland, OH 44114
(216) 579-9305

230 S. Broad Street
10th Floor
Philadelphia, PA 19102
(215) 545-3150

1108 17th Avenue South
Nashville, TN 37212
(615) 327-2958

2650 Fountainview, #325
Houston, TX 77057
(713) 972-1806

Two Dallas Communications
Complex
6309 N. O'Connor Road,
#111-LB 25
Irving, TX 75039-3510
(214) 869-9400

601 Valley Street, #200
Seattle, WA 98109
(206) 282-2506

Independent Casting Directors

Casting directors are involved in just about every area of the entertainment industry, from plays to musicals, feature films, and radio and television programs. Their primary function is to bring to the attention of producers and directors those performers who most typify particular characters in a play, a show, or in fact, any kind of show business production at all. To accomplish this purpose, casting directors will get in touch with performers whose work they personally are familiar with, or they will let the industry know, through casting calls or by contacting agents and press representatives, that a certain role is being cast. Auditions are then arranged for performers who seem most right for the part. Casting directors will sometimes cast just one part in a production, and other times may cast all roles, from top to bottom, from stars to walk-on parts.

The casting director is employed by the producer of a play, musical, feature film, commercial, or radio/TV program—including soap operas, pilots, series, mini-series, movies-of-the-week and specials. The casting director then presents the appropriate performer for the specific project. This is accomplished through auditions and meetings with the producer along with the director, writer, and other members of the creative staff.

Not too many years ago the profession of casting director did not even exist. It was up to the producer or director to cast a role. Producers tend to use the same performers over and over again. As the performing unions grew stronger—Actors' Equity in particular—hundreds of people *had* to be seen, and it became an unwieldy and time-filling task for the director and producer to handle alone. A new profession was born, and the producer put his show in the hands of a trusted person whose taste and wisdom he could rely upon.

Back Stage contacted some of the top professionals on the Broadway scene in order to define exactly what a director does and/or how he or she chooses the actors that he/she will work with. All agreed that their primary goal is to work for the actor's best interest and to connect it to the director's best interest. Here are some of those responses:

Geoffrey Johnson: "I rely on my knowledge of the actors and actresses that I have seen perform and have liked in the many varieties of theater, film, and television available to me (i.e., showcases, scene nights, soap scenes, etc.). I also go back to the notes I keep on actors who have auditioned for me. However, just because I've liked an actor's work, it does not mean I feel they are right for the project I am currently casting . . . .

"Treat every audition you get as a business appointment. Be professional, try to learn as much as you can beforehand about the project and the people you are auditioning for without being bothersome. The results, even though you may not get the role (next time you will!) will be rewarding to the casting director, the project, and yourself."

Joanna Merlin: "A casting director must use intuition and be imaginative. Often an actor may unconsciously limit himself, whereas when a casting director reads him, he or she can envision him doing something he has never done before. If the casting director can convince the actor to experiment a little, guide him into a new way of thinking, it becomes a creative experience for both of them."

Pat McCorkle: "A casting director is only a funneling system of sorts. You look at a character and you say, 'What do I need to make this come alive? Who do I need?' The creative juices flow and you start searching."

Stuart Howard: "In seeing the hundreds of pictures and resumes that come into the office, I will always give a second look to those who have gone to college . . . I root for the one who is well-prepared and willing. If he doesn't get my job, I'm sure going to hold on to his name or refer him to someone else."

Julie Hughes: "Objectivity is truly difficult. If asked, our casting firm will give our opinion, and if we have developed a trusting relationship with the producer or director, we can be helpful in pinpointing a problem. Producers are not as experienced as they were in the days of David Merrick and Kermit Bloomgarden. Most are businessmen—we are grateful for their interest, but sometimes they do not have the life experience we have."

Warren Pincus: "Actors should look into themselves as to why they didn't get a particular part. Did they do their homework? Did they dress properly? Do they have an attitude? Will they do things differently next time? Believe me, if I have learned one thing in this business, it's simply keep on trying. You just never know."

Independent Casting Directors

New York City

The following is a listing of some of the casting directors in New York City and Los Angeles. Note that we have not included phone numbers, since most of these offices request that initial contact be made through picture/resumes, by mail only.

JOSEPH ABALDO
CASTING
450 W. 42nd St.
New York, NY 10036

ACTORS UNLIMITED
CASTING SERVICE
1 Times Square
11th Fl.
New York, NY 10036

AQUILA/PEMRICK
CASTING
1633 Broadway
Suite 1801
New York, NY 10019

JAY BINDER CASTING
513 W. 54th St.
New York, NY 10019

JANE BRINKER
51 W. 16th St.
New York, NY 10011

DEBORAH BROWN
CASTING
250 W. 57th St.
New York, NY 10107

BURNS & FAHEY
CASTING
121 W. 27th St.
Suite 503
New York, NY 10001

KATE BURTON
39 W. 19th St.
New York, NY 10011

CTP CASTING
22 W. 27th St.
New York, NY 10001

CAST-AWAY! CASTING
SERVICE
14 Sutton Place South
New York, NY 10022

CENTRAL CASTING OF
NY
200 W. 54th ST.
New York, NY 10019

BOB COLLIER
ENTERPRISES, INC.
1650 Broadway
Suite 509
New York, NY 10036

COMPLETE CASTING
240 W. 44th St.
New York, NY 10036
Mailing address only

CONTEMPORARY
CASTING, LTD.
41 E. 57th St.
Suite 901
New York, NY 10022

MERRY L. DELMONTE
CASTING & PROD'N. CO.
460 W. 42nd St.
New York, NY 10036

DONNA DE SETA
CASTING
424 W. 33rd St.
New York, NY 10001

LOU DIGIAIMO
ASSOCIATES, LTD.
P.O. Box 5296, FDR Station
New York, NY 10150

HERMAN & LIPSON
CASTING
24 W. 25th St.
New York, NY 10010

STUART HOWARD
ASSOCIATES, LTD.
215 Park Ave. So.
Suite 1806
New York, NY 10003

SYLVIA FAY
71 Park Ave.
New York, NY 10016

LEONARD FINGER
1501 Broadway
Room 1511
New York, NY 10036

MAUREEN FREMONT
CASTING
641 W. 59th St.
Room 21
New York, NY 10019

GINGER FRIEDMAN
Mailing address: Actors
Outlet, 120
W. 28th St.
New York, NY 10001

GODLOVE, SEROW,
SINDLINGER CASTING
151 W. 25th St.
New York, NY 10001

GOLDEN CASTING
133 W. 72nd St.
Room 601
New York, NY 10023

MARIA GRECO
ASSOCIATES
1261 Broadway
Suite 308
New York, NY 10001

JUDY HENDERSON &
ASSOCIATES CASTING
330 W. 89th St.
New York, NY 10024

HUGHES MOSS CASTING
311 W. 43rd St.
Suite 700
New York, NY 10036

HYDE-HAMLET CASTING
165 W. 46th St.
Room 1115
New York, NY 10010

JOHNSON-LIFF CASTING
1501 Broadway
Suite 1400
New York, NY 10036

KASHA/LIEBHART
275 Central Park West
Suite 2C
New York, NY 10024

KELLY & CASE CASTING
ASSOCIATES
155 W. 13th St.
New York, NY 10011

JODI KIPPERMAN CASTS
211 Thompson St.
Suite 1C
New York, NY 10012

LYNN KRESSEL
CASTING
111 W. 57th St.
Suite 1422
New York, NY 10019

JASON LAPADURA
CASTING
39 W. 19th St
12th Floor
New York, NY 10011

LEHNER/STEPHENS
CASTING
156 Fifth Ave.
Suite 1208
New York, NY 10010

MCL CASTING, LTD.
165 W. 46th St.
New York, NY 10036

McCORKLE CASTING,
LTD.
264 W. 40th St.
Ninth Floor
New York, NY 10018

D. LYNN MEYERS
CASTING
c/o Burns
330 W. 42nd St.
32nd Floor
New York, NY 10036

MYERS/TESCHNER
333 W. 52nd St.
New York, NY 10019

NAVARRO/BERTONI
CASTING CO., LTD.
101 W. 31st St.
Room 2112
New York, NY 10001

JOANNE PASCIUTO, INC.
1457 Broadway
Suite 308
New York, NY 10036

JEFF PASSERO
47 Perry St.
Suite 10
New York, NY 10014

IRMA PUCKETT
CASTING
39 W. 19th St.
12th Floor
New York, NY 10011

REED & MELSKY
CASTING
928 Broadway
Suite 300
New York, NY 10010

REED/SWEENEY/REED
INC.
1780 Broadway
New York, NY 10019

RICHMOND/
MUSSENDEN, INC.
141 Fifth Ave
Suite 5S
New York, NY 10010

CHRISTINE ROELFS &
ASSOCIATES, LTD.
850 Seventh Ave.
Suite 1005
New York, NY 10019

MIKE ROSCOE CASTING,
LTD.
153 E. 37th St.
Suite 1B
New York, NY 10016

MARCIA SHULMAN
Mailing address: 80 Eighth
Ave.
Suite 303
New York, NY 10011

SHERIE L. SEFF
CASTING
400 W. 43rd St.
New York, NY 10036

SHIRLEY SENDER
CASTING
92 Horatio St.
Room 5H
New York, NY 10014

BARBARA SHAPIRO
111 W. 57th St.
Suite 1420
New York, NY 10019

SIMON & KUMIN
CASTING
1600 Broadway
Suite 609
New York, NY 10019

TODD THALER
130 W. 57th St.
Suite 12E
New York, NY 10019

DAVID TOCHTERMAN
CASTING
311 W. 43rd St.
Suite 604
New York, NY 10036

JOY TODD, INC.
Two W. 32nd. St.
New York, NY 10001

URELL CASTING
641 W. 59th St.
Room 10
New York, NY 10019

JOY WEBER CASTING
250 W. 57th St.
New York, NY 10019

SUSAN WILLETT
CASTING
1170 Broadway
Suite 1008
New York, NY 10001

BILL WILLIAMS
CASTING
119 W. 25th St., PH
New York, NY 10001

MARJI CAMNER WOLLIN
& ASSOCIATES
233 E. 69th St.
New York, NY 10021

RONNIE YESKEL
CASTING
268 W. 84th St.
New York, NY 10024

JEFFREY ZEINER
451 W. 43rd St.
New York, NY 10036

Los Angeles

BCI (Barbara Claman)
6565 Sunset Blvd., #412
Los Angeles, CA 90028

BENGSTON/COHN
11365 Ventura Blvd., #119
Studio City, CA 91604

BROWN/WEST
7319 Beverly Blvd., #10
Los Angeles, CA 90036

THE CASTING COMPANY
7319 Beverly Blvd., #One
Los Angeles, CA 90036

CHAMPION/BASKER
CASTING
7060 Hollywood Blvd.,
#808
Los Angeles, CA 90028

RACHELLE FARBERMAN
Kushner/Locke
10850 Wilshire Blvd.
Los Angeles, CA 90024

FENTON/FEINBERG/
TAYLOR CASTING
Universal Studios
100 Universal City Plaza
Bungalow 477
Universal City, CA 91608

HENDERSON/HANLEY
CASTING
8125 Lankershim Blvd.
North Hollywood, CA 91605

JUDITH HOLSTRA
CASTING
3518 Cahuenga Blvd. West
Los Angeles, CA 90068

CARO JONES
5858 Hollywood Blvd.
Suite 220
Los Angeles, CA 90028

LIBERMAN/HIRSCHFELD
CASTING
Sunset/Gower Studios
1438 N. Gower Ave.
Suite 1410
Los Angeles, CA 90028

MCLEAN/DIMEO &
ASSOCIATES
12725 Ventura Blvd.
Suite H
Studio City, CA 91604

BOB MORONES
733 N. Seward St.
Los Angeles, CA 90038

ONORATO/FRANKS
CASTING
1717 N. Highland Ave.,
#904
Los Angeles, CA 90028

PAGANO/BIALY
1680 N. Vine St., #904
Los Angeles, CA 90028

THE PART COMPANY
7080 Hollywood Blvd.,
#606
Los Angeles, CA 90028

PENNY PERRY CASTING
11350 Ventura Blvd., #210
Studio City, CA 91604

BARBARA REMSEN
CASTING
Raleigh Studios
650 N. Bronson Ave.
Los Angeles, CA 90004

REUBEN CANNON &
ASSOCIATES
Paramount Studios
Gloria Swanson Bldg., #306
5555 Melrose Ave.
Los Angeles, CA 90038

ROBINSON/ELLERS
COMPANY
451 N. La Cienega Blvd.
Los Angeles, CA 90048

LYNN STALMASTER &
ASSOCIATES
9911 W. Pico Blvd., #1580
Los Angeles, CA 90035

WALLIS NICITA &
ASSOCIATES
Paramount
5555 Melrose Ave.
Dressing Room Bldg., #200
Los Angeles, CA 90038

Auditioning for Commercials

by Rorri Feinstein

Acting in commercials can be a very lucrative business. In 1987, according to statistics provided by the Screen Actors Guild, New York area actors earned over $300 million in commercial session fees and residuals, and that figure increased in 1988. The question becomes: How can you have your earnings included in that statistic?

Although every spot is different, on the average, 40–50 actors per character are seen for on-camera work. This figure is not set in stone. There are some commercials where the client sees every model in the NY area and some where only five actors are seen. So the odds of getting a commercial once you've got the audition are not bad, considering what the odds are of getting a role from an Equity principal audition or an open call.

AUDITION TIPS

The majority of SAG/AFTRA commercial casting is done through agents' submissions to agency or independent casting directors. The casting director videotapes the preliminary auditions and presents a tape which is then reviewed by the production company, the agency creative team (producer, copy writer, art director) and the client. These three parties decide on who gets called back and who gets cast.

When you get a call for a commercial audition, find out from your agent as much information as possible about the character, the product and what you should wear. Casting people provide this information because they want you to do well. They are on your side! They want to put together the best audition tape possible. The better you look, the better they look to their clients.

Commercial directors are impressed with actors who make an extra effort to dress the part they are up for. If you are reading for a pharmacist, wear a white jacket; if you'll be playing a yuppie, think Brooks Brothers. In general, keep your wardrobe choices simple. Pale to medium shades are best. Try to avoid red, black, and white (except for uniforms), because these colors pose problems to the video camera. Actresses should keep their makeup light, fresh and natural-looking.

Arrive at your audition with your picture and resume stapled together, and with enough time to look over the storyboard and the copy. Use your time in the waiting room productively. Don't give a cold reading—give a performance. This is a business and should be treated as such. Casting people like to see performers who are prepared, who know how to ask the right questions, and who can take direction.

Your audition begins the moment you walk through the door, not when you read the first line from the cue card. Project a positive, professional image. If you are late, don't make a big deal of it. Find out from the receptionist if it has upset the schedule; if not, don't mention it.

At some auditions actors aren't given scripts. Some directors like completely spontaneous auditions. They feel that performers do their best and funniest commercial work when they are just being themselves, when they don't try to act, but just enjoy the process and have fun at the audition. Often the copy hasn't been finalized and the original storyboard can be shaped and enriched by the performers who are auditioning.

So how does one have fun at auditions? By approaching every commercial you read for in an original way. Take a sympathetic point of view, and try to be natural and believable. You don't have to go for a hard sell. Instead, be creative; try to establish your character with a single word or gesture. Although it's easier said than done, take the pressure off yourself. Don't think about who you are competing with or whether or not you'll be called back. If you are right for the role, you'll get it. Your job is simply to give a good audition, do the best work possible, and then leave. Casting decisions in commercials are made too whimsically for actors to be concerned with. You have to be satisfied with your performance. The casting director determines who gets to audition and be seen on the audition tape, that is all. Rarely does a casting director make the final casting decision. Often it is not the actor who gave the best performance who books the spot anyway. That is because looks are a major consideration and everyone has a different idea of what kind of mommy, daddy, executive or grandma the spot calls for. So you can give a great reading and the casting director and the director can love you. But you still won't book the spot if the client wants someone else.

ACTING COURSES AND COMMERCIAL TECHNIQUES

If you are new to the commercial world, it probably would benefit you to take a commercial acting course. What you learn will help you feel comfortable on camera, and you'll get a chance to build a technique that will prepare you for most audition situations. Being familiar with the process can help boost your self-confidence. There are technical things you need to know, such as how to hit a mark, read from a cue card and hold a product.

There are schools that specialize in helping actors prepare for working in commercials. At these schools actors have the opportunity to work with copy and be video-taped in a professional studio that simulates the audition experience.

Before you sign up for a course in a school, you should audit a few. A good school should have professional quality video equipment and should employ instructors who are professionals in the business (i.e. casting directors, commercial actors, directors). Classes must be small so that each student receives personal attention and gets to work in every session. Some of the staff from a few of the New York Commercial schools offer some advice on acting in commercials below.

Ruth Lehner of Lehner/Stephens stresses the importance of being yourself in front of the camera. She notes that a commercial is a one-to-one situation and that you have to make the copy believable and show that you care about the product. In addition to working on technique, Lehner also deals with the business side of commercials. In these classes, the SAG/AFTRA standard contract is explained, so that performers are knowledgeable enough to talk to their agents rather than just to listen to them.

Ed Barron of the Weist-Barron School of TV Acting stresses the art of communication in his classes and encourages his students to think of sharing information rather than selling. In this way you really can find the "commercials" in your own life; for example, when you tell a friend about a movie you really liked, or about a new restaurant, you employ the same techniques you use in a commercial: you like a product (movie or restaurant), and you want others to use the product.

Teacher Ruth Nerken of the William Esper Studio compares performing for the camera to talking on the telephone. She notes that we are all very comfortable talking to our friends and business associates on the telephone, but we are in fact talking into a mechanical device. She invites actors to find the essence of each spot and make acting choices that illustrate the point at hand. If the commercial is for a time-saving product, she suggests that you present yourself as a brisk businesslike character. If you are advertising perfume, you should present a softer, more sensual image. Above all, says Nerken, project a winning attitude, and at every audition, bring in something that makes you special.

Bob Collier of Bob Collier TV Success seminars, teaches his students that the secret to success is a positive mental attitude. In his classes a lot of work is done to achieve that goal, including the use of creative visualization and daily affirmations. Students are given a Polaroid of themselves doing a commercial (in the classroom), which is taken from the monitor screen. This helps students see themselves literally and in their minds' eyes to see themselves as working commercial actors.

Wendy Dillon, who teaches at the Bob Collier school advises actors to approach the business with the idea that people like you and want you to do well. Because actors are rejected so often, they often expect failure rather than success. Dillon emphasizes the importance of networking and talking about what you are doing in your career with people who have similar goals. She stresses that it is helpful both personally and professionally to exchange information with friends and to look for opportunities for your friends as well as for yourself.

ON THE SET

When you are cast in a commercial, you will have to deal with an entire set of unfamiliar production elements. Camera, sound, lighting, props, and so on have to be perfect, so you may be asked to do take after take even though your reading is just fine.

Because there are so many chiefs on a commercial set, you may get directional input from all sides. This can be a problem. The only person you should take direction from is the director. So nod politely to the client, the agency and production people, and try to tune them out. Your object is to maintain a good relationship with your employers while fulfilling your responsibilities to the director.

SOME CLOSING THOUGHTS

It has often been said that one should never read the reviews of a show while performing in it, because if you believe the good ones you have to believe the bad ones, too. The point here is to trust your own evaluation of your work. What is important is that you feel you have done a good job in an audition or on a shoot, because they may not use your best take, or you may not get the job where you gave a terrific reading. On the other hand, you could book a national spot on an off day.

Ad Agency Casting Directors

ALLY & GARGANO, INC.
805 Third Ave.
New York, NY 10022
(212) 688-5300
Rhoda M. Karp, Casting Dir. On-camera casting thru casting dirs. Voice-over casting thru agents. Voice-over tapes accepted from SAG and/or AFTRA members. No phone calls.

N W AYER, INC.
1345 Ave. of the Americas
New York, NY 10105
(212) 708-5960
Sally Howes Kandle, VP/Casting; Renee Howley, Maureen Chilton, Casting Dirs.; Joe Ann Brennan, Janet Eisenberg, Marilyn Zitner, Asst. Casting Dirs.; Emily Norton, Casting Coord. Send pix & resumes, will call if type is needed.

BACKER SPIELVOGEL BATES
405 Lexington Ave.
New York, NY 10174
(212) 297-1000
Nancy Fields, VP/Casting; Roger Sturtevant, Stephen DeAngelis, Casting Dirs. No solicitations or pix accepted.

BATTEN, BARTON, DURSTINE & OSBORN, INC.
1285 Ave. of the Americas
New York, NY 10019
(212) 459-6705
Terry Berland, Cabrina Carnevale, Heads of Casting; Eileen A. Powers, Asst. Pix & resumes accepted. No phone calls.

LEO BURNETT CO., INC.
950 Third Ave.
New York, NY 10022
(212) 759-5959
Casting thru Chicago office: Leo Burnett USA, Prudential Plaza, Chicago, IL 60601

CAMPBELL-MITHUN-ESTY
100 E. 42nd St.
New York, NY 10017
(212) 692-6200
Mary Tibaldi, Casting Dir.: Janine Minunno, Assoc. Casting Dir.: Pix & resumes accepted. Do not phone or visit.

D'ARCY MASIUS BENTON & BOWLES
909 Third Ave.
New York, NY 10022
(212) 758-6200
Linda Ferrara, Casting Dir.; Susan Bastian, Casting Asst. Casts thru files and agents. Do not call.

DELLA FEMINA, MCNAMEE, WCRS
350 Hudson St.
New York, NY 10014
(212) 886-4100
Linda Tesa, VP dir./TV & radio broadcasting; Eric Herrmann, Sr. Prod'r.; Debbie Lawrence, Prod'r.; Brendan O'Malley, Stephanie Slade, Asst. Prod'rs. Works thru production houses and casting agents. Do not phone.

GREY ADVERTISING, INC.
777 Third Ave.
New York, NY 10017
(212) 546-2000
Jerry Saviola, VP; Barbara Bennett, Assoc.; Claudia Walden, Madeline Molnar, Michael O'Gara, Arista Baltronis, Dolores Fisher, Casting Dirs.; Ted Sluberski, Lisa Weinberg, Casting Assts. Send pix & resumes for files. No calls accepted.

HOLLAND & CALLAWAY
767 Third Ave.
New York, NY 10017
(212) 308-2750
Carol Parrino, Broadcast Mgr., Casting; Arthur Wright, Russ Keiser, Prod'r./Casting. Pix & resumes accepted.

JORDAN, McGRATH, CASE & TAYLOR
445 Park Ave.
New York, NY 10022
(212) 326-9100
*Vicki Goggin, Casting Dir.; Karen Apicella,
Asst. Accepts pix & resumes.*

KORNHAUSER & CALENE, INC.
228 E. 45 St.
New York, NY 10017
(212) 490-1313
*Pamela Maytheny, Head of Prod'n.; Robert
Litt, VP Prod'r.; Tracy Dennis, Janice Ent-
wistel, Assts. Casts thru agents only. Accepts
pix & resumes by mail. No phone calls.*

LAURENCE, CHARLES, FREE &
LAWSON, INC.
260 Madison Ave., 4th floor
New York, NY 10016
(212) 213-4646
*Ellen Goldschmidt, Exec. Prod'r; Matthew
Messinger, Casting Dir. Casts only as required per commercial. Casts thru agents
only. Accepts pix & resumes from SAG extras
only. No phone calls.*

LINTAS/NY
1 Dag Hammarskjold Plaza
New York, NY 10017
(212) 605-8290
*Steve Schaefer, VP/Head; Barbara Blom-
berg, Casting Supv.; Susan Mattheiss, Casting Asst. Will call if type needed. Do not
phone.*

LOWE MARCHALK CO., INC.
1345 Ave. of the Americas
New York, NY 10105
(212) 708-8800
*Sharry Sabin, Casting Dir.; casts primarily
thru agents. No pix & resumes accepted. No
extra casting. Do not phone.*

McCANN-ERICKSON USA
485 Lexington Ave.
New York, NY 10117
(212) 697-6000
*John Cavoto, Dir. of Casting; Jeannie
Savino, Casting Dir. Send picture postcards
only. Do not send pix & resumes. Do not
phone.*

OGILVY & MATHER
2 E. 48 St.
New York, NY 10017
(212) 907-3400
*Daisy Sinclair, Casting Mgr./VP; Barbara
Herzog, Casting Dir.; J. B. Sutherland,
Print Casting Dir.; Kelly Barlow, Asst.
Casting done thru agents and files. Pix &
resumes for extras; appt. thru agents only for
interviews. Do not phone.*

ROSENFELD, SIROWITZ, HUMPHREY &
STRAUSS, INC.
111 5th Ave.
New York, NY 10003
(212) 505-0200
*Judy Keller, Casting Dir.: Jane Sircus, Ross
Kronman, Prod'rs. Casts thru agents and
from files. Send pix & resumes. Will call if
type is needed. Do not phone.*

SAATCHI & SAATCHI DEF COMPTON
375 Hudson St.
New York, NY 10014
(212) 463-2000
*Leslee Feldman, Tina Sperber, Casting
Dirs.; Kirsten Walther, Debi Gochman,
Assts. for extra work send pix & resumes.*

J. WALTER THOMPSON CO.
466 Lexington Ave.
New York, NY 10017
(212) 210-7000
*Evangeline Hayes, Casting Dir.; Heather
Aust, 2nd Asst. Casting Dir. Scale casting
done by production firms and independent
casting dirs.; principal, overscale and voice-
over casting done by the agency. Voice-over
types accepted.*

YOUNG & RUBICAM, INC.
285 Madison Ave.
New York, NY 10017
(212) 210-3000
*Barbara Badyna, Senior VP/Dir. of Casting;
Ann Batchelder, Sybil Trent, Cindy Bielak,
Janet Shahbenderian, Casting Dirs.: Brenda
Bareika, Talent Negotiator; Sue Barnes,
Thomas Winslow, Assts. Extras. Send pix &
resumes. Do not phone.*

Personal Managers

by Joseph Rapp

The right personal manager can sometimes really help a career take off. Many artists, though possessing the talent that can propel them all the way to the top, still require that extra nudge that the expert counsel of a resourceful personal manager can give them. A skillful personal manager can provide invaluable career planning and can manage a career all the way to superstardom.

Many in the entertainment industry are not really clear about what a personal manager does. Essentially, a personal manager is engaged in the occupation of advising talent and personalities. Personal managers also help to develop new talent. Moreover, personal managers act as liaison between their clients and theatrical agents, as well as all others in the industry.

Although entertainers do need the services of lawyers, accountants, publicity directors, choreographers, arrangers, theatrical agents, etc., they still need overall guidance. For such guidance it is the personal manager to whom they turn. The personal manager is the person who assists artists in their creative endeavors; the one who nurtures, grooms, guides, befriends and, at all times, is the driving force in the forefront—the one who can break through the barriers of frustration and difficulty that performers constantly encounter.

Obviously, to succeed in this undertaking, the personal manager must have the broadest of experience, must stay alert and keep abreast of the constant changes occurring in the industry.

AGENTS VERSUS MANAGERS

The fundamental difference between agents and managers has to do with the degree of *personal* attention they give their clients. According to the laws of New York City and State, theatrical agents are licensed as "Employment Agencies," to obtain "employment." Because of the number of clients they represent, agents cannot give performers the same personal service that the personal manager does. However, the separation between managers and agents should not be a competitive one—they should work together to enhance the careers of their clients.

In selecting a personal manager, you, the artist must use common sense, ask questions, check on the background of the manager, and speak to other entertainers. Be sure to read thoroughly and understand a management contract before signing it—in fact you should seek *legal* advice regarding such a contract. Word-of-mouth recommendations by other artists can be an invaluable aid in helping you select a personal manager. You should feel comfortable with your manager. You need to know that you can depend on this person, and that your manager has necessary contacts and an in-depth knowledge of the entertainment industry.

THE NCOPM

The National Conference of Personal Managers (NCOPM) was organized as a non-profit organization 32 years ago. Its purpose is to help personal managers expand their knowledge of the entertainment industry, to exchange information among its members, and to maintain a data and information library. Its National newsletters outline the activities of its members and chapters. Strict requirements must be met before an applicant can be accepted into the NCOPM, and applicants are required to list personal management as their primary occupation.

The NCOPM has reached a position of strength and prestige within the entertainment industry through adherence to a strict code of ethics and business practices among its members. NCOPM considers it an important part of its function to acquaint performers with the unethical practices of some companies and individuals within the industry.

Personal Managers

Listed below are members of the National Conference of Personal Managers. The name of the company is listed first, followed by the owner/manager's name. Associate members are listed below each phone number. The numbers in parentheses at the bottom of each listing indicate the different fields of entertainment in which a member is engaged. These numbers correspond to the seven categories listed here, i.e., (1) equals Actors/Actresses, and so on. (In some cases, a specific explanation is given next to a number.)

1) Actors/Actresses
2) Directors, and/or Producers, and/or Writers
3) Children, and/or Teenagers
4) Newscasters, and/or Sports Personalities
5) Variety, and/or Comedy Acts
6) Music: Performers, and/or Composers, and/or Recordings, and/or Concerts, and/or Lounge and/or Rock & Roll Acts
7) Miscellaneous: Anything not mentioned above (Artists, Photographers, and so on)

EAST COAST CHAPTER

The East Coast chapter of the Conference of Personal Managers is headed up by Joseph Rapp, executive director, 1650 Broadway, New York, NY 10019; (212) 265-3366.

ROGER AILES
COMMUNICATIONS
ROGER AILES
456 W. 43rd St.
New York, NY 10036
(212) 563-1970
Contact:
Mickey Harmon,
Judy Laterza
(1,2,4,5,6)

FOX-ALBERT
MANAGEMENT ENT.,
INC.
ADRIENNE ALBERT
1697 Broadway, Suite 1210
New York, NY 10019
(212) 581-1011
Contact:
Jean T. Fox
(1,3)

R. J. ALFREDO TALENT
MGMT.
RICHARD ALFREDO
320 E. 73rd St.
(212) 517-4169
New York, NY 10021
(1)

WORLD OF CULTURE,
LTD.
MARK HALL AMITIN
463 West St., Suite 509
New York, NY 10014
(212) 243-0292
(1,2,3,5)

JEMAVA INC.
DEE ANTHONY
40 E. 94th St., #27A
New York, NY 10128-0709
(212) 410-7200
(6,7)

MAHALO MGMT.
JEFFREY ARSENAULT
P.O. Box 2629
New York, NY 10009
(212) 473-4906
John Essay
(1)

FASTBREAK MGMT.
BUD AYERS
1775 Broadway, 7th Floor
New York, NY 10019
(212) 247-2990
Bob Rowland
(1,5,6)

TIN-BAR AMUSEMENT
CORP.
TINO BARZIE
11 W. 69th St., Suite 2B
New York, NY 10023
(212) 586-1015
(2,5,6,7)

HARVEY BELLOVIN
410 E. 64th St.
New York, NY 10021
(212) 752-5181
(1,2,6)

NEW PERSONALITIES,
INC.
MARK BELSKY
272-60 Grand Central
Parkway
Floral Park, NY 11005
(718) 631-3636
(1,3)

BENNU TALENT MGMT.
INC.
JOANNE BERKMAN
165 Madison Ave.
New York, NY 10016
(212) 213-8511
Contact:
Ron Uva
(1,6)

BOBBY BERNARD
40 Central Park South
New York, NY 10019
(212) 753-9843
(2,5,6)

MGMT. VII
VIC BERI
1811 N.E. 53rd St.
Ft. Lauderdale, FL 33308
(305) 776-1004
(1,5,6)

CLINTON FORD BILLUPS
JR.
101 River Road
Collinsville, CT 06022
(203) 693-1637
(5)

PHIL BOUGHTON
60 E. 42 St., Suite 524
New York, NY 10165
(212) 818-9531
(7: Scriptwriters)

NYLE BRENNER
20 W. 64th St.
New York, NY 10023
(212) 362-2735
(1,2)

LEONA BUDILOVSKY
2 S. 635 Ave. Vendom
Oak Brook, IL 60521
(312) 963-2611
(1,6)

TOP DRAWER
ENTERTAINMENT
ANTONIO CAMACHO
7742 164th St.
Flushing, NY 11366
(718) 591-1508
(5)

RAZOR SHARP PROD.,
INC.
DAVID CAMPBELL
60 W. 57th St.
New York, NY 10019
(212) 496-2057
(1,2)

RON COMENZO
320 W. 37th St., 4th Floor
New York, NY 10018
(212) 279-5198
(1)

THOMAS CURRIE
215 E. 29th St.
Suite 4
New York, NY 10016-8248
(212) 532-1476
(7: Directors)

PODESOIR INT'L
MGTMT.
K. CHARISSE DICKS
401 Schenectady Ave.
Suite 7E, 5th floor
Brooklyn, NY 11213
(718) 756-4016
(1,3,5,6)

MICHELE DONAY
TALENT MGMT.
MICHELE DONAY
236 E. 74th St.
New York, NY 10021
(212) 744-9406
(1,3)

KARLEKEN
INTERNATIONAL INC.
NILDA ECKERT
423 Middlessex Ave.
Metuchin, NJ 08840
(201) 548-6273
(6)

THINK TANK TALENT
JOEL FELTMAN
225 E. 79th St., Suite 5D
New York, NY 10021
(212) 570-9421, or (914) 570-9424
Contact:
Grace White
(1,4)

VICTORIA FRANKMANO
84-01 53rd Ave.
Elmhurst, NY 11373
(212) 593-4764
(1,3)

DISCOVERY TALENT
MGMT., LTD.
ESTELLE FUSCO
72 Moriches Road
Lake Grove, NY 11755
(212) 877-6670
or (516) 467-7574
(1,3)

GEKIS MGMT.
THEODORE GEKIS
240 W. 44th St., Suite 8
New York, NY 10036
(212) 302-2556
(1,3)

YOUNG TALENT, INC.
TOBE GIBSON
301 E. 62nd St., Suite 2C
New York, NY 10021
(212) 308-0930
(1,3,6)

BOBBIE GILES MGMT.
ADALINE R. GILES
340 Albany St.
New York, NY 10280
(212) 945-3608
(1)

FRESH FACES MGMT.
AGGIE GOLD
2911 Carnation Ave.
Baldwin, NY 11510
(516) 223-0034
(1,3: Ethnic)

GOLD STAR TALENT
MGMT.
SID & STEVEN GOLD
246 Fifth Ave., Suite 202
New York, NY 10001
(212) 213-1707
(3: Infants)

GMS MGMT
DICK GRASS
585 Ellsworth St., Suite 2G
Bridgeport, CT 06605
(203) 334-9285
Contact:
Danny Scarpone
(2,5,6,7)

LLOYD GREENFIELD
1140 Ave. of the Americas,
17th Fl.
New York, NY 10036
(212) 245-8130
(5,6)

GREEN KEY MGMT.
SETH R. GREENKY
251 W. 89th St., Suite 4A
New York, NY 10024
(212) 874-7373
(1,2,5,6,7)

MARC HOFFMAN
119 Langham St.
Brooklyn, NY 11235
(212) 460-7906
(1,6)

SHANDEILA
ASSOCIATES, INC.
VAL IRVING
30 Park Ave.
New York, NY 10016
(212) 685-5496
(1,2,4,5)

JOHN N. JENNINGS
881 10th Ave., Suite 1A
New York, NY 10019
(212) 581-0377
or (201) 224-5974
(1,3,5,6)

MURIEL KARL TALENT
MGMT., INC.
MURIEL KARL
888 Eighth Ave.
New York, NY 10019
(212) 245-3770
(1,3)

ANDREA KAUFMAN
1012 Atlantic Ave.
Atlantic City, N.J. 08401
(609) 347-8839, (609)
348-6736
(5,6)

KEYS-CO.
ENTERPRISES, INC.
BEVERLY M. KEYS
PO Box 110423
Nashville, TN 37211
(615) 331-KEYS
(1,5,6)

CARROLL L. KNOWLES
220 E. 63rd St.
New York, NY 10021
(212) 832-1135
(1)

LLOYD KOLMER
ENTERPRISES
LLOYD KOLMER
65 W. 55th St.
New York, NY 10019
(212) 582-4735
(1)

JENNIFER LAMBERT
1600 Broadway, Suite 1001
New York, NY 10019
(212) 315-0665; 315-0754
(1,3,5,6)

LANDSTAR PRODNS,
INC.
ALISON LANDES
253 W. 73rd St., Suite 8B
New York, NY 10023
(212) 874-5700
(7: Speakers)

DICK LEE
230 Sycamore Court
Chanticleer
Cherry Hill, NJ 08003
(609) 424-5354
(1,4,6)

LEVITON MGMT.
ABBE LEVITON
1650 B'way, Suite 304A
New York, NY 10019
(212) 541-5460
(1,5)

JOSEPH LODATO
264 W. 35th St., Suite 1003
New York, NY 10001
(212) 967-3320
(1,5,6: Rec. Prod.)

CREATIVE MGMT.
NETWORK INC.
SANDRA LORD
P.O. Box 515
New York, NY 10185
(212) 633-9548; 724-2800
(1,2,3,5,6)

RICK MARTIN
PRODUCTIONS
RICK MARTIN
125 Fieldpoint Rd.
Greenwich, CT 06830
(203) 661-1615
(1,5,6: Rec. Prod.)

McGOVERN/GOODWIN
THEATRICAL MGMT.
ARLINE McGOVERN
9 Layton Ave.
Hicksville, NY 11801
(212) 860-7400
or (516) 681-2723
Contact:
Lois Goodwin
(1,3)

SANDI MERLE
101 W. 57th St.
New York, NY 10019
(212) 489-1578
(4,5,6)

BURT MILLER
ASSOCIATES, INC.
BURT MILLER
308 Fern St.
W. Hartford, CT 06119
(203) 236-1983
(6)

J. MITCHELL MGMT.
JEFF MITCHELL
88 Bleecker St.
New York, NY 10012
(212) 777-6686
(1,3)

DONNA MOLLO
1143 West Broadway
Hewlett, NY 11557
(516) 569-3253
(3)

F.J.M. PRODUCTIONS,
INC.
FRED J. MONTILLA, JR.
7305 W. Sample Rd.,
Suite 101
Coral Springs, FL 33063
(305) 753-8591
(6)

MOORE
ENTERTAINMENT
GROUP
BARBARA MOORE
11 Possum Trail
Upper Saddle River, NJ
07458
(201) 327-3698
(1,2,3,6)

WILL MOTT
481 W. 22nd St., Suite 1
New York, NY 10011
(212) 924-1444
(1)

DEE-MURA
ENTERPRISES INC.
DOREEN NAKAMURA
269 West Shore Drive
Massapequa, NY 11758
(516) 795-1616
(2,5)

ROSELLA OLSON MGMT.
ROSELLA OLSON
2130 Broadway, Suite 1610
New York, NY 10023
(212) 874-7436
(1,5,6)

CATHY PARKER
MANAGEMENT, INC.
CATHY PARKER
PO Box 716
Voorhees Township, NJ
08043
(609) 354-2020
(1,3)

MORNING STAR MGMT.
MARIE PASTORE
1635 August Rd.
N. Babylon, NY 11703
(516) 243-1121; 243-1123
(1)

PRODUCTIONS &
MANAGEMENT GROUP
ALLAN S. PORTNOY
122 W. 75th St., Suite 1B
New York, NY 10023
(212) 877-2038
(1,2,6)

GERARD W. PURCELL
ASSOC., LTD.
GERARD W. PURCELL
210 E. 51st St.
New York, NY 10022
(212) 421-2670
Contact:
Faith Ball,
Donald B. Tabler
(2,5,6: TV, Records)

VIC RAMOS MGMT.
VICTOR RAMOS
49 W. 9th St., #5B
New York, NY 10011
(212) 473-2610,
(212) 673-9191
(1)

CHARLES RAPP
ENTERPRISES, INC.
HOWARD RAPP
1650 Broadway, Suite 609
New York, NY 10019
(212) 247-6646
(1,2,4,5)

JOSEPH RAPP
ENTERPRISES, INC.
JOSEPH RAPP
1650 Broadway, Suite 705
New York, NY 10019
(212) 265-3366
(5,6: TV, Records)

REAVESTOCK MGMT.
PATRICK REAVES
302 W. 79th St., Suite 3D
New York, NY 10024
(212) 580-1130
(1,2)

EDIE ROBB TALENT
WORKS INC.
EDIE ROBB
301 W. 53 St., Suite 4K
New York, NY 10019
(212) 245-3250
or (215) 947-5361
Contact:
Charles Worthington
(1,3)

CONNECTIONS
PEGGY ADLER ROBOHM
45 Lawson Dr.
Madison, CT 06443
(203) 245-4448
(1,3)

JACK ROLLINS
130 W. 57th St.
New York, NY 10019
(212) 582-1940
(1,2,5,6: TV, Film)

TALENT & COMEDY
MGMT.
JOAN M. ROSENBERG
3 Adam St.
Floral Park, NY 11001
(718) 343-9530
(1,3,5)

ROBIN SADIN
150 E. 39th St., P/H-D
New York, NY 10017
(212) 725-0972
(1,2)

SUZELLE ENTERPRISES
SUSAN SCHACHTER
182-06 Midland Parkway
Jamaica Estates, NY 11432
(718) 380-0585
(1,3)

PETER DUCHIN ORCH.
MGMT.
OTTO SCHMIDT
150 Cypress Club Dr., #503
Pompano Beach, FL 33060-
9245
(305) 771-4863
(5,6)

TED SCHMIDT &
ASSOC., INC.
TED SCHMIDT
2149 N.E. 63rd St.
Fort Lauderdale, FL 33308
(305) 771-7282,
(212) 751-0200
(5,6)

EDIE F. SCHUR, INC.
EDIE F. SCHUR
176 E. 71st St.
New York, NY 10021
(212) 734-5100
(1,2,3,4,7)

CHERYL SCOTT MGMT.
CHERYL A. SCOTT
25 Breezy Hill Rd.
Collinsville, CT 06022
(203) 693-0891/8270
(6: Rock)

SEA-MANAGEMENT
MARY H. SEAMAN
2548 N. Lincoln St.
Burbank, CA 91504
(818) 953-7149
(1,3)

JACK SEGAL
ENTERPRISES
JACK SEGAL
10 Park Ave.
W. Orange, NJ 07052
(201) 731-8801
(5)

SID SEIDENBERG
1414 Ave. of the Americas
New York, NY 10019
(212) 421-2021
(6)

EARL SHANK
Six Hibiscus Dr.
Ormond Beach, FL 32074
(904) 441-3768
(1,5)

SCOTT EDEN CREATIVE
MGMT.
MARTIN SIEGEL
4 Vails Lane
Millwood, NY 10546
(914) 941-8684
or (212) 953-1379
(1,3)

NO NAME MGMT.
C. WINSTON SIMONE
1780 Broadway, Suite 1201
New York, NY 10019
(212) 974-5322
(5,6,7: Rec. Prod.)

CUZZINS MGMT.
HELENE SOKOL
250 W. 57th St., Suite 1632
New York, NY 10019
(212) 586-1573
(1,3)

FULL CIRCLE MGMT.
JASON MERRICK
SOLOMON
460 W. 57th St.
New York, NY 10019
(212) 757-0213; 678-7400
(1,5)

SOMMERVILLE MGMT.
GRETSCHEN
SOMERVILLE
538 E. 14th St., Suite 21
New York, NY 10009
(212) 614-9286
(1,5)

CHRISTOPHER GROUP
PROD.
CHRISTOPHER SPIERER
1775 Broadway, 7th fl.
New York, NY 10019
(212) 601-1951
(1,6)

FONDA ST. PAUL MGMT.
MS. FONDA ST. PAUL
3811 Multiview Drive
Los Angeles, CA 90068
(213) 876-6161
(1)

BURT STRATFORD
221 W. 57th St.
New York, NY 10019
(212) 757-2211
(1,2,5)

LARRY TUNNY
ENTERPRISES, INC.
LARRY TUNNY
30 Lincoln Plaza
New York, NY 10023
(212) 582-2023
(6)

BARTON G. WEISS
MGMT., LTD.
BARTON G. WEISS
425 E. 58th St., Suite 18A
New York, NY 10010
(212) 751-9788; 614-9577
(1,5,6)

DWYER & WEISSMAN
MGMT.
MARCIA WEISSMAN
270 Lafayette St., Suite 808
New York, NY 10012
(212) 925-3300
(1)

TERRY WHATLEY
315 E. 57th St.
New York, NY 10022
(212) 308-9682
(1,2)

ZAZZA TALENT MGMT.
FRANK M. ZAZZA
Astoria Studios
34-12 36th St.
Astoria, NY 11106
(718) 729-9288
(1,2)

WEST COAST CHAPTER

The West Coast chapter of the Conference of Personal Managers is headed up by Tami Lynn, executive director, 4527 Park Allegra, Calabasa Park, CA 91302; (818) 888-8264.

RICHARD ALAN
ASSOCIATES
RICHARD ALAN
10817 Whipple Street, No. 7
North Hollywood, CA 91602
(818) 761-6689
(1)

TAP, INC.
TOMMY AMATO
1907 Villa Way South
Reno, NV 89509
(702) 826-5899

DAVID BUFFUM
3681 Berry Drive
Studio City, CA 91604
(818) 769-2811
(1,2,5)

FRANK CAMPANA
20121 Ventura Blvd.,
Suite 343
Woodland Hills, CA 91364
(818) 999-4834
(1,2,5,6)

PAUL CANTOR
ENTERPRISES, LTD.
PAUL CANTOR
14332 Dickens St., Suite 1
Sherman Oaks, CA 91423
(818) 907-5224
(6)

LAMBERT TALENT
MGMT.
PEG LAMBERT CAPONE
18992 Florida St., #7
Huntington Beach, CA
92648

J. C. MGMT.
JAN CUMMINGS
1501 N. Kings Road
Los Angeles, CA 90069
(213) 654-7189
(3)

JOEL DIAMOND
8733 Sunset Blvd.,
Suite 102
Los Angeles, CA 90069
(213) 659-0599

SUANNE B. DIAMOND
8250 Blackburn Ave., #1
Los Angeles, CA 90048
(213) 655-0445

LAKA & COMPANY
MICHAEL DODD
1860-A Kamani Place
Honolulu, HI 96818
(808) 833-4228

GEORGE DURGOM
ASSOCIATES
BULLETS DURGOM
999 North Doheny,
Suite 702
Los Angeles, CA 90046
(213) 278-8820; 275-6382
(1,5)

HILLARD ELKINS
ENTERTAINMENT CORP.
HILLARD ELKINS
8306 Wilshire Blvd.,
Suite 438
Beverly Hills, CA 90211
(213) 650-8306
(1,2,4,5,6,7)

EVANS MGMT.
STANLEY EVANS
10707 Camarillo St.,
Suite 308
North Hollywood, CA 91602
(818) 766-0114
(1,2,4,5,6)

MIXED MEDIA
MICHAEL GLYNN
4116 Warner Blvd., Suite B
Burbank, CA 91505
(818) 846-2111
(1,5,7)

CARMAN
PRODUCTIONS, INC.
JOE GOTTFRIED
15456 Cabrito Road
Van Nuys, CA 91406
(213) 873-7370;
(818) 787-6436
(1,2,5,6)

HOWARD HINDERSTEIN
PRODUCTIONS
HOWARD HINDERSTEIN
6430 Sunset Blvd., #1018
Hollywood, CA 90028
(213) 262-7140; 464-4300
(1,2,3,5)

INTERNATIONAL
TALENT MGMT.
BILL HUX
829 N. San Vincente
Suite Two
Los Angeles, CA 90069
(213) 652-1662

HEPHAESTUS
PRODUCTIONS
LES JANKEY
1790 North Orange Grove
Ave.
Los Angeles, CA
90046-2149
(213) 850-5607
(1)

JONES ENTERPRISES
MGMT.
ROSE ANDREA JONES
10834 DeFoe Ave.
Pacoima, CA 91331
(818) 896-1800
(1,3)

TRANS-WORLD MGMT.
RACHEL KAE
9161 Beachy Ave.
Arleta, CA 91331
(818) 897-2060
(1)

HARVEY KALMENSON
5730 Wish Ave.
Encino, CA 91316
(818) 342-6499
(1)

INA KESTEN
17730 Lassen, #127
Northridge, CA 91325
(818) 993-6454
(1,3)

RICHARD O. LINKE,
PERSONAL MGMT.
RICHARD LINKE
4445 Cartright Ave., #305
North Hollywood, CA 91602
(213) 760-4988; 760-2500
(1,5)

JEFFREY C. LOSEFF
4521 Colfax Ave., Suite 205
North Hollywood, CA 91602
(818) 505-9468

TAMI LYNN MGMT.
TAMI LYNN
4527 Park Allegra
Calabasa Park, CA 91302
(818) 888-8264
(3,4)

PRISCILLA LAMARCA
2655 W. 230th Place
Torrance, CA 90505
(213) 325-8708
(1,5)

NM MGMT.
NINA MARINO
1131 Alta Loma, Suite 229
Los Angeles, CA 90069
(213) 657-3588
(6)

JAN MARLYN MGMT.
JAN MARLYN
955 North Beverly
   Glen Blvd.
Bel Air, CA 90077
(213) 474-6350
(1)

MRM ENTERTAINMENT
CORP.
DAVID MARTIN
4370 Tujunga Ave.,
Suite 150
Studio City, CA 91604
(818) 980-8600
(1,2,4,5,6)

STEPHEN METZ
RAPP/METZ
ENTERTAINMENT CORP.
4370 Tujunga Ave.
Studio City, CA 91604
(818) 980-8600
(1,2,6)

ARNOLD MILLS &
ASSOCIATES
ARNOLD MILLS
8961 Sunset Blvd., Suite F
Los Angeles, CA 90069
(213) 278-2025
(4,5,6)

STAN MORESS
2114 Pico Blvd.
Santa Monica, CA 90405
(213) 450-9797
(5,6)

DEBORAH S. McMANUS
3918 Willow Crest
Studio City, CA 91404
(818) 569-3079
(1)

PAGE MGMT.
JEAN PAGE
5315 Oakdale Ave.
Woodland Hills, CA 91364
(818) 703-7328
(1,3)

OPM MGMT.
CHRISTINA PHILLIPS
8033 Sunset Blvd.,
Suite 4058
Los Angeles, CA 90046
(213) 654-4683
(1)

RIBEIRO PRODUCTIONS,
INC.
MICHAEL RIBEIRO
19122 Halsted St.
North Ridge, CA 91324
(818) 349-0334
(1)

BUD ROBINSON
PRODUCTIONS, INC.
BUD ROBINSON
1100 N. Alta Loma Road,
#707
Los Angeles, CA 90069
(213) 652-3242
(1,2,5,6)

BETTE ROSENTHAL
1300 San Ysidro
Beverly Hills, CA 90210
(213) 276-8924
(3,5,6)

JEFF ROSS
4470 Ventura Canyon Ave.
Sherman Oaks, CA 91423
(818) 788-6841
(1,2,5)

JOE SCANDORE
12411 Magnolia Blvd.,
Suite 311
North Hollywood, CA 91607
(818) 505-8588
(5)

ENTERTAINMENT
CONTRACTOR
J. SCHWARTZ
P.O. Box 65151
Los Angeles, CA 90065
(213) 256-9613
(1,3)

BARBARA J. SILVER
3300 Red Rose Drive
Encino, CA 91436
(818) 906-3544
Contact:
Wendy Phillips

TELESIS
ENTERTAINMENT
WESLEY STAPLES
P.O. Box 69919
Los Angeles, CA 90069
(213) 654-6061
(1,3,5)

CMT MGT.
CORETHA TIMKO
5013 W. Carson St.
Torrance, CA 90503
(213) 540-2724; 316-0304
(1,3)

TOLKIN TALENT MGMT.
JEWEL TOLKIN
6088 James Allen St.
Cypress, CA 90630
(714) 827-8525,
(714) 995-4673
Contact:
Al Tolkin
(3,7)

MIMI WEBER MGMT.,
LTD.
MIMI WEBER
9738 Arby Drive
Beverly Hills, CA 90210
(213) 278-8440;
(818) 954-1736
(1,7: Production)

HALLMARK
ENTERTAINMENT INC.
HOWARD B. WOLF
8033 Sunset Blvd.,
Suite 1000
Los Angeles, CA 90046
(213) 650-2245
(6)

Auditioning for the Musical Theater

by Fred Silver

A few decades ago there were actually jobs in the musical theater that went begging. Performers had their pick of Broadway and Off-Broadway musicals, national company productions, dinner theater and summer stock companies, night club revues, industrial shows, and variety shows. Actors could get needed experience in performing while building their careers, eventually establishing themselves as veteran Broadway performers.

As the result of economic attrition and the competition of television for the audience's attention, opportunities for performers have decreased to the point that actors no longer have the same chance to gain the necessary experience as performers. This makes it more difficult for them to effectively showcase themselves and their talent when they audition.

An audition is a live performance, given before potential employers, and the actors must create the impression that they are capable and worthy of being hired. There are some guidelines that you can rely on to help you do your best. They could well be called the *Ten Commandments of Auditioning for a Musical*, and should be reviewed before every audition.

1. Dress up for the occasion: An audition is a job interview. Since success breeds success you want to look prosperous and not down at the heels. Wear your Sunday best.

2. Select audition material that shows off who you are: Unless you are specifically requested to do so, don't select material from shows that are current, because everyone else will be singing the same material. Try to choose older goodies that you can bring something to. Avoid signature songs, those songs that are identified with the famous performers who created them. Keep away from character songs that are identified with a well-known character from a musical, such as "The Soliloquy" (Billy Bigelow from *Carousel*), "Hello Young Lovers" (Anna from the *King and I*), or "Shy" (Winifred from *Once Upon a Mattress*). You don't want the people you are auditioning for to see you as being limited to playing only the characters you show them, so it is important that you select material that allows your unique personality to come through.

3. Be prepared: Don't sing material that you learned a few days ago just for this audition. It takes at least three weeks of living with a piece before you can make it your own. You can iron the kinks out of new material by using it for auditions that you don't care about, those that are for jobs you wouldn't consider taking. Otherwise, singing something new for the people who can give you a job is one of the surest causes of stage fright. *Note:* It's also important to make sure that the people giving the audition have your picture and resume. Give it to them before you walk over to the pianist so they have something to look at while you are going over your music.

4. Practice ahead of time: Rehearse how you're going to enter the room, what you are going to say to the people who are there, and where you are going to stand. Rehearse what you are going to tell the pianist, who will need to know where or when to begin, and the tempo of your song.

5. Be sure your music is in order: Since you are at the mercy of the accompanist it is wise to be sure your music is attached in such a way that it is easy for the pianist to turn pages. Make sure any repeats or stops are clearly marked, and that transpositions and chord changes are clearly written out. If you are using separate music sheets paste them on rigid cardboard so they won't fall off the piano's music rack.

6. Don't look at anyone while you sing: Avoid making eye contact with your auditors: they are not your acting partners. Rather they are voyeurs watching you give a performance to an imaginary partner. If you look at them you deprive them of their role and they will have to look away, and not at you. Instead, select a spot a foot over the head of the central person you are auditioning for and place your imaginary acting partner there.

7. Keep your performance from becoming static: By all means use your hands and don't keep them down at your sides. Mannequins become boring to look at after a few measures. Don't be afraid to move downstage or to the side between sections of the song. Such devices can help you to control the attention of your auditors.

8. Don't leave before you are dismissed: Many actors lose jobs because they walk out of the room immediately after they finish singing. Perhaps they thought they hadn't gotten a response, or perhaps they believed they hadn't given a good performance. There is a moment of silence, almost a pregnant pause, after a performance during which the auditors are trying to decide whether they want to have the performer read or sing another song. If you make your exit at this moment you make it difficult for them to go after you and call you back. There just isn't time. Stand there, face them, and wait for them to dismiss you.

9. Keep a diary: It is important that you remember whom you sang for, for what show, what you sang, and what you wore. If you get a callback, they are going to remember you by what you wore and what you sang so don't change anything you did unless you are specifically requested to do so. Keep the same hairstyle, wear the same clothes (laundered of course) and sing the same material.

10. Radiate confidence: If you were earning five thousand dollars a week in a soap how would you walk? How would you dress? How would you feel? How would you look? Obviously, the answer to all those questions is, "self-confident." Although it might be difficult to go through a whole day acting out such a role, almost anyone can pull it off for a few minutes during an audition. People are often treated the way they feel they deserve to be treated. Believe you deserve the best.

Succeeding in Los Angeles

by Susan Goldstein

The business of show business is conducted differently in Los Angeles than any-where else in the world. Spread out geographically over many miles, L.A. is nonethe-less a small town when you're on the "inside." Because of this, the formula for getting cast for a show, a film, or in television is different here than anyplace else. The traditional means of waiting for your agent or manager to submit you will not work in this city. Being "merely" a good actor will not get you the job either, although it can help. No, to get hired in Los Angeles, you must become skilled at something called "networking."

Networking essentially means that you keep up with what is happening inside the industry among filmmakers, stars, producers, directors, packagers, other perform-ers, and anyone connected with the industry. Networking also includes "schmooz-ing," that is, hanging out and going to screenings, seminars, and workshops in order to meet and talk to filmmakers and other entertainers. Networking is extremely important to success in L.A. So, if possible, never turn down a networking opportu-nity. If the American Film Institute, USC, UCLA, or the Independent Feature Proj-ect/West are having a screening—go! Try to make this a hard-and-fast rule that you break only in the event that you are working or in case of extenuating circumstances.

Why go to a screening? For several reasons: 1) Filmmakers might be present, which will give you an opportunity to schmooze; 2) you might meet other actors with whom you can share information and leads; and 3) you'll learn more about your chosen profession—about performing and acting, and about what goes on "behind" the camera: directing, producing, cinematography, art direction, editing, etc. Actors who understand a film crew's responsibilities are more valuable professionally than those who don't. Such understanding lends actors and performers a veneer of profes-sionalism which can be an asset in acquiring work.

Another way to keep up with what is happening in the film-theater-video com-munity is to keep abreast of current industry news. Consult the "hot lines." These are telephone messages recorded by SAG, AFTRA, and Equity of up-to-date casting information. Also, call up the larger theaters in and around Los Angeles; many of them see new actors on a regular basis. Read all the local papers and the trade papers, too. Read the *Los Angeles Times* and/or the *Los Angeles Herald Examiner*, (and, if you live in the San Fernando Valley, aka "The Valley," you might want to read *The Daily News)*. Then there are the *L.A. Weekly*, the *L.A. Reader, Drama-Logue, Movieline*, and, of course "the trades," i.e., *The Hollywood Reporter* and the *Daily Variety*.

If this sounds like a lot of reading, think of it as an investment in your success rather than as an obligation. Once you understand how Hollywood operates, your anxiety level will be reduced, you'll have more confidence, and you'll be in greater control of your L.A. destiny. Your reading will keep you up-to-date on everything from who's buying what property, or which star just left what film due to "creative differences," to who's being "spun off" into their own series. By keeping attuned to such information, you are actively participating in building your own success; managers and agents find it easier, more exciting, and more fulfilling to promote artists who are knowledgeable and well-informed.

It is important to keep an eye on the "properties" that are discussed in the daily trades. These properties often consist of the rights to books that are best sellers or real-life stories. These properties can be interesting and many times are widely covered by the media. Talk to your agent or manager about possible roles in these properties. Also, keep a lookout for upcoming films and work with your agent and/or manager to contact the people involved. Then stay in contact up until and including the casting stage.

Once you have found work you need to know how to promote yourself. The best way to get hired for future productions is to combine good work with a good promotional effort. This means that in addition to the publicity done for you by your publicist (if you have one), that you must also promote yourself. For example, when you get a role in a play, you should have a printer make up some postcard-size fliers (in L.A. they are called "zed" cards) for you. These should be sent to producers, directors, casting directors (plus agents and managers, if you are currently seeking one or both). All the pertinent information should be included on the card (about both the play and you), as well as a good photograph reduced to fit the postcard. You can buy pre-addressed labels at stores where industry-related books and magazines are sold. (Larry Edmunds and Samuel French bookstores have the best selections of these at their Hollywood locations.) After your initial mailing make a timely follow-up phone calls. If the play and/or you get a favorable review then it may be a good idea to send out new zed cards quoting the review(s).

At any one time there are at least 100 plays being performed in Los Angeles. Casting persons in particular are always on the lookout for new talent, but you have to tell them where you are, and often they need a reminder. The competition for their attention is stiff since in L.A. most theaters only perform Thursday through Sunday. In addition, casting directors get bombarded with requests to see friends, acquaintances, and other performers. Therefore, they have to make a choice. Your job is to help them make "the right choice" by mailing them an invitation they can't refuse, either because your card is cleverly written; or because the play has a good or well-known cast, director, or producer; or because of great reviews; or because of a performance on a Special Industry Night.

The trade papers offer one of the best opportunities for promoting yourself. They are read by almost everybody and are very effective if you can afford it. The information in the ad should be similar to the information on your zed card and could, in fact, duplicate it exactly. The size of the ad will depend on your current finances, but it could cost as little as $200 for a one-liner. While investigating the trades, look into the possibility of getting yourself a blurb in the *Hollywood Reporter* or the *Daily Variety*. You might also try to get listed in *Drama-Logue*. This is a weekly publication specializing in small theater activity. It also includes casting notices for theater, film, television, and video (in addition to interesting information about what's happening in New York and San Francisco).

Developing a demo reel is an excellent way of promoting yourself. Even if you haven't been cast in a feature film, there are other ways to get good footage of yourself. Each week *Drama-Logue* has numerous listings of student films and low-budget features that are looking for acting talent and crew members. Remuneration for these projects often consists of only meals and a copy of the finished product, which may not be a bad bargain if you are just looking for experience and a demo. Not only will you learn something about how a film is put together, but you will get that prized footage for your demo.

Self-promotion is not only an investment in your career, it also accomplish two important goals: 1) it will continue to keep your name and face in front of the industry; 2) it will make you look busy (which is very important to an industry filled with insecure people—a busy actor is presumed to be a talented one).

Actors, dancers, singers, and entertainers arrive in L.A. from all over the world to become movie stars. Stardom is one definition of success. But perhaps a more practical definition is simply working—being able to pay your rent (and car insurance payments!) by performing. Considering that Screen Actors Guild statistics show that at any one time 85 percent of its members are out of work, performers who work steadily should consider themselves quite fortunate. Trying to succeed in Los Angeles can be taken as a challenge, a challenge that can be exciting and gratifying if approached in a professional, competent manner.

PART FOUR

Getting a Show on the Road

Producing Your Own Show

by Bill Ervolino

Playwrights struggling to have their plays produced have one course of action they can always fall back upon—they can produce their work themselves. And one of the best options open to those playwrights who are willing to shoulder the responsibilities of a self-produced venture is an Equity Approved Showcase. An Equity Approved Showcase production must meet the standards set by the AEA Showcase Code and must be approved by AEA. (Although Equity Showcase productions are unique to New York City, there are similar opportunities in other communities throughout the United States. Those who would like to undertake such a production outside of New York should contact an AEA liaison person in their area.) There are, of course, many factors to consider before beginning such an undertaking, such as time, money, energy, organizational ability and business acumen. Some of the obstacles facing producers of plays are described below, and the requirements of an Equity Showcase production are outlined.

SHOULD YOU OR SHOULDN'T YOU?

The golden rule in show business has always been: Never use your own money. Film director Francis Coppola found that out the hard way and lost his empire in the process. Countless others who have produced their own films, plays, and record albums have learned the same lesson. Certainly it's admirable to believe so strongly in something that you are willing to put yourself on the line for it, financially speaking. But there are risks involved. One danger in producing your own show is that it could be identified as a "vanity production"; this could cause others not to take your show seriously.

Many ask whether it is possible to be creative and also have a good business sense. It is very possible—and also very preferable! The costs of Broadway and Off-Broadway productions are astronomical, but it is possible to mount your own Equity Showcase production for $5,000 or less. Although this is for a limited run (16 performances maximum), and the chances of recovering your investment are slim, there are, nevertheless, still advantages to undertaking such a production yourself.

First off, the very fact that you are doing an Equity Showcase lends a certain amount of prestige to your project. A reading is one thing, but a showcase lets those people you've invited know that someone is serious enough about your work to put real money into it, even if that someone is you. (And no one has to know that, unless you tell them.) "Those people" includes potential backers and producers as well as critics. And good reviews from New York critics can only help your chances of luring even more potential backers and producers. Producing a play is also a bit like spending a summer doing rep. You probably won't be painting scenery, but you'll more than likely be doing everything else. And, what you don't know, you'll learn. Very quickly.

Finally—and this may be the toughest lesson of all—you may discover that despite what your friends have been telling you, your play really isn't as marvelous as you thought. Audiences may not respond to it, critics may not respond to it, and producers may not respond to it. If you can be objective enough to accept this, then your showcase can save you a lot of time, aggravation, postage and misery.

All of which brings us back to our basic question: "Should you or shouldn't you produce your own work?" As with so many of life's basic questions, the only person who can decide this is you. There are, however, a few other questions which should be considered before producing a show of your own. They are:

Can you come up with the money to mount the production? And, most importantly, can you afford to lose that money?
If you cannot answer in the affirmative to both of these questions, you may be well-advised to postpone a self-produced show. It could be very frustrating to be forced to abandon a project in midstream or to have to overlook aesthetic considerations because of budgetary pressures.

Is the play ready to be produced?
One way to find out is to try a staged reading. If you have already staged a reading and have gotten a positive response, then a showcase could be the next logical step.

Do you have the right cast? And the right director?
Never underestimate the importance of these factors. If your production is weak, there are those who will think your play is weak (including critics and some potential backers and producers). A theatrical showcase, just like a department store showcase, is a sales tool—it should be as attractive as possible.

Do you have a space?
A space could mean anything from a loft in SoHo to the Radio City Music Hall. And booking it could turn out to be the toughest part of the entire project.

Do you have the time to devote to producing?
If your time is already at a premium, producing a showcase could be extremely trying. Perhaps you already have a demanding job. Maybe you're even juggling two. Are your hours flexible? Could you take off from work if you were needed at the theater? Will your boss complain about the inevitable phone calls you'll be making and receiving on company time?

FURTHER CONSIDERATIONS

As you probably already know from your playwriting experience, the ability to visualize a finished work is 50 percent of the battle. This same skill that makes you a competent writer can also make you a competent producer. Your ability to come up with ideas, to visualize a finished product and to organize your thoughts effectively will serve you well during the pre-production period, when you are called upon to carry out certain steps, often simultaneously, and pull them all together.

As a producer you have many responsibilities. You have to hire a cast. You have to hire a director. You have to find a space. You have to work with the landlord. You have to consult an attorney. You have to sign contracts. You have to purchase insurance. You have to arrange for publicity. You have to hire a ticket agent. You have to arrange for rehearsal time. You have to put together a comp list (a list of people who will receive complimentary tickets). You have to make sure all the right people are invited. You have to contact critics. You have to have programs made. And that's before you even open!

Once you do open, you have to deal with your cast. Then you have to deal with your director. Then you have to deal with problems between your cast and your director. And problems between your director and your landlord. And problems between your landlord and your audience.

WHERE TO BEGIN?

Since so many things have to be done at the same time and since you probably won't have much help doing any of it, you have a dilemma on your hands. You need a cast. You need a space. And, you need a cast that's available when the space is available. So you're going to have to find a way to bring all these elements together.

If you've already done a reading of your play, chances are you already have a cast and director in mind. If you haven't done a reading, then you should do one. A reading of your play will allow you to see and hear your work performed, assess dialogue and structure, and get some feedback from an audience as well as the performers and director. (Often, playwrights will direct this kind of reading themselves, but having someone else involved will free you up so that you can really observe what is going on.)

In preparation for the reading, find someone you think might be a good director. Allow that person a few days to read and digest your play and then sit down and talk it over. Listen to this person's ideas and see if the two of you are in accord over interpretation, key characters, and the situations you have placed them in. Make sure this is not just some idle chat over coffee. When your meeting is over, you should be able to walk away from it with some idea of whether or not this is the person you want to be your director. Just as importantly, how do the two of you get along? Is this someone you can work with, someone who inspires confidence, and who shares your enthusiasm for the work? Your relationship with your director is crucial. Don't select someone simply because you can't find anyone else.

When you've found a director you're comfortable with, discuss casting possibilities together. Between the two of you, you will have to come up with actors for the reading. Many actors who are between projects will gladly give their time for a reading. All you have to do is find them.

Once you have assembled your director and cast, set a date, find a place and do the reading. Three rehearsals should be sufficient for this type of informal reading—actors with books in hand and an audience of your friends. Some rough blocking will liven things up a bit, but don't go crazy. You're looking for feedback here, not a Tony Award.

On the night of the reading, pay close attention to what the actors are doing, how they're doing it, and how your audience is responding. There's going to be a lot of visualization going on, but the essence of the play should come across loud and clear. Take notes along the way and when the reading is over, discuss the play with the audience and the actors. How did it sound? How did it feel? (A tape recording of the reading might be a good idea, too.)

At this point you'll have to decide whether the time is right to attempt your showcase. Perhaps you'd like more time to work on the play. Perhaps you'd rather put together a *staged* reading. Get as much feedback as you can and give the matter plenty of thought. If you don't feel totally comfortable with the work, then a staged reading—in which the actors are fully blocked, off-book, and working with major props—will probably be the best way to go. When you feel that the play is ready (either before or after a staged reading) it is time to move on to the next phase of production.

SETTING A DATE

It's going to be necessary for you to set a target date for your showcase. If your work has a seasonal theme, you may wish to have it performed during that particular season. Summer is generally a bad time for a play to open because so many people are out of town, but, for whatever reasons, summer may be best for your play. Weigh your decision carefully, and then start looking for a space.

Call anyone you know who has ever been involved in an Equity Showcase, and find out where it was produced. Keep in mind that the Equity Showcase Code states that "AEA members may not rehearse or perform on any premises which lack adequate sanitary facilities or which do not comply with New York City and State fire codes." Also bear in mind that productions mounted under the terms of this code shall not be presented in any theater, auditorium or hall which is listed by AEA as a contract house. This eliminates large theaters from your list of possibilities. Seating for your showcase may not exceed 100, and that number is firm.

Speak to as many landlords as you can, and ask them what their spaces go for and when they are available. And don't be shy about it. If the rental seems steep to you, try to negotiate. In addition to finding out the cost of the space per night, find out what it will cost per week, and whether it is possible for you to get a per-night rate should you opt for a rental of three or four weeks. (Equity will allow your showcase to run for 12 performances with the option of adding another four. These performances need not be held on 16 consecutive evenings. Your total run, however, may not exceed a four-week period.)

You will need answers to the following questions from your prospective landlord: Does this space rent by the evening, the week, or by the hour? Is the theater yours all day? Can you sublet the space? Will any other party have use of the space during your run? Will it be necessary to strike the set every night?

When you have found a space that looks right, ask to inspect the premises. Take along your director and one or two members of your cast. Check out the dressing rooms for size and sanitary conditions. Walk across the stage and try to visualize your play on it. Look at the backstage area. Is there enough room for the sets and props you need? What is the seating like? Are the chairs in decent condition or are they broken and uncomfortable? How are the sightlines? Also check out the light board and ask for a demonstration. If you aren't technically adept, bring someone with you who is.

There's no way you'll think of everything when you walk into an unknown theater, but be prepared to experience the space from the standpoint of your actors as well as your audience. Ask plenty of questions, but try to keep your meeting cordial and professional. If the landlord is interested in theater and proud of what he has to offer you, chances are he'll be only too willing to give you a grand tour of the place. If he's cold and indifferent, think twice before entering into an agreement with him. Ask to see a sample contract and if there is anything you don't understand, ask the landlord to explain it to you. *Sign nothing.* If the landlord wants a deposit, make sure it is refundable. If it isn't, say you'd prefer to speak to an attorney first and will get back to the landlord as soon as possible. If you're getting a hard-sell ("I have someone else who wants to rent it on the same days you want it.") proceed with caution. If you're sure you want the space and are afraid you might lose it, go with your instincts.

EXAMINING YOUR CONTRACT

No matter what the landlord tells you, there is no standard rental agreement for what you are doing, so don't assume that everything's going to be okay just because it looks good to you on paper. If you don't have a lawyer, find one who has a background in theater.

Yes, your agreement lists performance dates—but what about rehearsal dates? You're going to want your cast to have at least some rehearsal time in the theater. What will that cost? And how will it be paid? In advance? Per night? If the landlord offers a certain amount of rehearsal time at no cost, make sure this appears in the final agreement you sign. (When renting by the hour make sure that the times your cast may enter and must leave the theater are clearly stated. And this, of course, goes for rehearsal days and performance days. If you're planning on an 8 o'clock curtain, make sure your cast and stage manager are allowed at least an hour to prepare.)

Also find out what is included in the rent. If there is a fee for lights, make sure you're aware of it. If you are running during summer months, you are most probably going to want air conditioning. Is there any in the theater? Will it be automatically turned on or do you have to pay for that too?

The rental contract should outline terms of payment. Your landlord will probably want the entire amount in advance, plus security. If that is going to present a problem to you, try to negotiate the matter. Chances are if you're doing the full 16 performances Equity allows, you're going to have to lay out a hefty amount of cash.

A few other things that must be in the contract are: time involved for you to vacate the premises at the end of your run and to restore the space to its original condition; your responsibility for damages; policies concerning cancellation of any performances, including the entire run. Whatever you do, don't sign away the rights to your play; your landlord has no right to future percentages or options.

EQUITY APPROVAL

Now that you have your cast, your director, your space, and your dates, it is time to seek AEA approval for your showcase production. The AEA Showcase Code, available by contacting Actors' Equity Association, is an 11-page document that spells out certain provisions you *must* follow. For a copy, contact the union at 165 West 46th Street, New York, NY 10036 or call (212) 869-8530. Michael LaValley is the business rep in charge of showcase productions.

As stated within the code, an application must be made to AEA 14 days prior to casting and must include the producer's name, the title of the production, the type of production (musical revue, dramatic play, and so on) and information concerning previous productions. In the application you must also include basic information about the theater, a statement of financial backing and a proposed production budget. (For what Equity deems "a one-shot producer," the total budget must be under $15,000.)

Prior to casting, the producer must furnish Equity with a copy of the cast breakdown indicating the roles available, the dates of rehearsals and performances, and the address at which pictures and resumes will be accepted; these will be posted at the Equity offices. At least half of the total number of performances must be presented on a weekday (Monday through Friday) with no more than one two-performance day per week. The producer may not cut the number of performances without the unanimous written consent of the AEA members in the production.

The AEA Showcase Code allows for 12 performances over a period of four weeks with an option of four additional performances. (AEA cast members must be reimbursed at $5 per member for each additional performance beyond the initial 12.) The theater may seat up to 100 people and admission can be no more than $8 per ticket. (AEA members are to be comped, on a standby basis, upon presentation of a membership card.)

Your cast and crew are working for reimbursement of their expenses, and what is commonly defined as public transportation for each rehearsal and performance. Keep in mind that this is *their* showcase, too. Their photos must be prominently displayed in the lobby of the theater. Their bios must appear in the program. And their guests—casting agents, other producers, anyone in a position to cast them in something else—are automatically comped. (As a courtesy, you should make a certain number of personal comps available to the cast as well. Four is a nice, round number.)

THE COST OF AN EQUITY SHOWCASE
No matter how hard you try to keep costs down, you're going to find new expenses every day as you get closer to opening night. Keep track of everything!

The following is a budget sample, like the one you must send to Equity, for a five-character show (with minimal as in "bring your own" sets, props and costumes) running the full 16 performances:

Theater rental (performances)	$3,200
Theater rental (rehearsals)	$ 220
Security	$ 100
Insurance	$ 750
Ticket agent	$ 84
Postage	$ 140
Printed Cards/Flyers	$ 60
Set/props/costumes	$ 150
Carfare for cast, director and stage manager	$ 320
Miscellaneous paper	$ 15
Equity/LORT Trust Fund	$ 150
Total	$5,189

As new expenses are incurred, add them to your list. You'll need adequate records for tax purposes. Accordingly, make sure that your reservations book is legible and accurate.

WHO'S IN CHARGE HERE?

As your production comes together, problems are bound to come up. As producer, you will have to recognize when you should be involved, when you should keep your mouth shut and when you should step in and resolve something.

In the center of your production is the director, who is supposed to be the person guiding the creative end. If you undermine the director's authority you're going to have a major mess on your hands, one that is bound to get worse and worse as you come closer to opening. Once rehearsals have commenced (and you can rehearse your cast a maximum of four weeks), if you feel that the play is moving in the wrong direction, speak to the director privately and try to correct it.

There are also bound to be problems between landlord and staff, if one exists, and your cast and crew. Props may have been moved onstage. Personal items may be missing from the dressing room. Whatever the problem, it's bound to fall in your lap sooner or later. Be prepared, and do your best to handle whatever comes up as painlessly and diplomatically as possible.

TICKET AGENTS

You can hire a ticket agent for all four weeks of your run for under $100. And, while you could just as easily handle it yourself, a ticket agent does offer certain advantages. A ticket agent will have representatives on staff who have all the information in front of them that a caller might request; they will provide you with the names and numbers of callers every evening before you go to the theater. What's easier than that?

Unless you're completely strapped, and have no other options available, don't use your own phone number. It won't look good for you and it won't look good for the production.

ARE YOU IN GOOD HANDS?

Regardless of what kind of insurance your landlord may have on the building, you are probably going to wind up purchasing your own. Concerning this matter, the AEA Showcase Code reads as follows:

"The producer shall cause to be provided liability insurance at all interviews, auditions, rehearsals and performances. He shall make the name of the insurance carrier available to the actors at the place of the interview, audition, rehearsal and performance. In the event of an injury, the producer shall advise the actor of the procedure for filing a claim." Without the proper insurance, Equity can close down your production. That's nowhere near the loss you could face, however, if one of the actors is injured and you are held responsible. (If the landlord insists that his or her coverage will apply to your actors, consult your attorney. Generally, the landlord's policy will apply to members of your audience who may fall on a stairwell, or trip getting into their seats. Make sure this is clear, approved by your attorney, and approved by Equity!)

MISCELLANY

Here are some miscellaneous pointers relating to expenses and production.

1. The Equity Showcase Code requires a contribution from the producer to the Equity-LORT Subsidiary Rights Trust Fund in the amount of $150 per play ($350 maximum per season—July 1 to June 30).

2. To keep from being labeled a vanity production ("John Smith presents: *Saturdays at Seven* by John Smith"), it's a good idea to come up with a name for your company. ("Sentinel Productions presents: *Saturdays at Seven* by John Smith"). Use your production company name in publicity announcements, on the program and when you apply for insurance.

3. No taping, filming or recording of any rehearsal or performance of an Equity Showcase production may be made without the written permission of Equity.

4. A performance is defined by Equity as "any presentation before an audience, invited or paid, including previews and/or rehearsals." If you are planning a special performance of some kind, remember that it must be included in the performance schedule you agreed to.

5. Don't forget to copyright your play. Contact the Copyright Office in Washington, D.C., 202-287-9100, and ask for Pack 119. The cost is $10.)

6. Opening nights and closing nights are the responsibility of the producer. You don't need to plan anything too fancy, of course, unless you have the money, but some champagne would be nice. If you can't afford to take the whole gang out on closing night, an inexpensive house party will suffice.

7. You're going to require some kind of house staff: someone who can take the money at the door, a coat-room person (if the theater has a coat room) and, depending on whether or not you have designated seating, an usher. For these tasks enlist your friends—don't do these jobs yourself.

8. Make sure you purchase two notebooks at the beginning of your run—one for reservations, the other for your guest list. All guests should sign in with their addresses, so you can add them to your ever-growing mailing list.

PROGRAMS

You will undoubtedly want the people who come to see your play to receive a program. But, whether you do or not, Equity says you have to, so start typing.

Certainly, if you have the money, a slick, printed program isn't going to turn anybody off. If you are on a tight budget, however, you'll probably wind up doing what most showcase producers do: Type it all up on a typewriter or word processor and make photocopies on colored paper.

Some things to keep in mind:

1. Don't call your program a Playbill or use the name of any other established publication. There are laws against that—the same kind of laws that protect *your* work.

2. The most common format consists of: the title of the work and some kind of artwork (page 1); the lists of scenes and characters, as well as the actors playing them (page 2); the "Who's Who in the Cast," consisting of the actors' bios (page 3); bios of the director, tech people and author (page 4); The AEA program bio and logo, to be supplied by Equity, must also appear somewhere on the program.

3. The actors may wish to have their addresses and phone numbers included in their bios. Ask them first before printing this information! Bios should be uniform in structure and the information in them factual.

4. Cast members and tech people who are members of Equity must have an asterisk placed next to their name with the following note: "These actors and stage managers are members of Actors' Equity Association, appearing without benefit of contract or salary. The donation of their professional services is with the special permission of Actors' Equity Association."

6. Make sure that the name of the theater, its address, the telephone number of the ticket agent and the dates of your run are printed somewhere on the program.

PUBLICITY AND ADVERTISING

Cards and/or flyers are the best way to advertise your production. Mail these out to friends and business acquaintances. If your director or any members of your cast have access to mailing lists, make sure you take advantage of them, too. Then, go to the post office and discuss the different mail sizes you have in mind and how much postage will cost.

From the post office, go directly to a printer and ask to see some different paper stocks. Discuss your ideas for cards and flyers and get feedback on prices. Make sure you find out how large the paper is to start with. The printer should mention that you can print two or more cards on each piece of paper. Naturally, this would be a savings for you and is something you should consider.

The next person to speak with is an artist, preferably one of your close friends who won't charge you too much to make your cards up. You will require professional typography and perhaps some artwork or a logo incorporating the title of your play. The unfinished product should be easy to read, as sharp-looking as possible and should entice people to call up for reservations. The following information should appear on every card or flyer you make:

1. The name of the play, the names of the director, cast, and crew members.

2. The name and address of the theater, with directions how to get there if it is on some out-of-the-way corner.

3. The number to call for tickets, the price of the tickets, the dates of the run and the showtimes.

4. The words "Equity Approved Showcase," as well as asterisks next to the names of Equity people with a note that they are AEA members.

If you have sufficient funds you may consider hiring a professional publicist. (See "Hiring a Publicist" and "Creating Your Own Publicity," page 115.) Such a person deals with all of the newspapers and magazines on a regular basis and is more likely to be able to get a mention of your play into print.

If you can't afford a publicist, you'll have to create your own publicity. But you *are* a writer, and that at least gives you a jump on things. A well-written press release shouldn't be too much of a challenge, as long as you remember to keep it simple and include all the pertinent information.

A press release need be no more than a short blurb which adequately describes your play. For example: *Hanging from the Chandelier*, a new play by Goldie Candle-styx, is the touching and often hilarious story of four ex-college buddies who are unexpectedly reunited while standing on line to buy tickets for *Phantom of the Opera*.

You can use such a blurb in all the publicity you send out, from full-sized press releases to tiny column items. You may also try to pitch stories on members of your cast, your director and yourself, to local papers, magazines and radio and TV shows.

Approaching critics is more difficult, but not impossible. Keep in mind that critics receive countless invitations each week and yours is going to go into a pile with all the rest. For that reason, try to make your initial announcement and subsequent invitation as enticing as possible, and easy to read, and make sure to include all of the necessary information. A personal note won't hurt either. Critics like to know that you're familiar with their work and that you value their input on your work.

Certain publications may be willing to review your work, even though their reviews won't run until your showcase has ended. Welcome them with open arms, anyway. A review is a review and if it's a good one, it can only help your chances for mounting future productions.

Keep in mind also that photo breaks can work miracles for your show. Arrange to have some good pictures taken and send prints to any publication that prints photos. Make sure the shots you send out are clear, interesting and tasteful and, whatever you do, don't send every newspaper in town the same picture.

Listings are another way to publicize your production and many of them are free. Send your blurb, plus other pertinent information to any publication that runs play listings and keep your fingers crossed. For best results, write up each listing in the format of that particular publication. As with critics, a short personal note can be helpful.

As far as advertising is concerned, your main consideration is probably going to be financial. Print ads are extremely expensive and could easily increase your budget by 100 percent. Once again, unless someone involved in your production has some name recognition, you're probably better off waiting until you have some reviews to tout. Don't wait until the last minute, though, to plan out an advertising strategy. Find out the publications that run theatrical advertising, their rates, and their deadlines. If you do receive some positive reviews, an ad can substantially help increase the size of your audience.

IT'S A WRAP!
Well now you know all about producing an Equity Approved Showcase. Do you still want to produce your *own* play? Think you're ready for the strain? The headaches? The non-stop aggravation? If you are, then more power to you. Even if the production isn't sensational, even if producers don't start beating your door down, even if the critics don't praise you to the heavens, and even if you lose a couple of thousand dollars, it could be the wisest investment you'll ever make of your time and your money. You'll learn a lot about your play. You'll learn a lot about yourself. And you'll learn a lot about the business—more than any six-month course could possibly teach you. Who knows? Once you have acquired experience as a producer, you may be motivated to go on and produce other works.

Choosing a Rehearsal Room

by Andrea Wolper

Performers in search of a rehearsal room will discover a variety of suitable spaces that are inexpensive and fall well within the budgetary limitations of struggling actors and entertainers. Whether you're looking for space in which to rehearse a play or to practice an audition piece, to teach dance classes or to coach actors, to hold auditions or to practice the tuba, you should be able to find a space that provides much, if not all, of what you need. Although the commentary presented here is based upon rehearsal spaces in Manhattan, the requirements of what makes an acceptable rehearsal space are generally the same everywhere. Performers in other cities should be able to adapt these guidelines to their own cities.

FINDING SUITABLE FACILITIES

The first thing to ask yourself when hunting for space is what kind of facility best meets your needs. There are the big, bright and beautiful *dance and/or rehearsal complexes* that feel entirely professional and just plain fun to be in. There are the *smaller, homier spaces* that aren't always so bright and beautiful but are quite good nonetheless. There are the *mid-sized dance studios*, where dance classes and rehearsals are scheduled around each other with a minimum of fuss. There are the smallish *private acting schools*, whose studios are rented to outsiders when classes aren't in session. There are the *little theatres*, often of the black box variety, usually accompanied by a studio or two that can be used as a rehearsal studio, dressing room, greenroom, etc. Whichever of these rough categories a space falls into (and there are a few that defy categorization), each is unique, and all of them, from the most humble to the most glorious, have something to offer.

COST

For many performers looking for rehearsal space, cost will be a primary consideration. Even those on the tightest of budgets can take heart: there are still a few places where, for little more than the cost of a movie, you can buy an hour's time. Of course, rock bottom rates won't buy a luxury space. They will buy, however, a workable space, and sometimes even some surprising amenities.

When you find a space you like, be sure to find out if the rental fee includes the use of everything you find in the room. Does it cover use of a reception area or waiting room? Will there be an added charge if you need a piano moved into the studio you're renting? And when, by the way, was that piano last tuned? Is there an extra charge for bringing in heavy film, video, or lighting equipment that might have an effect on the facility's utility bill?

STUDIO SIZE

Equally as important as cost is the size of the studio. If you make preliminary inquiries by phone, be sure to get actual room dimensions, and not just the square footage. A 900-square-foot room may turn out to be a nice square 30' by 30', just the right size for an acting class. On the other hand, it may turn out to be 45' × 20', which would be more appropriate for dance or exercise classes and for auditions. Depending upon your field of activity, ceiling height may also have some bearing. Be sure to check on the height and width of the doors if you'll be carrying set pieces or large props into the rooms.

You may need to take into consideration the size of the entire facility. If you're holding auditions there must be enough space outside the audition room to comfortably accommodate those waiting to be seen. If you're conducting an open call, this is a real priority. Not only will you need a large waiting space, you'll also need plenty of chairs or benches.

Be sure to check out the number and size of restrooms and changing rooms (especially for dance auditions, or any activity involving a lot of people) before renting a space. If you're going to be doing a production, the location and size of dressing rooms shouldn't be overlooked. You'll also want to be sure that restrooms and showers if available, are clean and in working order.

There are many questions that will present themselves as you look around the studio. Is the floor carpeted, hardwood, linoleum, or does it consist of some other kind of dance flooring? If it's not specifically a dance studio, is dancing allowed on those nice wood floors? Are there barres, good mirrors, piano, plenty of tables and chairs, rehearsal furniture, record player or tape recorder? Is there enough light? How's the natural light? Are there fans or air conditioning? Heaters? Are there enough electrical outlets? Be sure to let the studio manager know if you'll be building sets, playing musical instruments, or engaging in other noise-producing activities— you may require a studio that's soundproof.

THE EXTRAS

The little extras offered at some facilities may be important to you. A number of studios have vending machines; and a few even have snack bars. Some have lockers. Most have at least one pay phone; those that don't may let you use the office phone for a quarter. There are studios that have phones in every room hooked up through a central switchboard.

LOCATION AND SECURITY

The location of your rehearsal space should be convenient and safe. Look at the surrounding area. Are there subway stations, bus stops, and parking lots within walking distance? Will you feel reasonably safe walking in the area after a late night of work? What kind of security have the studio owners provided? If you're working earlier or later than regular business hours, is there a number you can call in case of emergency? Will you need a key to get in and out of the building? Is there a storage area in which you can safely leave props or costumes overnight?

RATES

While most studios rent space at hourly rates, some also offer discounts for weekly, monthly, or ongoing rentals and, in some cases, full-day rentals. At some studios, the discounted rate can be negotiated, while at others, regular and discounted rates are fixed. If you're renting for more than a half-day, be sure to ask about lower rates. For short-term use, some studios require that you rent a designated minimum number of hours. And some require full or partial payment in advance.

There are a number of studios that operate on a twenty-four hour basis. At some that are not generally open around the clock, it may be possible to make arrangements for access during off-hours. Frequently, rates go up for evening, night, or very early rentals; occasionally, however, you'll find that prices go down during these times.

EQUITY-APPROVED FACILITIES

Actors' Equity Association producers are required to find spaces that are clean and spacious, and that have adequate facilities and waiting space. Chorus and open calls, for example, must be held in spaces that have at least two changing areas and restrooms. Additionally there are some studios which, while meeting basic requirements, are approved only for certain specified uses. Equity does publish a list of approved spaces, although a studio that does not appear on the list should not be considered off-limits and in fact, Equity does not presently have an off-limits list. What might get a studio on such a list if one existed, are things like lack of cleanliness and proper ventilation.

CITY SERVICES AVAILABLE

New York City's Department of Cultural Affairs' Public Works Program can provide studio managers operating under non-profit status with janitorial services, clerical help, stage hands, and even graphic artists, free of charge. With such a service available, there is no reason for any non-profit theater, school, or rehearsal facility to be dirty. Anyone wishing to apply for such services should send information about their organization along with official proof of non-profit status, to Kathy Hughes, Program Dept., Dept of Cultural Affairs, 2 Columbus Circle, New York, NY 10019. Those who apply will be sent an application, which takes about two or three weeks to process.

The following list is a good sampling of rehearsal room space available in New York City; it is, however, by no means a complete summary of Manhattan studios. You'll find some of the busiest, most well-known facilities listed, as well as some of the newer, relatively unknown studios—and lots in between. Good luck!

Rehearsal Rooms in New York City

THE ACTING STUDIO
31 W. 21 St. (7th fl.)
(212) 206-8608
Owner: James Price
Mgr: Elyse Barbell

ACTORS' EQUITY
ASSOCIATION AUDITION
CENTER
165 W. 46th St., 2nd fl.
(212) 869-8530
Dir: Tony Nicosia
Assts: Karen Nothmann,
Jerry Alan Cole

THE ACTORS' SPACE,
INC.
250 W. 54 St., 10th fl.
(212) 757-5900
Mgr: Sheila M. Wood

SIDNEY ARMUS
54 W. 22nd St., 2nd fl.
(212) 243-2805
Mgr: Sidney Armus

THE CASTILLO CENTER
7 E. 20th St., 10th fl.
(212) 505-1070
Mgr: Gabrielle Kurlander

MICHAEL CHEKHOV
STUDIO
19 W. 36th St., 8th fl.
(212) 736-1544
Mgr: Jim Boerlin

CORNER LOFT STUDIO
99 University Place
(212) 228-8728
Mgr: Elaine Gold

THE CUBICULO
414 W. 51st St.
(212) 265-2139
Mgr: Mark Barreiro

DANCE CONCEPTS
231 W. 54th St., 4th fl.
(212) 757-1941
Mgr: Edvige Val

DANCE SPACE
622 Broadway, 6th fl.
(212) 777-8067
Mgrs: Michelle Miller,
James Garvey

DIA ART FOUNDATION
155 Mercer St.
(212) 431-9232
Mgr: Joan Duddy

18TH STREET
PLAYHOUSE
145 & 151 W. 18th St.
(212) 929-7907; 243-8643
(theater pay phone)
Mgr: Vivian

890 DANCE CENTER
890 Broadway, 6th fl.
(212) 475-2870
Mgrs: Tom Aberger,
Daryl Samuel

DOUGLAS FAIRBANKS
STUDIO
432 W. 42nd St.
(212) 564-3643
Mgr: Gail Bell

FAZIL'S TIME SQUARE
STUDIOS
143 8th Avenue
(212) 245-9504

FIRST-RUN STUDIOS
306 W. 40th St.
(212) 760-9310
Mgrs: Joe Lanteri,
Dan Wolgemuth

GENE FRANKEL
THEATRE WORKSHOP
24 Bond St.
(212) 777-1710
Mgr: Gerri May

HARBOR PERFORMING
ARTS CENTER
1 E. 104th St.
(212) 427-2244
Mgr: Ramon Rodriguez

HARLEQUIN STUDIOS
203 W. 46 St., 2nd fl.
(212) 819-0120
Mgr: Bob Sokoler

HEBREW ARTS SCHOOL
& ABRAHAM GOODMAN
HOUSE
129 West 67th St.
(212) 362-8060
Mgr: Paula Mayo

NAT HORNE MUSICAL
THEATRE
440 W. 42nd St.
(212) 736-7128
Mgr: Mark De Gasperi

JOHN HOUSEMAN
THEATRE CENTER
450 W. 42nd St.
(212) 967-7069
Mgrs: Eric Krebs,
John-Ann Washington

JOY OF MOVEMENT
400 Lafayette St., 2nd fl.
(212) 260-0453
Mgr: Audrey Phillips

THEA KOREK EXERCISE
2121 Broadway, 2nd fl.
(212) 724-8889
Mgr: Thea Korek

LE TANG SCHOOL OF
DANCE
109 W. 27th St., 8th fl.
(212) 627-1126/27
Mgrs: Ellie and Henry Le
Tang

LEZLY DANCE & SKATE
SCHOOL
622-626 Broadway, 4th fl.
(212) 777-3232
Dir: Lezly Ziering

MANHATTAN PUNCH
LINE
410 W. 42nd St., 3rd fl.
(212) 239-0827
Mgr: Steve Kaplan

SANFORD MEISNER
THEATRE
164 11th Avenue
(212) 206-1764
Mgr: Robert Coles

MINSKOFF REHEARSAL
STUDIO
1515 Broadway, 3rd fl.
(212) 575-0725
Mgr: Diane Johnson

MLT LOFT STUDIOS
40 W. 22nd St.
(212) 989-7274
Mgr: Walt Whitcover

MUSICAL THEATRE
WORKS
440 Lafayette St., 3rd fl.
(212) 677-0040
Mgr: David Schaap

NATIONAL
SHAKESPEARE
CONSERVATORY
591 Broadway, 6th fl.
(212) 219-9874,
1-800-472-6667
(out-of-state)
Mgr: Kent Adams

NEW YORK KARATE
ACADEMY
1717 Broadway, 2nd fl.
(212) 245-8055
Mgr. Aaron Banks

NEW YORK THEATRE
WORKSHOP
220 W. 42nd St., 18th fl.
(212) 302-7737
Mgr: Ben Pesner

NOLA REHEARSAL
STUDIOS
250 W. 54th St., 11th fl.
(212) 582-1417
Mgr: Phil Johann

OUR STUDIOS
622 Broadway
(212) 529-1111
Mgr: Peter Broderson

PERIDANCE CENTER
33 E. 18th St., 5th fl.
(212) 505-0886
*Artistic Director: Igal Perry
School Director: Miguel
ValdezMor*

PRODUCER'S CLUB
358 W. 44th St.
(212) 246-9069
Mgr: Benjamin Kolbert

R.A.P.P. ARTS CENTER
220 E. 4th St.
(212) 529-5921
*Mgrs: Phil Langer,
Jacqueline Hayes*

T. SCHREIBER STUDIO
83 E. 4th St.
(212) 420-1249
Mgr: Deborah Parker

STUDIO THEATRE 603
REHEARSAL SUITE 1404
311 W. 43rd St.
(212) 246-5877
Mgr: Michael Parva

STEPS 74TH
2121 Broadway, 3rd fl.
(212) 874-2410
Mgr: Caralynn Sandorf

TADA! THEATRE
120 W. 28th St., 2nd floor
(212) 627-1732
*Artistic Directors:
Janine Nina Trevens
James Learned*

T.O.M.I.
23 W. 73rd St., 16th fl.
(212) 787-3980
*Mgrs: Lisa Bottalico,
Vincent Arnone*

THEATER
COMMUNICATIONS
GROUP (TCG) INC.
355 Lexington Ave.
(212) 697-5230
Mgr: Penny Boyer

VIDEO PORTFOLIOS
142 W. 24th St., 11th fl.
(212) 989-3858
Mgr: Albert Dabah

CLYDE VINSON STUDIO
612 8th Ave., 3rd fl.
(212) 505-0529
Mgr: Madeleine Barchevska

THE VITAL ARTS
CENTER
33 E. 18th St., 3rd fl.
(212) 475-1065/1297
Mgr: Minet Garcilazo

DAN WAGONER DANCE
FOUNDATION
476 Broadway, 4th fl.
(212) 334-1880
Mgr: Rhonda Shary

WEIST BARRON
35 W. 45th St., 6th fl.
(212) 840-7025
Mgr: Valerie Adami

WESTBETH
151 Bank St.
(212) 691-2272
Mgr: Bob Anderson

WEST END ARTS
CENTER
302 W. 91st St.
(212) 769-9327, 724-2070
*Mgrs: Father Pappas
Anastasia Loizidis*

WESTSIDE DANCE
PROJECT/CITY MUSIC
SCHOOLS
220 W. 80th St.
(212) 580-0915
*Mgrs: Maris Zannieri,
John De Blass*

WEST 72ND ST. STUDIOS
131 W. 72nd St.
(212) 799-5433
*Owners: Patricia Ripley,
Shane Grier*

THE WORKING
THEATRE
400 W. 40th St.
(212) 967-5464
Mgr: Murray Rubenstein

THE WRITER'S
THEATRE
145 W. 46th St.
(212) 869-9770
Mgr: Barbara Tirrell

Hiring a Publicist

by Bill Ervolino

Public relations in one form or another has long been an integral part of the entertainment business. The reason, quite simply, is that PR sells tickets, whether it consists of spreading a message by word of mouth, or the behind-the-scenes activity involved in getting a three-line item placed in a newspaper column.

You've probably already had a brush or two with the power of PR. You may not have your own press agent—not yet, anyway—but chances are that you will eventually. Most professionals agree, in fact, that hiring a publicist is the most effective way of getting and keeping your name in the public eye. Short of being elected President or marrying Elizabeth Taylor or Eddie Murphy, it's probably the only way.

If the prospect of paying someone to get your name around makes you feel a little uncomfortable, you're not alone. Many individuals involved in the arts feel the same way. Hiring a publicist, they nervously insist, is too expensive, too confusing or will in some way tarnish their hard-earned reputation. All of these things can be true. But, they don't have to be.

It is true that hiring a publicist can be an expensive proposition. Some "names" actually spend thousands of dollars every month on press agents. It is important to note, however, that not all publicists cost that kind of money. Unless your biggest decision is whether or not to let *Life* do a cover story on you, such concerns needn't worry you. Getting some press for your soon-to-be opening club act, showcase or Off-Broadway play doesn't have to break your bank account. And, it could be the best investment you ever make.

The politics of publicity can be very confusing. Does the columnist you've just discussed your next project with expect an exclusive on this story? Should you attempt to drum up feature stories before you've been reviewed? What's the best way to get critics in to see you—and where do you seat them when they finally show up? All of these questions, and hundreds of others, confound even the men and women who do PR for a living. If you don't know the answers to these questions, in other words, if you don't have a handle on the politics involved, that's all the more reason to hire someone who does.

As for your reputation, yes, publicity can be damaging if it is mishandled. Countless serious artists have been hyped into oblivion, unable to live up to the tremendous media attention that was focused on them. Others have found themselves unable to draw the critics or have turned away audiences because their publicity has been bizarre, offensive or misleading.

Publicity doesn't have to be expensive, it doesn't have to be confusing and it doesn't have to be hype. Nor should it detract from your personal goals, artistic or otherwise. The best you can buy is the publicity that does what you want it to.

The cost of hiring a press agent varies. This is not surprising since performers' needs and press agents' services vary so widely. But unless you are mounting a Broadway play (which has a set rate, through the Association of Theatrical Press Agents and Managers, of $1,128 plus, per week), prices are flexible. For showcase,

Off-Off-Broadway and cabaret acts, there are some press agents who will tailor a budget to what you can afford.

Before we consider some very important questions, such as whether you are ready for a publicist, where you can find one, or what kinds of services press agents offer, perhaps we had better define our terms. For our purposes, the terms "press agent" and "publicist" are used interchangeably, as are "press," "publicity" and "public relations." Technically, there are subtle differences between these terms, but since the people who do it for a living can't seem to agree on what those subtle differences are, you need not worry about it either. Now let's get to those questions.

ARE YOU READY FOR A PUBLICIST?

Before you clean out your bank account and go publicist-shopping, it's important to know if the time is right. As with just about every other aspect of show business, timing can be everything. Having something good, whether it's an act, a play or whatever, doesn't mean that it or you are promotable. At least not yet.

For a performer, hiring a press agent too early can be disastrous. And a publicist who signs you on, strictly on your ability to pay, without really knowing who you are, what you've done and where you hope to go, isn't doing you any favors.

Press agent Penny Landau points out that the publicist's name goes with the client. "That's why I want to see them perform," Landau says; "I want to see what's there." Landau's firm, Maya Associates, handles a number of club performers and her clients include Jamie de Roy, Geri Jewell, Larry Amoros, Alison Steele and For Play, an improv company.

Seeing a performer in action is imperative, but it still isn't enough to convince her to climb aboard for the ride. Landau says, "I usually ask them: 'Have you done three runs? Have you gotten good response? Do you have some positive reviews?' I also want to know what they want to accomplish. Broadway? TV? Daytime? I have to gear what I'm doing. Some of them say they don't want TV. All they want is a 'package of reviews.' Others want the moon. And they want it yesterday."

Tony Origlio, whose Tony Origlio Media Relations company handles Karen Akers, *High-Heeled Women* and numerous cabaret performers, is quick to agree. "People who don't know the publicity game come in and expect a lot," says Origlio. He cited three reasons he would turn down a potential account. "The first is if I don't think I'm right for the project. For instance, I've had many authors and artists come to me and ask me to handle them, but the book world and the art world are not my expertise. The second reason I would say no is if my workload is too heavy at the moment and I don't think I could give them the attention they deserve. The third is if they're looking for maximum press and I don't think they have the talent to get it. I have to believe in their talent."

Your publicist's working relationship with the critics is extremely important. Publicists talk to critics on the phone, they send them mail every other day and chat with them at openings and social functions. The success of these working relationships depends largely on whether the critics feel they can rely on what the publicist tells them. A publicist who raves about you to a critic is putting a lot on the line for the both of you. As Penny Landau pointed out, her name and reputation goes with every client she recommends.

And, as an artist, your name goes with your reviews, so it is important to get good reviews. Negative reviews can be difficult to overcome. "Bad reviews can be very damaging," observes Tony Origlio. "Everything can stop there. It's very hard to get critics to come back again." Sometimes, according to press agent Francine Trevens, no news can be the best news. And no review, she stresses, "is better for the life of many a show—and company—than an out-and-out devastation in print."

Trevens has run FLT Press Representatives for more than ten years. Her present client list includes several Off- and Off-Off-Broadway productions and theater companies that include The Glines, The Quaigh, and TADA! Children's Theater. She notes that handling a play can be quite different from handling a performer. With a play, there usually is no production to see when she is called upon to do the press. But, there is a script. "I always read the script," Trevens said, "and see if I respond to it. If I don't respond to the script, I don't take it on. I don't like to sell something I don't like personally."

Trevens admits, however, that reading a script isn't foolproof. Press agent Jeffrey Richards wholeheartedly agrees: "Sure you try to work with clients you believe in. But, a lot can happen between page and stage." In addition to the American Jewish Theater, Richards' clients include the Hudson Guild Theater and WPA. He has also done the press for such memorable shows as *Scrambled Feet*, *American Buffalo* with Al Pacino, and *Three Guys Naked from the Waist Down*. Before taking on a client, he likes to see the material and also likes to get to know the people who are involved with it. "I want to know what their ambitions are and what their necessities are," he explains.

If your ambitions include bringing in major critics and outrunning *A Chorus Line*, you'll never do it without a press agent. But, if you've approached three or four and none of them are interested, have the good sense to ask them why. They aren't the last word on American Theater but they do have a working knowledge of the business. They know what sells and they know what doesn't and you can be sure that if they're turning away your money, they're doing it for a reason. Find out what that reason is.

If publicists tell you that your project isn't ready for a full-fledged publicity campaign, that doesn't mean that you should abandon it or give up hope that anyone will come to see it. It just means that you'll have to work at it a little longer. If the PR people think your press expectations are too high based on what you have to offer, give that some serious consideration too and come back down to earth. Then, weigh what you can afford to pay against the value of the publicity that press agents feel they can realistically deliver.

PROFESSIONAL PUBLICITY—CREDIBILITY GUARANTEED

It's not impossible to get some coverage without a press agent. Some editors, interviewers, and critics truly delight in "discovering" new talent and saying in a column, feature, or review, "Keep an eye on this performer!" and "Remember, you heard it here first!"

Having a professional handling your press gives your project a certain air of legitimacy that in-house publicity or do-it-yourself campaigns cannot. Some critics do review shows that do not have press representation, but most will not, unless someone they trust has offered a hearty recommendation.

American Jewish Theater productions, for example, received reviews regularly in the Jewish press. But it wasn't until the company hired a press agent that their press *noticeably* increased. "There's a certain prestige that comes from working with a first-rate agent," notes AJT artistic director Stanley Brechner. "The image that you want to project is a sense of quality: first-rate people doing first-rate work. A press agent helps for that to happen."

Another thing to consider is that PR can lend a certain credibility to your company that can help it obtain city, state, private, and corporate funding. "When you're in the paper," says Jim Learned, co-artistic director of TADA! Children's Theater, "and you have some press, it's sort of proof that you exist. When you include clips with a funding application, it lends you authenticity."

ADDITIONAL PUBLICITY

In addition to obtaining press and bringing in critics, there are many other services that press agents can provide. Not all publicists offer the same services, however, so it's important to determine what services they do offer during your initial meeting. Press agents, like FLT's Francine Trevens, offer clients a printed list outlining services they offer. On the same piece of paper, however, Trevens stresses that "all of the above are not done for every show, but they are among the things press agents can and will do at times." Among those services are the following:

Setting up invitations for the critics: The importance of this cannot be overstated. Critics, even those on smaller publications and monthlies, are literally inundated every week with more invitations than they know what to do with. If your opening or press preview falls on the same night as another opening a critic is already committed to, chances are you won't see that critic. Publicists keep track of what's going on and can advise you accordingly.

Constructing press packets: This is another very important service, one that can make a big difference with a critic. Your publicist knows the critics and knows what they want and don't want in a press package. Some critics, for example appreciate being given reviews you've already received. Others abhor the practice. Some critics need photos they can hand in with their stories. Others don't need these and will probably just throw them away. Your press agent will supply you with a professional package that is neat, contains correctly spelled names, and all other information that the critic requires.

Offering advice on which critics to approach: A review in one of the dailies can be a great way to bring in business, but not if the review is awful. Critics have their own tastes and preferences. How many times have you read three different reviews of the same show and found three entirely different points of view? Certain shows are virtually "critic-proof" on the basis of the talent involved but, unless you're Neil Simon or Andrew Lloyd Webber, it might be best not to risk inviting every critic right away. A bad review can cause a lot less damage if it comes after you've gotten some good ones and built an audience. Your press agent can tell you the critics who are most likely to be receptive to—and appreciative of—what you are doing.

Supervision of the ad campaign and schedule: This is a service that not all press agents offer. But those who will give you some input on ads are offering you the benefit of their considerable experience. A press agent can advise you on what to say or not say in your ad, how it should look, what are the best outlets for reaching your audience, and how often you should run the ad.

PUBLICITY AND THE DEVELOPMENT OF IDENTITY

In addition to helping you sustain an image, a press agent can help you to create one, providing, of course, that you are ready to do so. Some performers resent being categorized so blatantly as "the new James Dean," or "the new Bette Midler." During interviews, they invariably feel compelled to tell reporters, "I'm me, not the new someone else," when PR-inspired comparisons are made.

If being pegged in such a way bothers you, you may as well get used to it, for such comparisons are inevitable. After 25 years in the business, international acclaim, three Tony awards, an Oscar, an Emmy, and a Golden Globe, Liza Minnelli is still being compared, in print, to her mother! And Barbra Streisand was pegged, on the cover of her first album, as a cross between Helen Morgan, Fanny Brice, Beatrice Lillie, and a painting by Modigliani.

Such comparisons are even more likely when you're not known to the general public. Press agents use pegs to pitch you to writers. Writers use the same peg to pitch you to their editors. And the completed feature pitches the peg back to the readers.

Ellen Stewart's name may not be familiar to all, but in the past two decades Stewart has become a legend in the theater community. As the founder and guiding light of La Mama Experimental Theater Company, Stewart has made a name for herself as someone who discovers and nurtures talent, takes risks and presents provocative work in exciting and very theatrical ways. Stewart has made her reputation, and sustained it, by carefully choosing material and working with people who share her personal vision of what theater is. Through the years, her public relations strategy has developed just as carefully. Interviews with Stewart, features on La Mama and all advertising for the company have furthered La Mama's esoteric image, not detracted from it.

Image and identity can be thought of as a kind of shorthand—a quick way of saying what you do or what you're like, so that people will come and see for themselves. So you may as well learn to deal with the idea of a press-created image. As long as it's accurate, as long as it works, and as long as it allows you room to grow, if the image fits, wear it.

THE CLIENT-PUBLICIST RELATIONSHIP

Although it is important to work in cooperation with your press agent, there are some public relations stratagems on which you will need to draw the line. For occasionally, press agents get a little over-zealous in their work. If your publicist wants to call your walk-on appearance the most monumental event to hit the theater since Laurence Olivier or Fanny Brice, it's time for you to be raising an objection. This points to what is essentially a double-edged sword in the client-publicist relationship. This relationship must be based on trust, but you also have to establish limitations on that trust. It's a little like hiring an interior decorator, or a haircutter, or the accountant who prepares your tax return. You can't just give them money, close your eyes, and tell them to do whatever they feel like. Whether you handle your own press or not, you are still responsible for it and the way it develops.

Julie Sheppard's one-woman show, *Julie, Julie, Julie,* based on the life of Judy Garland, had a lengthy run at Don't Tell Mama. Julie Sheppard advises those who are about to hire a publicist to establish realistic goals about the show they are appearing in and to draw definite limitations on how their press should be handled. "I wanted desperately for *Julie, Julie, Julie* to be viewed as a theater piece," Sheppard said, and, sure enough, that description was stressed in all of her publicity. Because of the nature of the show, the actress knew she could upset a lot of people if the press was not handled just right. "I didn't want people to get the impression that I was dragging Judy Garland through the mud one more time for old time's sake. I wanted them to know that the show was respectful and I was lucky enough to have a press agent who believed in what I was doing."

Other performers Sheppard has known haven't been quite as lucky. "Any crazy scheme someone comes up with to get them on TV, they go along with because they want the exposure. But, it can be damaging," she says. Concerned that the public might construe her show as some kind of glorified drag act, Sheppard refused to release press photos of herself as Garland or to make TV appearances in her character role. "I refuse to this day to appear on TV that way," Sheppard said. "I won't even allow people in the audience to take photos during performances." Her reasoning? "I'm an actress. If I were going on *Live at Five* and I were Betty Buckley, they wouldn't ask me to come on as Grizabella the Cat."

Some stunts are destined to get press. Others, even the tiniest, most innocuous stunts, are not always so surefire. For a show called *Neckties,* publicist Francine Trevens had a whole batch of fliers made up that were shaped like little ties. It was a clever idea and people loved them. For another show called *T.N.T.,* Trevens sent critics their invitations in rolls of cardboard disguised as sticks of dynamite. The critics summed up the stunt the same way they summed up the play: a bomb.

If stunts of this type disturb you, or if any other aspect of PR is simply not right for you, make sure you discuss this with your publicist at the outset. If you find it difficult to have this sort of conversation, or get your point across, there is something very wrong with the relationship you are embarking on. Here are some comments by the press agents on the publicist/client relationship.

Tony Origlio: "I always tell people to look at a publicist's clients and at the results. Look at their reputation. But, there also has to be a special rapport. Without one, it's going to be difficult to work together."

Jeffrey Richards: "You must have confidence and trust in the person you are dealing with and tell them, up front, what you expect."

Francine Trevens: "It's a personal relationship. If it works, don't look any further. If it doesn't, look around and make a change."

Bruce Cohen: "Check references and above all, keep it real. It must be an honest relationship."

Penny Landau: "Honesty is important. You have to trust them and they have to trust you. And remember, the only guarantee is that there are no guarantees."

FINDING A PRESS AGENT
Once you've decided the time is right, that you believe in your project, and that you're ready for a full-fledged publicity campaign, you need to know how to find a press agent.

You could try the Yellow Pages, but a much better bet would be to ask people you trust for some referrals. Once you have a few of these, make some phone calls, set up some interviews and see what happens. Listen to what these publicists have to say; notice whether or not they're listening to what you have to say, and see if you have any rapport with them.

If your referrals don't pan out, then contact the Association of Theatrical Press Agents and Managers. Their address is 165 W. 46th St., New York, NY 10036. Send a letter directly to this union's business agent with a description of your project. Ask for suitable referrals and take it from there.

As you confer with various press agents, provide them with enough information about yourself and your project so that they can realistically assess your potential for publicity and their compatibility with the project. If they express interest in what you're doing, ask them about rates, the range of additional services they offer and specific terms (such as a month up front, a three-month trial, and so on.)

Don't sign anything until you've spoken to at least three press agents and given the matter plenty of thought. Base your decision on the data you've collected, personal recommendations and your own gut instinct.

Hiring a press agent is a major step in a career into which you have already invested a lot of blood, sweat, and tears. Make sure the step you take is the right one, correctly timed and fully thought out.

Creating Your Own Publicity

by Bill Ervolino

Performers who are unable to latch on to a publicist should not overlook the do-it-yourself option. Many entertainers have learned how to put together an effective publicity campaign with no previous experience. So if you're willing to do a little leg-work and some research you might want to explore this approach. Obviously, you won't gain the advantages of a full-scale promotional effort mounted by a major press agent, but you can do at least some of the public relations work that is so important to your career. A do-it-yourself PR campaign, if professionally prepared and well organized, can produce very positive results.

THE PRESS KIT

Start out by preparing a press kit. Here is a description of a really stunning press kit that was put together by a men's fashion designer: For a folder it had a photograph of one of the designer's sweaters printed on a rich textured cardboard. The first page had the designer's logo imprinted on a sheet of charcoal gray suede. A bio was included, as were some black and white fashion photos. An additional enclosure, a poster-sized calender, featured the designer's logo, full-color fashion photos, address, telephone and Telex numbers. The photographs were shot, on location, atop a snow-covered mountain. This press kit, was, of course, the work of a professional publicist and was very impressive. But a press kit doesn't have to be this slick to get the job done. In fact, if you're an unknown, too-slick a press kit could wind up turning people off. Your goal primarily is to produce a press kit that looks professional.

An effective press kit should contain a description of your project, bios of the people involved, clips and reviews, photographs of performers (or a scene from the production), and a personal letter.

Make sure that your PR is well written. Editors have eyes like eagles when it comes to spotting typos, poor grammar, and rambling sentences. There is nothing worse to send to an editor than a poorly written press kit.

Keep your bio short and sweet. If information is colorful, include it. If it's pertinent to your project, include it. If it incorporates anyone famous, include it! Everyone loves to see names so, if you studied with Uta Hagen, took gym class with Meryl Streep, or shared an apartment with anyone well-known, it will be of interest.

Your photographs are extremely important in publicizing your project and should be the best quality you can afford to buy. Unprofessional photos that are fuzzy or grainy or just plain awful will only hurt your publicity effort. If you're beautiful, make sure that your photos are beautiful. If you're funny, try a funny pose, perhaps with some props. Don't send out photos that are misleading.

The most effective cover letter is one that is personal and to the point. It should tell the editor or critic what you are doing, when you are doing it, and why you think it is of interest. If the editor recently wrote an article bemoaning how musicals aren't what they used to be, and you're in the middle of rehearsals for a real old-fashioned musical comedy, be sure to mention it. If you are a cabaret singer by night and a veterinarian by day, include this information in your letter and politely suggest a feature on moonlighting professionals.

A personal press agent would sit you down and interrogate you like Elliot Ness for any potential story angle that might emerge. Without a press agent, you'll have to discover these angles on your own. If you think about it long enough you're bound to come up with something interesting.

FINDING OUTLETS

Identifying all of the press outlets that are available to you will take time, patience, and all the resourcefulness you can muster. Start by making a list of all the dailies, weeklies, and monthlies you can think of that carry entertainment items. Then go to the largest newsstand you can find and do some browsing. After this, go to a library and ask for any guides they might have which list metro-area publications. Keep adding to your list and don't rule out the hometown papers. They can be excellent sources of publicity and could provide you with a nice feature you can clip out and stick in your press kit.

Once you have a list of possible outlets, make appropriate notations next to each publication with regard to the types of PR opportunities that exist in each. Some types of press outlets you may find are as follows:

Listings: Many newspapers and magazines list shows and events in their directories. Readers of these publications generally rely on such listings when planning a night on the town. Your best chance of being included in a directory is to study the format in each publication and then write up a listing that is compatible. Make sure you include all the pertinent information (who, what, where, when) and that your listing is neatly typed. Then call the publication you are interested in, ask for the listings or calendar editor, and inquire about deadline information. Address your listing to that particular editor, unless you are told otherwise. A handwritten note, accompanying the listing, probably won't hurt. ("Dear Mr./Ms. Smith: Thanks for the information the other day. Hope you can use this!")

Photo Submissions: Editors and art directors like attractive pictures and many publications use one or more on every page. When sending a photo to a publication, make sure to enclose a caption that contains all necessary information and correctly identifies, from left to right, the people in the photo. Also make sure that the photographer's credit is stamped or written legibly on the back of the photo. Your photo can be arty, comical, or provocative. The best tip concerning the submission of photos, however, is to study the publication you are sending them to and see the type of material they like. Once you're familiar with the publication, use some common sense and forward something appropriate.

Column Items: There are countless publications in which you can publicize your project. Look around, familiarize yourself with what's out there, and then be selective about where you send your material. If you have an especially good item, something involving a "name," for example, you may want to send it to Liz Smith, Page Six of the *New York Post*, or some of the other better-known columns. Keep in mind, however, that the bigger the column, the warier the columnist is likely to be about taking items from strangers. If you want to take a chance, write up the item in the style of the column, keep it brief, send it off, and follow up with a phone call. Be reminded, though, that major columnists are very busy, so don't tie them up with long-winded conversation. A simple, "Will you be using the item?" will do the job.

Features and Interviews: When pitching yourself as a feature subject, make sure you provide the editor or writer with as much information as possible, written as concisely as possible. Include who you are, what you're doing, and sell, sell, sell. If a prominent critic has said something wonderful about you, include it in your pitch. If you have worked with some famous people in the past, include that too. Perhaps you have a special skill or situation that might prove enticing to the editor. If so, try it, no matter how far out it might seem.

Don't be disappointed if your request for a feature or interview is turned down. Arranging press of this type definitely requires a talent for finding angles and pitching them. It is not unheard of for an unknown to grab this type of coverage, but this occurs rarely. Your best bet is to start with your hometown press and build slowly from there.

TELEVISION BOOKINGS

This one is really tricky. It isn't impossible, but it certainly isn't easy and it isn't always advisable. If you don't have a press agent, have never appeared on TV before and don't have a long-term publicity campaign mapped out, you may not be ready for a TV appearance. Of course, such an appearance could lead to all kinds of offers, but if you're not ready to hire an agent, you're probably not ready for David Letterman either.

According to Sandra Furton, the head talent coordinator for "Late Night with David Letterman," her office receives between 20 and 30 videotapes per day from performers who want to appear on the show. She receives another 70 letters or calls for appointments daily. The vast majority of performers, of course, will never appear on the show, but that doesn't stop them from trying.

If you are intent on trying for a TV appearance go right ahead. But without a publicist, your chances are very slim. "We feel more confident if there's a publicist involved," Furton noted, "especially if they have worked with us in the past and recommended someone [who appeared on the show]. You learn to trust certain publicists." Furton offers this advice to performers without publicists. "Send a letter, enclose as much information as you can, and, if you have a videotape, send that along, too. It gives us the opportunity to see you in a TV situation." Furton says that there are eight people currently working in the show's talent office and at least five of them review each request. Furton advises people who have been turned down "not to picket outside, not to call again for at least a few months, and not to disregard her 'no' and immediately approach someone else in her office."

As the Letterman show is taped in New York, many guests are local performers. Theater companies are rarely represented, unless an act is particularly unusual. One person who did make it onto the show and was invited back a couple of times, was neither a performer nor an artistic director. She was a Broadway house-usherette, who talked about her 45 years behind a flashlight.

Don't overlook *local* TV shows and cable TV programs. They are always looking for guests. Most prefer to deal with publicists, too, but they are bound to be more receptive than national programs. The local shows can also give you an opportunity to get your feet wet. If you've never been interviewed before on camera, it's best to keep it on the smallest scale possible. To book yourself on one of these shows, you should contact the talent coordinator, ask what the requirements are and then follow up with a letter. If you have a tape, send that as well. Sell yourself as best you can.

Your chances of obtaining exposure are better if you can do something different or unusual during your segment. If you have successfully dealt with a serious issue in your life, overcome a condition or illness or have anything else that you wouldn't feel uncomfortable talking about on TV, propose it as a segment. Discussing how you've dealt with dyslexia for example, could get you some exposure and help others in the process. Make absolutely sure that you feel comfortable with an appearance of this sort and that a personal issue does not get exploited.

CULTIVATING THE MEDIA

Without a press agent out there helping to develop a relationship with the media for you, you're going to have to do it yourself. This isn't easy, but it can be done.

Critics and editors are used to pushy people, but that doesn't mean they enjoy dealing with them. The more you socialize with friends in the business, the more likely it is that you will run into various members of the press. It is important for you to cultivate professional relationships with these people, so don't just stand there staring at them. If it's someone you don't know, wait for the right time, and go over and introduce yourself. When you run into writers or critics whom you have already met, by all means walk over and say hello. Mention what you've been up to and, if you happen to recall a recent article they've written, it probably won't hurt to comment on it. Be cordial. Be charming. And be quick about it. Don't be pushy, don't be obnoxious and don't take up too much of their time—just enough to remind them of who you are and what you are doing.

Other ways to remind the press that you're still alive include occasional notes ("I saw your article on such-and-such and found it very informative, and so on.") and cards ("Merry Christmas, Happy Hanukkah, Happy New Year, and hope you can catch my next show at Panache"). Also, follow-ups are important. Critics do appreciate thank-you notes for their reviews and, if you point out something they said that you felt was particularly on the mark, that's even better. You can even send a polite note for a negative review, thanking the critic for reviewing you, or for any positive comments or suggestions that were in the review.

In between writing all these notes, don't forget mailings to the people who have already seen you in performance. Many small theater companies and individual performers, make an address book available to members of the audience who want to be put on their mailing list. Anyone who came to see you and signed your address book is interested in what you are doing. Don't forget about those people. Send them flyers or newsletters and keep them posted on your present and future projects.

Publicity plays a major role in achieving success as a performer. It is hard work, but well worth the effort. Make the most of whatever PR options are available to you during the engagements for which you are hired. Some clubs and theaters have in-house publicity that could help you. Pay attention to what works and what doesn't and learn to be patient, letting your publicity build over time.

PART FIVE

Working in the Theater

Off and Off-Off-Broadway

by Victor Gluck

Off-Broadway theaters have always stood for an alternative to the Broadway stages. These small theaters located all over New York City are intimate spaces that allow for lower production costs and plays of specialized interest. Although a performer's ultimate goal may be Broadway, the majority of work in the New York theater is actually produced Off and Off-Off-Broadway. The Broadway theater's high rents are prohibitive, but these hundreds of theater companies away from the Broadway theater district are able to offer affordable space and endless opportunities to producers, directors, and performers at all levels.

Many well-known stage actors began their careers in Off- or Off-Off-Broadway productions. The staggering number of plays produced in this venue has provided New York theater with hundreds of opportunities that did not previously exist. Countless newcomers to the legitimate theater now gain performance experience on Off-Broadway stages. Meryl Streep, William Hurt, Al Pacino, Robert De Niro and Richard Dreyfuss are just a few of the stars who, at one time in their careers, were closely linked to the Off-Broadway theater scene. Legends were born in Off-Broadway that have permanently changed American theater—talents such as Ellen Stewart, Tom O'Horgan, Charles Ludlam, Julian Beck and Judith Malina, Joseph Chaikin, Harvey Fierstein, and Joseph Papp.

While *Off-Broadway* specifically refers to commercial productions in small theaters, *Off-Off-Broadway* refers to non-commercial, nonprofit productions which appear for limited engagements in even smaller theaters. The Off-Off-Broadway movement began with Caffe Cino in 1959 and the La Mama Experimental Theater Club in 1962 in a ferment of creativity that launched the careers of such playwrights as Leonard Melfi, Sam Shepard, Lanford Wilson, John Guare, Israel Horovitz, Robert Patrick, Maria Irene Fornes and Tom Eyen.

The last 25 years has seen the rise of Off-Off-Broadway nonprofit theater companies that have become an integral part of New York's cultural life. Because many Off-Off-Broadway companies specialize or play host to various kinds of theater, they offer newcomers to the acting profession valuable training and experience. Some theaters, like the York Theater Company, only perform revivals; others, such as the Classic Stage Company (CSC), offer new interpretations of the classics. Some theaters present house-style productions, such as the poetic realism practiced at Circle Repertory. Others may offer competitive one-act festivals, as does the Ensemble Studio Theater, thereby giving an actor a chance to be seen in several different plays at one time.

Some companies are run by various groups from the theater community. Playwrights Horizons is such a company. This theater has as its board of directors a group of playwrights. Often a collective of actors and directors will be formed for the purpose of showcasing the talents of its members. Still other companies, like the Negro Ensemble Company, the Jewish Repertory Theater, or the Pan Asian Repertory Theater, are the home of specific ethnic groups. These companies give work to actors that might not be found elsewhere. The Second Stage specializes in giving a second chance to plays that the company feels have been unjustly neglected. Manhattan Punch Line calls itself the "house of comedy", and makes use of actors' comedic gifts, while the Soho Repertory Theater even represents an alternative to Off-Off-Broadway, producing unusual plays with an emphasis on language and theatricality.

The theater space of Off-Off-Broadway may be a church, loft, school, warehouse, or basement. Off-Off-Broadway can, in fact, exist anywhere, from just outside the Broadway theater district to the outer fringes of New York City.

The seriousness with which non-Broadway productions are now taken can be measured by two facts. First, during the 1988–89 resident theater season, one-half to two-thirds of the plays chosen were originally produced Off-Broadway or by a nonprofit theater company. Second, the Pulitzer Prize, one of the most respected theater awards in America, has regularly recognized Off-Broadway achievement since 1970. It was in this year that the prize went to the New York Shakespeare Festival's production of *No Place to Be Somebody* by Charles Gordone. Since then, two other New York Shakespeare Festival productions have received Pulitzer Prices as Off-Broadway plays—*That Championship Season* in 1973, and *A Chorus Line* in 1976, (both of these plays had already moved to Broadway at the time of the awards).

Other theaters honored for initiating Pulitzer Prize-winning productions include the Theater for the New City for producing Sam Shepard's *Buried Child* in 1979; Circle Repertory Company for its production of Lanford Wilson's *Talley's Folly* in 1980; the Negro Ensemble Company for producing *A Soldier's Play* by Charles Fuller in 1982, and Playwrights Horizons for its production of *Driving Miss Daisy*, a first dramatic play by Alfred Uhry in 1988. The commercial run of Paul Zindel's *The Effect of Gamma Rays On Man-In-the-Moon Marigolds*, which ran Off-Broadway for several years, won the Pulitzer Prize in 1971 before becoming an acclaimed film.

The prestige of Off-Broadway productions today is incalculable. Major stars of stage and screen as well as big name producers are as likely to be working Off-Broadway as on. Many of Broadway's biggest hits were tried out at Off-Broadway theaters before risking larger and more expensive venues. Recent Tony winners *Torch Song Trilogy, The Elephant Man* and *I'm Not Rappaport* would not have been possible without the Off-Broadway tryouts that came first. All of these plays kept their original Off-Broadway casts when they moved to Broadway. Hit musicals like *Little Shop of Horrors, Joseph and the Amazing Technicolor Dreamcoat* and *The Best Little Whorehouse In Texas*, were given glamorous Broadway-style productions in Off-Broadway theaters away from the Great White Way.

Many Off-and Off-Off-Broadway box office hits go on to become hit movies— *Crossing Delancey, Fool for Love, Key Exchange, Little Shop of Horrors*, and *A Soldier's Story*, to name a few. Others have been seen on television, such as *Painting Churches* and *Lemon Sky*. Sometimes the original actors are signed to recreate their roles in these films. Even if they weren't given this opportunity, the very fact that they created the original roles increases their stock with casting agents, directors and playwrights immensely. For some playwrights, producers, directors, and performers, Off Broadway is the road to stardom.

Off- and Off-Off-Broadway Theater Companies

The following is a list of Off- and Off-Off-Broadway theatre companies in New York City. Some are non-Equity companies, some produce under Equity's Showcase or Tier Codes, while others may produce under an Equity contract.

THE ABOUT FACE COMPANY
442 W. 42nd St.
New York, NY 10036
(212) 866-6737
Sean Burke, Richard Corley, artistic dirs. Susan Geer, prod. dir.; Allison Jones, mng. dir.

THE ACTING COMPANY
PO Box 898, Times Square Station
New York, NY 10108
(212) 564-3510
Gerald Gutierrez, artistic dir.

THE ACTING GROUP
Box 1252, Old Chelsea Station
New York, NY 10011
(212) 645-1459
Celia Barrett, producing artistic dir.

ACTORS' ALLIANCE INC.
J.A.F. PO Box 7370
New York, NY 10116
(718) 768-6110
(718) 805-0099
Melanie Sutherland, Juanita Walsh, artistic dirs.

ACTORS OUTLET THEATRE
120 W. 28th St.
New York, NY 10001
(212) 645-0783
(212) 807-1590
Eleanor Segan, exec. dir.; Ken Lowstetter, artistic dir.

ACTORS REPERTORY THEATRE
303 E. 44th St.
New York, NY 10017
(212) 687-6430
Warren Robertson, artistic dir.

THE ACTORS' SPACE
250 W. 54th St., 10th fl.
New York, NY 10019
(212) 757-5900
Alan Langdon, artistic dir.

ALCHEMY THEATER COMPANY
515 E. 85th St.
New York, NY 10028
(212) 744-4275
Gita Donovan, artistic dir.; Geoffrey H. Dawe, mng. dir.

AMAS REPERTORY THEATRE
1 E. 104th St., 3rd fl.
New York, NY 10029
(212) 369-8000
Rosetta LeNoire, artistic dir.

AMERICAN ENSEMBLE COMPANY
PO Box 972, Peck Slip Station
New York, NY 10272
(212) 571-7594
Robert Petito, artistic dir. Theater address: 339 E. 28th St. New York, NY 10016

AMERICAN FOLK THEATRE
230 W. 41st. St., Suite 1807
New York, NY 10036
(212) 391-2330;
757-0608 (box off.)
Dick Gaffield, artistic dir.

AMERICAN INDIAN COMMUNITY THEATRE SPACE
842 B'way, 8th fl.
Theater Dept.
New York, NY 10003
(212) 598-0100
Gloria Miguel, artistic dir.

AMERICAN JEWISH THEATRE
307 W. 26th St.
New York, NY 10001
(212) 633-1588;
633-9797 (box off.)
Stanley Brechner, artistic dir.

THE AMERICAN LINE
810 W. 183rd St., #5C,
New York, NY 10033
(212) 740-9277
Richard Hoehler, artistic dir. Shakirah Wadud, managing dir.

AMERICAN PLACE THEATRE, INC.
111 W. 46th St.
New York, NY 10036
(212) 840-2960
Wynn Handman, artistic dir.; Mickey Rolfe, gen'l. mgr.

AMERICAN
PLAYWRIGHTS
REPERTORY
276 Fifth Ave., Suite 505
New York, NY 10001
(212) 362-3964
Sarah Emory, artistic dir.

THE AMERICAN
RENAISSANCE THEATRE
112 Charlton St.
New York, NY 10014
(212) 929-4718
Susan Egert, artistic dir.

THE AMERICAN
STANISLAVSKI THEATRE
485 Park Ave., #6A
New York, NY 10022
(212) 755-5120
Sonia Moore, artistic dir.

AMERICAN THEATRE OF
ACTORS
314 W. 54th St.
New York, NY 10019
(212) 581-3044
James Jennings, artistic dir.

ANY PLACE THEATRE
PO Box 2467
New York, NY 10185
(212) 956-2384
Lynn Middleton, artistic dir.

APPLE CORPS THEATRE
336 W. 20th St.
New York, NY 10011
(212) 929-2955
John Raymond, artistic dir.

ART & WORK
ENSEMBLE
870 6th Ave.
New York, NY 10001
(212) 213-0231
*Anthony DiPietro, artistic
dir.*

ARTS CLUB THEATRE
80 E. 3rd St., #10
New York, NY 10003
(212) 673-5636
Linda Pakri, artistic dir.

BARE STAGES
PO Box 6233
FDR Station
New York, NY 10150-1901
(212) 627-8495

BARROW GROUP
PO Box 2236
New York, NY 10108
(212) 512-1707
Seth Barrish, artistic dir.
David Diamond, gen'l. mgr.

BILLIE HOLIDAY
THEATRE
1368 Fulton St.
Brooklyn, NY 11216
(718) 857-6363
Marjorie Moon, prod'r.

BLACK SPECTRUM
THEATRE COMPANY
119th Ave. & Merrick Blvd.
Jamaica, NY 11434
(718) 723-1800
Carl Clay, artistic dir.

SUSAN BLOCH THEATRE
307 W. 26th St.
c/o Roundabout
100 E. 17th St.
(212) 420-1360
Ellen Richard, gen'l. mgr.

BLUE HERON THEATRE
645 West End Ave.
New York, NY 10025
(212) 787-0422
Ardelle Striker, artistic dir.

BOND STREET
THEATRE COALITION
2 Bond St.
New York, NY 10012
(212) 254-4614
*Joanna Sherman, artistic
dir.*

BONK
P.O. Box 1776, Peter
Stuyvesant Station
New York, NY 10009
Lisa Napoli, artistic dir.

BREAD AND PUPPET
THEATER
c/o. George Ashley
310 Greenwich St., #31-A
New York, NY 10013
(212) 964-0263
George Ashley, publicity

THE CAB THEATRE CO.
1729-31 1st Ave., #5C
New York, NY 10128
(212) 996-1959
Joann Carollo, mng. dir.

CACTUS THEATRE
91 Charles St.
New York, NY 10014
(212) 242-0709
Bo Brinkman, artistic dir.

CHICAGO CITY LIMITS
351 E. 74th St.
New York, NY 10021
(212) 772-8707
Paul Zuckerman, prod'r.

CIRCLE REPERTORY
COMPANY
161 Ave. of the Americas
New York, NY 10013
(212) 691-3210;
924-7100 (box office)
Tanya Berezin, artistic dir.
Theater Address: 99 7th
Ave. So.
New York, NY 10014

CIRCUS THEATRICALS
711 W. 171st St., #67
New York, NY 10032
(212) 529-7794
Jack Stehlin, artistic dir.

CSC REPERTORY, LTD.
The Classic Stage Co.
136 E. 13th St.
New York, NY 10003
(212) 677-4210
Carey Perloff, artistic dir.;
Ellen Novack, mng. dir.

CLASSIC THEATRE
200 Park Ave.
New York, NY 10166
(212) 636-4120
*Maurice Edwards, artistic
dir.; Nicholas John Stathis,
exec. dir.*

JEAN COCTEAU
REPERTORY
330 Bowery
New York, NY 10012
(212) 677-0060
Eve Adamson, artistic dir.

COMMON GROUND
210 Forsyth St.
New York, NY 10002
(212) 505-6047
Norman Taffel, artistic dir.

CONEY ISLAND, USA
Boardwalk & W. 12th St.
Coney Island, NY 11224
(718) 372-5159
Dick Zigun, artistic dir.

COURTYARD PLAYERS
PO Box 30952,
Port Authority Sta.
New York, NY 10011
(212) 496-4288
Bob Stark, artistic dir.
Theater Address: 39 Grove St.
New York, NY 10014

DEAR KNOWS
263A W. 19th St., Suite 149
New York, NY 10011
(212) 691-9622
Paul Walker, Christopher
Markle, artistic dirs.

DOUBLE IMAGE
THEATRE
444 W. 56th St., Rm 1110
New York, NY 10019
(212) 245-2489
Helen Warren Mayer, artistic
dir.

DRAMA COMMITTEE
REPERTORY THEATRE
118 W. 79th St.
New York, NY 10024
(212) 595-1733
Arthur Reel, artistic dir.

DRAMATIC RISKS
60 E. 4th St., #19
New York, NY 10003

ECCENTRIC CIRCLES
THEATRE
c/o Hopkins
400 W. 43rd St., #4N
New York, NY 10036
Rosemary Hopkins, Paula
Kay Pierce, Janet Bruders,
Barbara Bunch, artistic
dirs.

ECONOMY TIRES
THEATRE
DTW's Bessie Schonberg
Theater
219 W. 19th St.
New York, NY 10011
(212) 924-0077
David White, exec. dir.

ELYSIUM THEATRE
COMPANY
PO Box 20521
Tompkins Square
New York, NY 10009
(212) 260-6114
Gregori Von Leitis, artistic
dir.

EN GARDE ARTS
225 Rector Place, Suite 3A
New York, NY 10280
(212) 945-0336
Anne Hamburger, prod'r.

ENSEMBLE STUDIO
THEATRE
549 W. 52nd St.
New York, NY 10019
(212) 247-4982
Curt Dempster, artistic dir.

EQUITY LIBRARY
THEATRE
Business Office:
165 W. 46th St.
New York, NY 10036
(212) 869-9266
Theater:
310 Riverside Dr.
New York, NY 10025
(212) 663-2880
George Wojtasik, producing
dir.

THE FAMILY
9 Second Ave., 4th fl.
New York, NY 10003
(212) 477-2522
J.J. Johnson, artistic dir.

THE FIREDRAKE
COMPANY
PO Box 400
Richmond Hill, NY 11418
(718) 849-4864
Joanna Andretta, David
Gearino, co-artistic dirs.

FIRING SQUAD/COMEDY
REP ENSEMBLE
Mailing address: 121 E. 12th
St., Suite 7F
New York, NY 10003
(212) 473-0413
David Stamford, producing
dir.; Jackson Heath, artistic
dir.

FIRST AMENDMENT
COMEDY THEATRE
2 Bond St.
New York, NY 10012
(212) 473-1472
Barbara Contardi, artistic
dir.

FOLKSBIENE THEATRE
123 E. 55th St.
New York, NY 10022
(212) 888-0410
Ben Schechter, artistic dir.;
Morris Adler, chairman.

FOURTH WALL REP. CO.
79 E. 4th St.
New York, NY 10003
(212) 254-5060
John Harvey, artistic dir.

GOLDEN FLEECE, LTD.
204 W. 20th St.
New York, NY 10011
(212) 691-6105
Lu Rodgers, artistic dir.

HISPANIC
ORGANIZATION OF
LATIN ACTORS (HOLA)
250 W. 65th St.
New York, NY 10023
(212) 595-8286
Francisco Rivela, exec.
committee;
Carlos Carrasco, artistic dir.

HUDSON GUILD
THEATRE
441 W. 26th St.
New York, NY 10001
(212) 760-9810
Geoffrey Sherman, artistic
dir.

INTAR HISPANIC
AMERICAN THEATRE
PO Box 788
Times Square Sta.
New York, NY 10108
(212) 695-6134
Max Ferra, artistic dir.;
James Diapola, mng. dir.

INTERART THEATRE
549 W. 52nd St.
New York, NY 10019
(212) 246-1050
Margot Lewitin, artistic dir.

IRISH ARTS CENTER
553 W. 51st St.
New York, NY 10019
(212) 757-3318
Nye Heron, producing dir.;
Kurt Wagemann, gen'l. mgr.

IRONDALE ENSEMBLE
PROJECT
782 West End Ave.
New York, NY 10025
(212) 666-7856, 633-1292
James Niesen, artistic dir.

ITALIAN-AMERICAN
REPERTORY THEATRE
496A Hudson St.
Suite E-25
New York, NY 10014
(201) 836-0907
Gene Ruffini, artistic dir.

JEWISH REPERTORY
THEATRE
344 E. 14th St.
New York, NY 10003
(212) 674-7200
Ran Avni, artistic dir.

LA MAMA ETC
74-A E. 4th St.
New York, NY 10009
(212) 475-7710
Wesley Jensby, artistic dir.;
Ellen Stewart, founder.

LAMB'S THEATRE
COMPANY
130 W. 44th St.
New York, NY 10036
(212) 575-0300
Carolyn Rossi Copeland,
producing dir.

LATIN AMERICAN
THEATRE ENSEMBLE
PO Box 1259, Radio City
Sta.
New York, NY 10101
(212) 246-7478; 410-4582
Margarita Toirac, exec. dir.;
Mario Pena, Margarita
Toirac, founders.
Theater address: 172 E.
104th St.
New York, NY 10029

LION THEATRE
COMPANY
422 W. 42nd St.
New York, NY 10036
(212) 736-7930

THE LIVING THEATRE
800 West End Ave.
New York, NY 10025
(212) 864-0516
Judith Malina, Hanon
Reznikov, artistic dirs.

MABOU MINES
150 First Ave.
New York, NY 10009
(212) 473-0559
Collective artistic leadership.

MANHATTAN ARTS
THEATRE, FILM, &
VIDEO
145 W. 46th St., 3rd Floor
New York, NY 10036
(212) 678-7550
Robert Mooney, artistic dir.

MANHATTAN CLASS
COMPANY
PO Box 279
Times Square Sta.
New York, NY 10108
(212) 239-9033
Bob LuPone, Bernard
Telsey, exec. dirs.
Theater Address: 442 W.
42nd St.
New York, NY 10036

MANHATTAN
ENSEMBLE, INC.
100 W. 86th St.
New York, NY 10024
(212) 769-9240
Raymond Marciniak, artistic
dir.

MANHATTAN PUNCH
LINE
410 W. 42nd St., 3rd fl.
New York, NY 10036
(212) 239-0827
Steve Kaplan, artistic dir.

MANHATTAN
REPERTORY COMPANY
648 Broadway, Suite 700-B
New York, NY 10012
(212) 995-5582
Tom Chiodo, Peter DiPietro,
artistic dirs.
Also owns Murder A
LaCarte.

MANHATTAN THEATER
CLUB
453 W. 16th St.
New York, NY 10011
(212) 645-5590
Lynne Meadow, artistic dir.

MASS TRANSIT STREET
THEATRE
c/o Robin Beall
96 Wadsworth Terrace, #5E
New York, NY 10040
(212) 795-0028

MEAT & POTATOES
COMPANY
36 W. 44th St., Suite 1208
New York, NY 10036
(718) 403-0033
Herbert DuVal, artistic dir.

MEDICINE SHOW
THEATRE ENSEMBLE
Box 20240
New York, NY 10025
(212) 431-9545
Barbara Vann, artistic dir.

MERELY PLAYERS
P.O. Box 606
New York, NY 10108
(212) 799-2253

MERRY ENTERPRISES
THEATER
354 W. 45th St.
New York, NY 10036
(212) 582-7862

MIRROR REPERTORY
COMPANY
352 E. 50th St.
New York, NY 10022
(212) 888-6087
Sabra Jones, artistic dir.

MODERN TIMES
THEATRE
250 W. 65th St.
New York, NY 10023
(212) 563-3292
Denny Partridge, artistic dir.

MUSIC THEATRE GROUP
735 Washington St.
New York, NY 10014
(212) 924-3108
Lyn Austin, artistic dir.

MUSICAL THEATRE
WORKS
440 Lafayette St.
New York, NY 10003
(212) 677-0040
*Anthony J. Stimac, exec.
dir.;
Mark S. Herko, assoc. art.
dir.*

NAT HORNE MUSICAL
THEATRE
440 W. 42nd St.
New York, NY 10036
(212) 736-7128
*Nat Horne, chairman
A membership organization
See the About Face Co.
Manhattan Class Co., and
Peter Samelson Illusions.*

NATIONAL BLACK
THEATRE
2033 5th Ave.
New York, NY 10035
(212) 427-5615
*Tunde Samuel, prod'r. of
'88–89 season.*

NATIONAL
IMPROVISATIONAL
THEATRE
223 8th Ave.
New York, NY 10011
(212) 243-7224
Tamara Wilcox, artistic dir.

NEGRO ENSEMBLE
COMPANY
1560 B'way, Suite 409
New York, NY 10036
(212) 575-5860
*Leon Denmark, producing
dir.*

NEW FEDERAL
THEATRE
Henry Street Settlement
466 Grand St.
New York, NY 10002
(212) 598-0400
Woodie King, Jr., artistic dir.

NEW RUDE
MECHANICALS
PO Box 2611
Times Square Station
New York, NY 10036
(212) 730-2030
*Robert Hall, John Pynchon
Holmes, artistic dirs.*

THE NEW STAGECRAFT
COMPANY, INC.
496A Hudson St.,
Suite H-33
New York, NY 10014
(212) 757-6300 (service)
Daniel P. Quinn, artistic dir.

THE NEW THEATRE OF
BROOKLYN
465 Dean St.
Brooklyn, NY 11217
(718) 230-3366
*Deborah J. Pope,
Steve Stettler, artistic dirs.*

NEW YORK
COLLABORATION
THEATRE
c/o Eugene Pelfrey
317 13th St.
Brooklyn, NY 11215
(718) 768-5836

NEW YORK GILBERT &
SULLIVAN PLAYERS
251 W. 91st St., 4-C
New York, NY 10024
(212) 769-1000
Albert Bergeret, artistic dir.

NEW YORK
SHAKESPEARE
FESTIVAL
425 Lafayette St.
New York, NY 10003
(212) 598-7100
*Joseph Papp, artistic dir./
prod'r.*

NEW YORK STAGE &
FILM CO.
450 W. 42nd St., #21
John Houseman Theater
New York, NY 10036
(212) 967-3130
*Leslie Urdang,
Mark Linn-Baker,
Max Mayer, producing dirs.*

NEW YORK THEATRE
STUDIO
130 W. 80th St.
New York, NY 10024
(802) 388-3318
Joanna Gard, artistic dir.

NEW YORK THEATRE
WORKSHOP
220 W. 42nd St., 18th fl.
New York, NY 10036
(212) 302-7737
*Nancy Kassak Diekmann,
mng. dir.*

ON STAGE
PRODUCTIONS, LTD.
50 W. 97th St., #8H
New York, NY 10025
(212) 666-1716
Lee Frank, artistic dir.

ONTOLOGICAL-
HYSTERIC THEATER
325 Spring St.
Suite 225
New York, NY 10013
(212) 243-6153
*Richard Foreman, artistic
dir.;
George Ashley, mng. dir.*

THE OPEN EYE: NEW
STAGINGS
270 W. 89th St.
New York, NY 10024
(212) 769-4141
Amie Brockway, artistic dir.

OPEN SPACE THEATRE
PO Box 1018
Cooper Station
New York, NY 10003
(212) 254-8630
Lynn Michaels, artistic dir.

PAN ASIAN REPERTORY
THEATRE
47 Great Jones St.
New York, NY 10012
*Tisa Chang, artistic/prod.
dir.*

PAPER BAG PLAYERS
50 Riverside Drive
New York, NY 10024
(212) 362-0431
Judith Martin, artistic dir.

PEARL THEATRE
COMPANY
125 W. 22nd St.
New York, NY 10011
(212) 645-7708
Shepard Sobel, artistic dir.

PENGUIN REP
1497 York Ave.
New York, NY 10021
(212) 650-9384
Dan Finnegan, mgr./owner.

PHOENIX ENSEMBLE
135 W. 45th St.
New York, NY 10036
(212) 719-9148
Carter Inskeep, artistic dir.

PING CHONG &
COMPANY
253 Church St.
New York, NY 10013
(212) 966-0284
Ping Chong, artistic dir.

PLAYWRIGHTS
HORIZONS
416 W. 42nd St.
New York, NY 10036
(212) 564-1235
Andre Bishop, artistic dir.

POWER THEATRE
COMPANY
311 E. 90th St.
New York, NY 10128
(212) 534-8390
Anthony DeRiso, artistic dir.

PRIMARY STAGES
COMPANY
584 9th Ave.
New York, NY 10036
(212) 333-7471
Casey Childs, artistic dir.

PROJECT III ENSEMBLE
THEATRE
PO Box 1502
Ansonia Station
New York, NY 10023
(212) 678-7526
Charles Otte, artistic dir.

PROMETHEAN THEATRE
701 Seventh Ave.
Suite 9W
New York, NY 10036
(212) 719-9812
Dan Roentsch, artistic dir.

PROMETHEUS THEATRE
239 E. 5th St.
New York, NY 10003
(212) 477-8689
Fred Fondren, artistic dir.

PUERTO RICAN
TRAVELING THEATRE
141 W. 94th St.
New York, NY 10025
(212) 354-1293
*Miriam Colon Valle, artistic
dir.*

THE PYRAMID GROUP
THEATRE CO.
302 W. 91st St.
New York, NY 10024
(212) 877-5166
Nico Hartos, artistic dir.

QUAIGH THEATRE
205 W. 89th St.
New York, NY 10024
(212) 595-6185
Will Lieberson, artistic dir.

QUOTIDIAN
FOUNDATION
Suite 225
325 Spring St.
New York, NY 10013
(212) 243-6153
*Stuart Sherman, artistic
dir.;*
Vincent Renzi, bus. mgr.

RAPP THEATRE
COMPANY
220 E. 4th St.
New York, NY 10009
(212) 529-5921
*R. Jeffrey Cohen,
Alexis S. Cohen, artistic
dirs.*

THE REAL THEATRE
140 W. 69th St., #11-1B
New York, NY 10023
(212) 724-3764
(212) 994-0514
Jay Michaels, artistic dir.

REPERTORIO ESPANOL
Gramercy Arts Theater
138 E. 27th St.
New York, NY 10016
(212) 889-2850
*Rene Buch, artistic dir.;
Lilberto Zaldivar, exec.
prod'r.; Robert Weber
Federico, resident designer.*

THE RESTORATION
PROJECT THEATRE CO.
190 Washington Ave.
Brooklyn, NY 11205
(718) 624-0249
*Felix Van Dijk, artistic dir.
Rob Krakowski, managing
dir.*

THE RICHARD ALLEN
CENTER FOR CULTURE
AND ARTS (RACCA)
550 W. 155th St.
New York, NY 10032
(212) 281-2220
Shirley Radcliffe, prod'r.

RIDICULOUS
THEATRICAL COMPANY
1 Sheridan Square
New York, NY 10014
(212) 691-2271
Everett Quinton, artistic dir.

RIVERSIDE
SHAKESPEARE
COMPANY
West-Park Presbyterian
Church
165 W. 86th St.
New York, NY 10024
(212) 877-6810
Tim Oman, artistic dir.

RIVERWEST THEATRE
155 Bank Street
New York, NY 10014
(212) 243-0259
Nat Habib, artistic dir.

ROUNDABOUT THEATRE
COMPANY
100 E. 17th St.
New York, NY 10003
(212) 420-1360
*Todd Haimes, exec. dir.;
Gene Feist, artistic dir.*

ROYAL COURT
REPERTORY
300 W. 55th St.
New York, NY 10019
(212) 956-3500
Phillis Craig, artistic dir.

RYAN REPERTORY
COMPANY
2445 Bath Ave.
Brooklyn, NY 11214
(718) 373-5208
*Barbara Parisi, artistic dir.;
John Sannuto, acting artistic
dir.; Michelle Jacobs, mng.
dir.*

ST. BART'S PLAYHOUSE
109 E. 50th St.
New York, NY 10022
(212) 751-1616
*Christopher Catt, artistic
dir.*

SANDCASTLE PLAYERS,
INC.
PO Box 1596
Cathedral Station
New York, NY 10025
(212) 677-6200
Jeanne Kaplan, artistic dir.

THE SECOND STAGE
PO Box 1807
Ansonia Station
New York, NY 10023
(212) 787-8302
*Robyn Goodman, Carole
Rothman, artistic dir.;
Dorothy Maffei, mng. dir.*
Theater address: 2162
Broadway
New York, NY 10023

SECOND STORY
ENSEMBLE
PO Box 21020
Columbus Circle Station
New York, NY 10023
(212) 957-9712
Janis Powell, artistic dir.

THE SHALIKO COMPANY
151 2nd Ave., Suite 1-E
New York, NY 10003
(212) 475-6313
*Leonardo Shapiro, artistic
dir.*

SHELTER WEST
COMPANY
440 W. 42nd St.
New York, NY 10036-6805
(212) 673-6341
Judith Joseph, artistic dir.

ROGER SIMON STUDIO
105 Llewellyn Rd.
Montclair, NJ 07042
(212) JU6-6300 (service)
*Roger Hendricks Simon,
artistic dir.*
c/o Actors & Directors Lab,
412 W. 42nd St.
New York, NY 10036

SOHO REP
80 Varick St.
New York, NY 10013
(212) 925-2588
*Marlene Swartz, Jerry
Engelbach, artistic dirs.*

SOUPSTONE PROJECT,
INC.
309 E. 5th St., #19
New York, NY 10003
(212) 473-7584
Neile Weissman, artistic dir.

SOUTH STREET
THEATRE CO.
424 W. 42nd St.
New York, NY 10036
(212) 564-0660
*Jean Sullivan, Michael
Fischetti, artistic dirs.*

SPECTRUM THEATRE
1 E. 104th St., #9B
New York, NY 10029
(212) 475-5529
Benno Haehnel, artistic dir.

SPIDERWOMAN
THEATRE WORKSHOP,
INC.
77 7th Ave., #8S
New York, NY 10011
(212) 243-6209
Muriel Miguel, artistic dir.

SPUYTEN DUYVIL
16 W. 16th St., #11FN
New York, NY 10011
Collective artistic leadership.

STAGE LEFT, INC.
PO Box 3251
New York, NY 10185
(212) 989-4682
*Patricia Vanderbeck, artistic
dir.*

STARET . . . THE
DIRECTORS COMPANY,
INC.
311 W. 43rd St., Suite 1404
New York, NY 10036
(212) 246-5877
*Michael Parva, artistic/
producing dir.*

TRG REPERTORY
c/o Marvin Kahan
60 E. 8th St.
New York, NY 10003
(212) 757-6315
Marvin Kahan, artistic dir.

THALIA SPANISH
THEATRE
PO Box 4368
Sunnyside, NY 11104
(718) 729-3880
Sylvia Brito, artistic dir.

THEATRE FOR THE NEW
CITY
155-157 First Ave.
New York, NY 10003
(212) 254-1109
*George Bartenieff, Crystal
Field, artistic dirs.*

THEATRE IN ACTION
46 Walker St.
New York, NY 10013
(212) 431-1317
Lev Shekhtman, artistic dir.

THEATRE OFF PARK
224 Waverly Place
New York, NY 10014
(212) 627-2556
Albert Harris, artistic dir.

THEATRE 22
54 W. 22nd St.
New York, NY 10011
(212) 243-2805
Sidney Armus, Sidney Salters, prod'rs.

THEATREWORKS/USA
890 Broadway
New York, NY 10003
(212) 677-5959
Jay Harnick, artistic dir.

THECO
99 Chrystie St.
New York, NY 10002
(212) 219-2450
Roberts Johnson, David Michael Kronick, co-artistic dirs.

THIRD STEP THEATRE
COMPANY
1179 Broadway
New York, NY 10001
(212) 545-1372
Al D'Andrea, artistic dir.; Melody Brooks, mng. dir.; Margit Ahlin, literary mgr.

13TH STREET THEATRE
REPERTORY COMPANY
50 W. 13th St.
New York, NY 10011
(212) 675-6677
Edith O'Hara, Terry Brogan, artistic dirs.

TRIANGLE THEATRE
CO.
316 E. 88th St.
New York, NY 10128
(212) 860-7245
Michael Remak, Molly O'Neil, artistic dirs.

THE USUAL SUSPECTS
THEATRE CO.
2819 W. 12th St., #9P
Brooklyn, NY 11224
(718) 946-4891
Robert Liebowitz, dir.

VIETNAM VETERANS
ENSEMBLE THEATRE
COMPANY
c/o HBO
1100 Ave. of the Americas,
13th Fl.
New York, NY 10036
(212) 512-1960
Thomas Bird, artistic dir.

VILLAGE PLAYERS
103 Great Oaks Rd.
East Hill, NY 11577
(516) 621-0694
Gloria Poraino, artistic dir.

VILLAGE THEATRE
COMPANY
Shandol Theater
137 W. 22nd St.
New York, NY 10011
(212) 243-9504
Susan Farwell, Randy Kelly, Marjorie Feenan, David McConnell, and Howard Thoresen, artistic directorship

THE VINEYARD
THEATRE
309 E. 26th St.
New York, NY 10010
(212) 683-0696
Doug Aibel, artistic dir.

WPA THEATRE
519 W. 23rd St.
New York, NY 10011
(212) 206-0523
Kyle Renick, artistic dir.

WESTBANK CAFE
Downstairs Theater Bar
407 W. 42nd St.
New York, NY 10036
(212) 695-6909
Rowan Joseph, exec. dir.

WESTBETH THEATRE
CENTER
151 Bank St.
New York, NY 10014
(212) 691-2272
Arnold Engelman, prod. dir.

WESTSIDE COMMUNITY
REPERTORY THEATRE
252 W. 81st St.
New York, NY 10024
(212) 874-7290
Allen Schroeter, artistic dir.

THE WILLOW CABIN
THEATRE CO.
10 Manhattan Ave., #1E
New York, NY 10025
(212) 662-0077
Edward Berkeley, artistic dir.

WINGS THEATRE
COMPANY
521 City Island Ave.
Bronx, NY 10464
(212) 645-9630
Jeff Corrick, artistic dir.

WOMEN'S PROJECT AND
PRODUCTIONS, INC.
220 W. 42nd St., 18th Floor
New York, NY 10036
(212) 382-2750
Julia Miles, artistic dir.

THE WOOSTER GROUP
33 Wooster St.
New York, NY 10013
(212) 966-9796
Elizabeth Le Compte, artistic dir.

WORKING STAGES
316 W. 93rd St.
New York, NY 10025
(212) 866-5759
Terry Adrian, artistic dir.

THE WRITERS THEATRE
145 W. 46th St.
New York, NY 10036
(212) 869-9770
Linda Laundra, artistic dir.

VORTEX THEATRE
COMPANY
164 11th Ave.
New York, NY 10014
(212) 206-1764
Robert Coles, artistic dir.

YORK THEATRE
COMPANY
2 E. 90th St.
New York, NY 10028
(212) 534-5366
Janet Hayes Walker, artistic dir.

THE YUEH LUNG
SHADOW THEATRE
34-71 74th St.
Jackson Heights, NY 11372
(718) 478-6246
Jo Humphrey, artistic dir.

The following theaters may
be used to house showcase
productions by the various
companies listed above and
by other independent
producers.

ACTORS' OUTLET
THEATRE
120 W. 28th St.
New York, NY 10001
(212) 807-1590

JUDITH ANDERSON
THEATRE
422 W. 42nd St.
New York, NY 10036
(212) 736-7930

HAROLD CLURMAN
THEATRE
412 W. 42nd St.
New York, NY 10036
(212) 594-2828

18TH STREET
PLAYHOUSE
145 W. 18th St.
New York, NY 10011
(212) 243-8643

ERNIE MARTIN STUDIO
THEATRE
311 W. 43rd St.
New York, NY 10036
(212) 397-5880

SANFORD MEISNER
THEATRE
164 11th Ave.
New York, NY 10011
(212) 206-1764

PERRY STREET
THEATRE
31 Perry St.
New York, NY 10014
(212) 255-7190

Los Angeles-Area 99-Seat Theaters

The following is a listing of theaters in the Los Angeles area, all of which house 99 seats or less. These spaces have been approved by Actors' Equity Association as 99-Seat (formerly Equity Waiver) theaters. Members of Equity or its sister unions may only perform in these theaters under the Los Angeles 99-seat Theater Plan.

ACTORS ALLEY
4334 Van Nuys Blvd.
Sherman Oaks, CA 91403
(818) 986-7440
Jordan Charney
Seating: 65

ACTORS CENTER
THEATRES
11969 Ventura Blvd.
Studio City, CA 91604
(818) 505-9400

ACTORS FORUM
3365½ Cahuenga Blvd. West
Los Angeles, CA 90068
(213) 850-9016
Audrey Marlyn/
Shawn Michaels
Seating: 50

ANTA WEST
1406 No. Lake Ave.
Pasadena, CA 91106
(213) 465-5315
Michael Potter

ATLANTIC & PACIFIC
RENAISSANCE THEATRE
6724 Hollywood Blvd.
Los Angeles, CA 90028
(213) 465-1282
Manu Tupou
Seating: 70

ATTIC THEATRE
6562½ Santa Monica Blvd.
Los Angeles, CA 90038
(213) 469-2051
Bill Sorrells
Seating: 51

BACK ALLEY THEATRE
15231 Burbank Blvd.
Van Nuys, CA 91411
(818) 780-2240
Laura Zucker/Allan Miller
Seating: 65

RICHARD BASEHART
21028-B Victory Blvd.
Woodland Hills, CA 91367
(818) 703-9623
H.M. Wynant

BEVERLY HILLS
PLAYHOUSE
254 So. Robertson Blvd.
Beverly Hills, CA 90211
(213) 652-6483
Eric Leonard
Seating: 99

BFA'S LITTLE THEATRE
(Bilingual Foundation of
the Arts)
421 No. Avenue 19
Los Angeles, CA 90031
(213) 225-4044
Margarita Galban
Seating: 78

BROADWAY PLAYHOUSE
550 W. Broadway
San Gabriel, CA 91776
(818) 282-5462
Fred Vaugeois

BURBAGE THEATRE
2330 Sawtelle Blvd.
Los Angeles, CA 90064
(213) 478-0898
Ivan Spiegel
Seating: 99/45

BURBANK LITTLE
THEATRE
1100 W. Clark Ave.
Burbank, CA 91510
(818) 848-7791

CALIFORNIA COTTAGE
THEATRE
5220 Sylmar Ave.
Van Nuys, CA 91401
(818) 990-5773

CALLBOARD THEATRE
8451 Melrose Place
Los Angeles, CA 90069
(213) 852-9205
Seating: 99

CAMINITO THEATRE
(Los Angeles City College)
855 No. Vermont Ave.
Los Angeles, CA 90029
(213) 669-4336/669-5528
Norman Mennes/
Cliff O'Connell
Seating: 99

CARPET COMPANY
STAGE
5262 W. Pico Blvd.
Los Angeles, CA 90019
(213) 932-9321
Sidney Friedman
Seating: 40

C.A.R.T. THEATRE
(California Artists Repertory
Theater)
10701 Magnolia Blvd.
No. Hollywood, CA 90601
Mail: 6612 Whitley Terrace
Los Angeles, CA 90068
(818) 760-9212
Peggy Webber McClory/
Sean McClory
Seating: 99

CASSANDRA GAYLOR
THEATRE
6543 Santa Monica Blvd.
Los Angeles, CA 90038
(213) 462-7644
Mark Madison
Seating: 25

CAST THEATRE
804 No. El Centro Ave.
Los Angeles, CA 90038
(213) 462-0265/462-9872
Ted Schmitt
Seating: 65

CAST-AT-THE-CIRCLE
800 No. El Centro Ave.
Los Angeles, CA 90038
(213) 462-0265/462-9872
Cast Theatre
Seating: 99

CELEBRATION THEATRE
426 No. Hoover
Los Angeles, CA
Mail; 1765 No. Highland
    Ave., #536
Hollywood, CA 90078
(213) 876-4257
Chuck Rowland
Seating: 40

CELEBRITY CENTRE
THEATRE
5930 Franklin Ave.
Los Angeles, CA 90028
(213) 464-0411
Seating: 64

CENTURY CITY
PLAYHOUSE
(Burbage Theatre Ensemble)
10508 W. Pico Blvd.
Los Angeles, CA 90064
(213) 478-0898
Ivan Spiegel
Seating: 95

CHAMBER THEATRE
3759 Cahuenga Blvd., West
No. Hollywood, CA 91604
(818) 760-9708
John Milford

CHURCH IN
OCEAN PARK
235 Hill Street
Santa Monica, CA 90405
(213) 399-1631

CITY HALL THEATRE
(Manhattan Pier Players)
1400 Highland Ave.
Manhattan Beach, CA 90266
(213) 545-5621/545-9192
Pat Gray Carroll
Seating: 94

CITY STAGE
464 E. Fourth St.
Los Angeles, CA 90013
(213) 489-3269

COAST THEATRE
8325 Santa Monica Blvd.
Los Angeles, CA 90069
(213) 654-8781/654-8780
Seating: 99

COMMONWEALTH
THEATRE
(1st Cong. Ch. of L.A.)
540 S. Commonwealth
Los Angeles, CA 90020
(213) 385-1241
Eleanor Logan
Seating: 99

COMPANY OF ANGELS
Mail: P.O. Box 3480
Los Angeles, CA 90038
(213) 464-9674
Seating: 50

CORONET STUDIO 3
368 No. La Cienega Blvd.
Los Angeles, CA 90048
(213) 652-4241
Frieda Gellis

COURT THEATRE
722 No. LaCienega Blvd.
West Hollywood, CA 90069
(213) 465-0070

COURTYARD THEATRE
550 Deep Valley Dr.
Rolling Hills Estates, CA
    90274
Rochelle K. Abrams

DEJA VU COFFEEHOUSE
1705 No. Kenmore Ave.
Los Angeles, CA 90027
(213) 666-0434
J.F. Smith
Seating: 40

ROLAND DUPREE'S
STUDIO THEATRE
8115 West 3rd St.
Los Angeles, CA 90048
(213) 655-1276/655-6895
Roland Dupree
Seating: 99

GENE DYNARSKI
THEATRE
5600 West Sunset Blvd.
Los Angeles, CA 90028
(213) 465-5600
Gene Dynarski
Seating: 99

EAGLE THEATRE
182 No. Robertson
Beverly Hills, CA 90211
(818) 249-2926
Gene Wallace

EAST WEST PLAYERS
4424 Santa Monica Blvd.
Los Angeles, CA 90029
(213) 660-0366
Mako/Janet Mitsui
Seating: 99

EN SCENE THEATRE
11305 Magnolia Blvd.
No. Hollywood, CA 91601
(818) 762-2276

FIFTH ESTATE THEATRE
1707 Kenmore Ave.
Los Angeles, CA 90027
(213) 666-0434
J.K. Smith
Seating: 40

FIG TREE THEATRE
6539 Santa Monica Blvd.
Los Angeles, CA 90038
(213) 463-6893
Peter Flynn
Seating: 50/60

THE FOUND THEATRE
1154 East 7th St.
Long Beach, CA 90813
Cynthia Galles

FOUNTAIN THEATRE
5060 Fountain Ave.
Los Angeles, CA 90029
(213) 663-1525
*Jerry & Penny Krompier
Holland*
Seating: 85

MAIN STAGE THEATRE
2135 Riverside Dr.
No. Hollywood, CA 91607
(818) 508-0786
J. Bratchell
Seating: 97

MARILYN MONROE
THEATRE
(Lee Strasberg Institute)
936 Santa Monica Blvd.
(213) 461-4333
Terri Kenneally
Seating: 99

MATRIX THEATRE
(Actors for Themselves)
657 Melrose Ave.
Los Angeles, CA 90046
(213) 653-3279
Joe Stern
Seating: 99

McCADDEN PLACE
THEATRE
1157 No. McCadden Place
Los Angeles, CA 90038
(213) 462-9070
Zy Donohue/Joy O'Neil
Seating: 49

MELROSE THEATRE
733 No. Seward St.
Los Angeles, CA 90038
(213) 465-1885
Paul Kent
Seating: 80

NEW PLAYWRIGHTS
FOUNDATION
5111 W. Olympic Blvd.
Los Angeles, CA 90048
(213) 935-4874
Jeff Bergquist

NOSOTROS
1314 No. Wilton Pl.
Los Angeles, CA 90028
(213) 465-4167
Loyda Ramos
Seating: 60

ODYSSEY THEATRE
ENSEMBLE
12111 Ohio Ave.
Los Angeles, CA 90025
(213) 826-1626
Ron Sossi
Seating: 1–99/2–95/3–82

OFF HOLLYWOOD
SHOWCASE THEATRE
11373 Ventura Blvd.
Studio City, CA 91604
(818) 760-9006 or
(213) 656-9385
Steve Oakley
Seating: 49

THE OFF-MAIN STREET
THEATRE
208 Pier Ave.
Santa Monica, CA 90405
(213) 396-8410

OFF RAMP THEATRE
1953 No. Cahuenga
Los Angeles, CA 90068
Mail: 6395 Ivarene Ave.
Los Angeles, CA 90068
(213) 469-4343/465-8059
Ken Rose

OLIO
3709 Sunset Blvd.
Los Angeles, CA 90026
(213) 667-9556/664-5909
Karen Desmond
Seating: 99

ON STAGE THEATRE
139 No. Golden Mall
Burbank, CA 91502
(818) 842-1072
Dean Brooks/Josh Taylor
Seating: 99

OPEN DOOR THEATRE
122 So. Golden Mall
Burbank, CA 91502
(818) 842-1051
Kenneth Mitchell

PACIFIC THEATRE
ENSEMBLE
705½ Venice Blvd.
Venice, CA 90291
(213) 306-3943

PLAYBOX THEATRE
1953 Cahuenga Blvd.
Hollywood, CA 90068
(213) 469-9434
Kenneth Rose

POWERHOUSE THEATRE
3116 Second St.
Santa Monica, CA 90405
(213) 306-1219
Paul Linke
Seating: 60

RICHMOND SHEPARD
THEATRE STUDIOS
(& Theatre III)
6468/74/78 Santa Monica
Blvd.
Los Angeles, CA 90038
(213) 462-9399
Richmond Shepard
Seating: 49/49/49

ROSE THEATRE
318 Lincoln Blvd.
Venice, CA 90291
(213) 392-4911
Tom Provenzano

RUTH ST. DENIS STUDIO
THEATRE
3433 Cahuenga Blvd. West
Los Angeles, CA 90068
(213) 850-9497
Valentine Oumansky
Seating: 99

SANTA MONICA
PLAYHOUSE
1211 4th St.
Santa Monica, CA 90401
(213) 394-9779
Evelyn Rudie/
Chris DeCarlo
Seating: 88

2nd STAGE THEATRE
6500 Santa Monica Blvd.
Los Angeles, CA 90038
Mail: % Lewis & Priven
14541 Hamin St.
Van Nuys, CA 91411
(213) 465-6029
Paul Fagen
Seating: 48

THE "SHOW" PLACE
THEATRE
12655 Ventura Blvd.
Studio City, CA 91604
(818) 766-5500
Mary Lansing
Seating: 50

SKYLIGHT THEATRE
(Beverly Hills Playhouse)
1816½ No. Vermont Ave.
Los Angeles, CA 90027
(213) 666-2202/652-6483
Milton Katselas
Seating: 96

FOUNTAIN THEATRE
ANNEX
(See Fountain Theatre,
above)
Seating: 35

FRIENDS & ARTISTS
THEATRE ENSEMBLE
1761 No. Vermont
Los Angeles, CA 90027
(213) 664-0680
Michael Nehring

GALAXY STAGE
5421 Santa Monica Blvd.
Hollywood, CA 90028
Mail: 1341 No. Mariposa
Ave.
Los Angeles, CA 90027
(213) 462-9616/469-6605
Alexander Lehr
Seating: 49

GARDNER STAGE
1501 No. Gardner
Los Angeles, CA 90046
(213) 475-3369
Seating: 99

JOHN GARFIELD
THEATRE
(Lee Strasberg Institute)
7936 Santa Monica Blvd.
Los Angeles, CA 90046
(213) 650-7777
*Connie Belna/
Jerry Kenneally*
Seating: 99

GLOBE PLAYHOUSE
(Shakespeare Society of
America)
1107 No. King Rd.
Los Angeles, CA 90069
(213) 654-5623
R. Thad Taylor
Seating: 99

GNU THEATRE
10426 Magnolia Blvd.
Toluca Lake, CA 91601
(818) 508-5344
Jeff Seymour
Seating: 48

G.P.B. STUDIO OF
ACTING
14515 Ventura Blvd.
Sherman Oaks, CA 91403
(818) 905-7336

GROUNDLINGS THEATRE
7307 Melrose Ave.
Los Angeles, CA 90046
(213) 934-9700/934-4747
Tom Maxwell
Seating: 99

GROUP REPERTORY
THEATRE
10900 Burbank Blvd.
No. Hollywood, CA 91601
(818) 760-9368
Lonny Chapman

GYPSY PLAYHOUSE
(Professional Dancers Studio)
3321 West Olive
Burbank, CA 91505
(818) 954-8458
Sylvia Lewis

HARMON THEATRE/
HARMON ALLEY
THEATRE
522 No. La Brea
Los Angeles, CA 90036
(213) 931-8130
Seating: 99

HELIOTROPE THEATRE
660 S. Heliotrope Dr.
Los Angeles, CA 90004
(213) 660-4247
Robert J. Linden

HIDDEN HILLS
PLAYHOUSE
2459 Long Valley Rd.
Hidden Hills, CA 91302
(818) 716-6600

INGLEWOOD
PLAYHOUSE
400 West Beach Ave.
Inglewood, CA 90302
(213) 412-5451/412-5508
Cepheus Jaxon
Seating: 57

INTERNATIONAL CITY
THEATRE
4901 E. Carson
Long Beach, CA 90808
(213) 420-4275

JIMSON THEATRE
1049 Havenhurst
West Hollywood, CA 90046
(213) 650-6649
Jim Prejean

THE JUDAIC T
8906 W. Pico Bl
Los Angeles, CA
(213) 272-7223

L.A. CONNECT
COMEDY REPE
THEATRE
13442 Ventura Bl
Sherman Oaks, (
(818) 784-1868/7
Kent Skov
Seating: 49/60

THE LEX
6760 Lexington A
Hollywood, CA 9
(213) 464-9151
Elaine Ellison

LITTLE VICTOI
THEATRE
3324 Victory Blv
Burbank, CA 915
(818) 843-9253/84
Seating: 48

THE LIVING RO
(The Unitarian C
3744 Barrington
Los Angeles, CA
Mail: 13953 Panay
Marina del Rey, C
(213) 821-2009
Jack Strand
Seating: 55

LOFT STUDIO T
ON LA BREA
130 So. La Brea
Los Angeles, CA
(213) 933-9888
William Traylor/Pe
Seating: 70

LOS ANGELES II
CITY CULTURAL
CENTER
1308 S. New Ham
Ave.
Los Angeles, CA 9
(213) 387-1161
C. Bernard Jackso
Seating: 99/75/40

MAIN FLOOR TH
1219 No. Vermont
Los Angeles, CA 9
(213) 669-9047/656
Max Rubinchik
Seating: 99

STAGE/LEE STRASBERG
(Lee Strasberg Institute)
7936 Santa Monica Blvd.
Los Angeles, CA 90046
(213) 461-5333
Jerry Kenneally
Seating: 49

STAGES THEATRE
CENTER
1540 No. McCadden Pl.
Los Angeles, CA 90028
(213) 465-1010/463-5356
Paul Verdier
Seating: 99/49

STARDUST STUDIOS
6419 Hollywood Blvd.
Los Angeles, CA 90028
(213) 465-5224
James Albright
Seating: 49

STUDIO JACK KOSSLYN
666 No. Robertson Blvd.
West Hollywood, CA 90069
(213) 855-9242
Jack Kosslyn
Seating: 45

STUDIO STRAS
(Lee Strasberg Institute)
7936 Santa Monica Blvd.
Los Angeles, CA 90046
(213) 461-4333
Jerry Kenneally
Seating: 49

STUDIO THEATRE
(Long Beach
   Community Players)
5021 E. Anaheim St.
Long Beach, CA 90804
(213) 494-1616/494-1014
*Elaine Herman/
Jerry Halbert*
Seating: 98

STUDIO THEATRE
PLAYHOUSE
(The Colony)
1944 Riverside Dr.
Los Angeles, CA 90039
(213) 665-3011/667-9851
Barbara Beckley
Seating: 99

TEATRO JORGE
NEGRETE
3665 Whittier Blvd.
Los Angeles, CA 90022
(213) 268-6401

THEATRE EAST
12655 Ventura Blvd.
Studio City, CA 91604
(818) 760-4160
Seating: 90

THEATRE EXCHANGE
11855 Hart St.
North Hollywood, CA 91605
(818) 765-9005
Rob Zapple/Matthew Faison
Seating: 50

THEATRE 40
241 Moreno Dr.
Beverly Hills, CA 90212
Mailing: P.O. Box 5401
Beverly Hills, CA 90210
(213) 277-4221
Seating: 99

THEATRE OF ARTS
4128 Wilshire Blvd.
Los Angeles, CA 90010
(213) 380-0511
Valmar Oleska
Seating: 90

THEATRE RAPPORT
(Hollywood Theatre Club)
1277 No. Wilton Pl.
Los Angeles, CA 90038
Crane Jackson

THEATRE/THEATRE
HOLLYWOOD
1713 No. Cahuenga Blvd.
Los Angeles, CA 90028
(213) 871-0210/850-6941
Jeff Murray
Seating: 85

THEATRE III
607 S. Park View St.,
   4th fl.
Los Angeles, CA 90057
(213) 383-9888
G.P. Hansen

THIRD STAGE
2811 W. Magnolia Blvd.
Burbank, CA 91505
(818) 842-4755
Seating: 50

TIFFANY THEATRES 1&2
8532 Sunset Blvd.
West Hollywood, CA 90069
(213) 854-3684
Paula Holt
Seating: 99/99

TRACY ROBERTS
THEATRE
141 So. Robertson Blvd.
West Hollywood, CA 90048
(213) 271-2730
Tracy Roberts/Allen Nelson

21st STREET THEATRE
(21st Street Theatre Co.)
11350 Palms Blvd.
Los Angeles, CA 90066
(213) 827-5655
Seating: 50

VENTURE THEATRE
Burbank, CA 91505
(818) 846-5323
Richard Fulvio
Seating: 60

VICTORY THEATRE
(Also see: Little
Victory Theatre)
3326 West Victory Blvd.
Burbank, CA 91505
(818) 843-9253/841-4404
Maria Gobetti/Tom Ormeny
Seating: 82

WEST COAST
ENSEMBLE
6240 Hollywood Blvd.
Hollywood, CA 90028
(213) 871-1052/871-8673

WEST END PLAYHOUSE
7446 Van Nuys Blvd.
Van Nuys, CA 91405
Michael Bell
Seating: 84

WHITEFIRE STAGE
13500 Ventura Blvd.
Sherman Oaks, CA 91423
(818) 990-2324
Lee Crook/David Beaird
Seating: 99

ZEPHER THEATRE
7456 Melrose Ave.
Los Angeles, CA 90046
(213) 653-4667
Lee Sankowich
Seating: 99

Resident Theaters

by Victor Gluck

If any theatrical group can lay claim to the title of national theater in America, then it must surely be the 200 nonprofit theater companies spread across the United States. Started in 1963, the resident theater movement began with the founding of the Tyrone Guthrie Theater in Minneapolis. As a result of the success of the Guthrie, other cities began taking steps to build their own resident theater companies. These companies eventually coalesced into the League of Resident Theaters (LORT), all members of which now have a working agreement with Actors' Equity Association. LORT companies provide work and opportunity to performers, directors, and playwrights and bring the experience of live theater to audiences in almost every state in the union.

LORT companies each have a unique house style and artistic policy. Heavily supported by subscribers, LORT companies are able to take risks that commercially backed theater ventures dare not attempt. LORT companies may, therefore, run a variety of productions during a typical season, drawing on chestnuts from the repertoire, experimenting with the avant-garde, or presenting works-in-progress. Performers, directors, and playwrights are given not only a chance to hone their crafts while under salary, but they are also offered exciting roles and challenges that they would not ordinarily encounter. Casting directors are well aware of the diversified experience that performers gain in resident theater and take special note when they see a LORT company listed on a resume.

Many in the industry see in resident theater the chance to develop and grow with an ensemble. Not only do members of a LORT company work at developing their crafts, but they work side by side with some of the greatest talents in the industry, including stars, and are engaged in a collaboration that leads to invaluable networking and the possibility of future work. Some resident theater productions may tour statewide, nationally, or may even end up on Broadway. This can mean important exposure, and in some instances, can even lead to stardom.

Some major playwrights prefer to work away from the spotlight of New York City, and many innovative directors feel that they are given more freedom to experiment in the less commercially pressured atmosphere of resident theater. Home to such playwrights and directors are such prestigious and trendsetting LORT companies as the Arena Stage in Washington, D.C., the Mark Taper Forum in Los Angeles, the Long Wharf Theater in New Haven, the Goodman Theater in Chicago, the Actors Theater in Louisville, the Magic Theater in San Francisco, and of course, the Tyrone Guthrie Theater in Minneapolis.

In recent years, LORT productions have brightened Broadway and Off-Broadway stages with such comedy and dramatic hits as *Children of a Lesser God, Agnes of God, Getting Out, The Foreigner, How I Got That Story, Crimes of the Heart, True West, Fool for Love, Sexual Perversity in Chicago,* and *American Buffalo.* Further attesting to the quality of LORT presentations are the Pulitzer Prize winners. Since 1977, the following LORT productions have been granted Pulitzer awards: *The Shadow Box, The Gin Game, Buried Child, Crimes of the Heart, 'night Mother, Glengarry Glen Ross,* and *Fences.*

Resident Theaters

The following is an up-to-date list of theaters operating under Equity's League of Resident Theaters (LORT) contract. They are listed alphabetically according to state and then by city within each state and then by theater within each city. The letter that follows the name of each theater (A, B, B+, C or D) indicates the category in which that theater operates. These categories are based on the certified actual weekly box office gross of each theater. The breakdown is as follows: D = $15,999.99 and below; C = $16,000–$29,999.99; B = $30,000–$49,999.99; B+ = $50,000 and above. There are no box office gross figures for A theaters. The names under the listings are those of the artistic director and/or managing director.

ALABAMA

ALABAMA
SHAKESPEARE
FESTIVAL (B/C) (D)
P.O. Box 20350
Montgomery, AL
36120-0350
(205) 272-1640
Martin Platt,
James Volz

ARIZONA

ARIZONA THEATER
COMPANY (C)
56 W. Congress
P.O. Box 1631
Tucson, AZ 85702
(602) 884-8210
Gary Gisselman,
Susan Goldberg

CALIFORNIA

BERKELEY REP.
THEATER (C)
2025 Addison St.
Berkeley, CA 94704
(415) 841-6108
Mitzi Sales,
Sharon Ott

BERKELEY
SHAKESPEARE
FESTIVAL (D)
Box 969
Berkeley, CA 94701
(415) 548-3422
Michael Addison,
Susan Duncan

SOUTH COAST REP.
THEATER (B) (D)
Box 2197
Costa Mesa, CA 92626
(714) 957-2602
David Emmes,
Paula Tomei

LA JOLLA PLAYHOUSE
(B/C) (D)
P.O. Box 12039
La Jolla, CA 92037
(619) 452-6760
Des McAnuff,
Alan Levey

L.A. THEATER CENTER
(D)
514 S. Spring St.
Los Angeles, CA 90013
(213) 627-6500
William Bushnell,
Don Hill

MARK TAPER FORUM
LOS ANGELES MUSIC
CENTER (A)
135 North Grand Ave.
Los Angeles, CA 90012
(213) 972-7384
Gordon Davidson,
Steve Albert

CALIFORNIA MUSICAL
THEATRE (B)
30 N. Raymond Ave.
Suite 608
Pasadena, CA 91103
(818) 792-0776
Gary Davis

PASADENA PLAYHOUSE
(B)
39 S. El Molino
Pasadena, CA 91101
(818) 792-8672
Susan Dietz,
Lars Hansen

OLD GLOBE THEATRE
(B) (B+) (C)
P.O. Box 2171
San Diego, CA 92112
(619) 231-1941
Jack O'Brien,
Thomas Hall

AMERICAN
CONSERVATORY
THEATRE (A)
450 Geary St.
San Francisco, CA 94102
(415) 771-3880
Edward Hastings,
Diane Prichard

SAN JOSE REPERTORY
CO. (C)
Box 2399
San Jose, CA 95109-2399
(408) 294-7572
Timothy Near,
Shannon Levak-Leskin

SANTA BARBARA
THEATRE FESTIVAL (B)
33 E. Canon Perdido St.
Santa Barbara, CA 93101
(805) 963-0761
Paul Blake,
Esther Newitt

COLORADO

DENVER CENTER
THEATRE CO. (C) (D)
1050 13th St.
Denver, CO 80204
(303) 893-4200
Donovan Marley,
Sarah Lawless

CONNECTICUT

GOODSPEED OPERA
HOUSE (B+) (D)
East Haddam, CT 06423
(203) 873-8664
Michael Price,
Sue Frost

HARTFORD STAGE CO.
(B)
50 Church St.
Hartford, CT 06103
(203) 525-5601
Mark Lamos,
David Hawkanson

LONG WHARF THEATRE
(B) (C)
222 Sargent Drive
New Haven, CT 06511
(203) 787-4284
Arvin Brown,
M. Edgar Rosenblum

YALE REPERTORY
THEATRE (C) (D)
Yale School of Drama
222 York St.
New Haven, CT 06520
(203) 432-1515
Lloyd Richards,
Benjamin Mordecai

EUGENE O'NEILL
MEMORIAL THEATRE
CTR. (C)
National Playwrights Conf.
305 Great Neck Road
Waterford, CT 06385
(203) 443-5378
Lloyd Richards

DISTRICT OF COLUMBIA

ARENA STAGE (B) (B+)
(D)
6th & Maine Ave., SW
Washington, DC 20024
(202) 554-9066
Zelda Fichandler,
William Stewart

FOLGER THEATRE
GROUP (C)
201 E. Capitol St., SE
Washington, DC 20003
(202) 547-3230
Michael Kahn,
Mary Ann Di Barbieri

FLORIDA

CALDWELL THEATRE
CO. (C)
P.O. Box 277
Boca Raton, FL 33432
(305) 368-7509
Michael Hall

THE HIPPODROME
STATE THEATRE (D)
25 Southeast 2nd Pl.
Gainesville, FL 32601
(904) 373-5968
Mary Hausch,
David Black

COCONUT GROVE
PLAYHOUSE (B) (D)
P.O. Box 616
Miami, FL 33133
(305) 442-2662
Arnold Mittelman,
Jordan Bock

ASOLO THEATRE
FESTIVAL (C)
P.O. Box Drawer E
Sarasota, FL 33578
(813) 355-7115
John Ulmer,
Donna Gerdes

GEORGIA

ALLIANCE THEATRE CO.
(B) (D)
1280 Peachtree St., N.E.
Atlanta, GA 30309
(404) 898-1119
Robert Farley,
Edith Love

ILLINOIS

GOODMAN THEATRE
CO. (B+/B) (D)
200 S. Columbus Dr.
Chicago, IL 60603
(312) 443-3811
Robert Falls,
Roche Schulfer

THE NORTH LIGHT REP
THEATRE, INC. (D)
2300 Green Bay Rd.
Evanston, IL 60201
(312) 869-7732
Russell Vandenbroucke,
Susan Medak

INDIANA

INDIANA REP. THEATRE
(B) (D)
140 W. Washington St.
Indianapolis, IN 46204
(317) 635-5266
Tom Haas,
Victoria Nolan

KENTUCKY

ACTORS THEATRE OF
LOUISVILLE (B) (D)
316-320 W. Main St.
Louisville, KY 40202
(502) 584-1265
Jon Jory,
Alexander Speer

MAINE

PORTLAND STAGE CO.
(D)
P.O. Box 1458
Portland, ME 04104
(207) 774-1043
Barbara Rosoff,
Mark Somers

MARYLAND

CENTER STAGE
700 North Calvert St.
Baltimore, MD 21202
(301) 685-3200
*Stan Wojewodski,
Peter Culman*

MASSACHUSETTS

**HUNTINGTON THEATRE
CO. (B)**
Boston University Theater
264 Huntington Ave.
Boston MA 02115
(617) 353-3320
*Peter Altman,
Michael Maso*

**SHAKESPEARE &
COMPANY BOSTON
SHAKESPEARE (D)**
52 Saint Botolph St.
Boston, MA 02116
(617) 267-5630
*Tina Packer,
Dennis Krusnick*

**AMERICAN REP
THEATRE CO. (B) (D)**
Loeb Drama Center
64 Brattle St.
Cambridge, MA 02138
(617) 495-2668
*Robert Brustein,
Robert Orchard*

**SHAKESPEARE &
COMPANY THE MOUNT
(C)**
Lenox, MA 01240
(413) 637-1197
*Tina Packer,
Dennis Krusnick*

**MERRIMACK REGIONAL
THEATRE (D)**
P.O. Box 228
Lowell, MA 01853
(508) 454-6324
Daniel Schay

STAGEWEST (C) (D)
Springfield Theatre Arts
Assoc.
1 Columbus Center
Springfield, MA 01103
(413) 781-4470
*Gregory Boyd,
Val Pori*

**BERKSHIRE THEATRE
FESTIVAL (B)**
Main Street
Stockbridge, MA 01262
(413) 298-5536
*Richard Dunlop,
Carol Dougherty*

MICHIGAN

**MEADOW BROOK
THEATRE (B)**
Oakland University
Rochester, MI 48063
(313) 377-3300
*Terence Kilburn,
James Spittle*

MINNESOTA

**THE GUTHRIE THEATRE
(A)**
725 Vineland Pl.
Minneapolis, MN 55403
(612) 347-1100
*Garland Wright,
Edward Martinson*

**ACTORS THEATRE OF
ST. PAUL (D)**
28 W. 7 Pl.
Saint Paul, MN 55102
(612) 297-6868
*Michael Andrew Miner,
Martha Richards*

MISSOURI

**MISSOURI REP
THEATRE (B)**
Univ. of MO at Kansas City
5100 Rockhill Rd.
Kansas City, MO 64110
(816) 363-4300
*George Keathley,
Robert Thatch*

**THE REP THEATRE OF
ST. LOUIS (B) (D)**
130 Edgar Rd.
Saint Louis, MO 63119
(314) 968-7342
*Mark Bernstein,
Steven Woolf*

NEW HAMPSHIRE

**AMERICAN STAGE
FESTIVAL (C)**
P.O. Box 225
Milford, NH 03005
(603) 673-4005
*Larry Carpenter,
Richard Rose*

NEW JERSEY

**NJ SHAKESPEARE
FESTIVAL (D)**
Science Hall
Drew University, Route 24
Madison, NJ 07940
(201) 377-5330
*Paul Barry,
Richard Yarnell*

**THE WHOLE THEATRE
CO. (D)**
544 Bloomfield Avenue
Montclair, NJ 07042
(201) 744-2996
*Olympia Dukakis,
Scott Clugstone*

**GEORGE ST.
PLAYHOUSE (D)**
9 Livingston Ave.
New Brunswick, NJ 08901
(201) 846-2895
*Gregory Hurst,
Michael Gennaro*

**McCARTER THEATRE
CO., INC. (B+)**
Princeton University
91 University Place
Princeton, NJ 08540
(609) 683-9100
*Nagle Jackson,
John Herochik*

NEW MEXICO

NEW MEXICO
REPERTORY THEATRE
(D)
P.O. Box 789
Albuquerque, NM 87103
(505) 243-4577
Andrew Shea,
John Beauchamps

NEW YORK

CAPITAL REPERTORY
CO. (D)
P.O. Box 399
Albany, NY 12201-0399
(518) 462-4531
Peter Clough,
Bruce Bouchard

STUDIO ARENA
THEATRE (B)
710 Maine St.
Buffalo, NY 14202
(716) 856-8025
David Frank,
Raymond Bonnard

ACTING COMPANY (C)
Touring (B)
420 W. 42nd St., 3rd fl.
New York, NY 10036
(212) 564-3510
Margot Harley,
Mary Beth Carroll

CIRCLE IN THE SQUARE
(A)
1633 Broadway
New York, NY 10019
(212) 307-2700
Theodore Mann,
Paul Libin

LINCOLN CENTER
THEATRE CO. (A) (B)
165 W. 65th St.
New York, NY 10023
(212) 362-7600
Gregory Mosher,
Steve Callahan

NEGRO ENSEMBLE
COMPANY (D)
165 W. 46th St.
New York, NY 10036
(212) 575-5860
Douglas Turner Ward,
Leon Denmark

NY SHAKESPEARE
FESTIVAL (B)
The Public Theater
425 Lafayette St.
New York, NY 10003
(212) 598-7100
Joseph Papp,
Bob MacDonald

ROUNDABOUT THEATRE
CO. (B) (D)
100 E. 17th St.
New York, NY 10003
(212) 420-1360
Gene Feist,
Todd Haimes

GEVA THEATRE (C)
75 Woodbury Blvd.
Rochester, NY 14605
(716) 232-1366
Howard Millman,
Thomas Pechar

LONG ISLAND STAGE (D)
Box 9001
Rockville Centre, NY 11571
(516) 546-4600
Clint Atkinson

SYRACUSE STAGE (C)
John D. Archbold Theater
820 East Genesee St.
Syracuse, NY 13210
(315) 423-4008
Arthur Storch,
James A. Clark

NORTH CAROLINA

CHARLOTTE
REPERTORY THEATRE
(D)
Spirit Square
110 E. 7th St.
Charlotte, NC 28202
(704) 375-4796
Mark Woods,
Keith Stevens

PLAYMAKERS
REPERTORY CO. (D)
206 Graham Memorial 052A
Chapel Hill, NC 27514
(919) 962-1122
Margaret Hahn,
David Hammond

NORTH CAROLINA
SHAKESPEARE
FESTIVAL (D)
P.O. Box 6066
High Point, NC 27262
(919) 841-6273
Lou Rackoff,
Pedro Silva

OHIO

CINCINNATI PLAYHOUSE
IN THE PARK (B) (D)
P.O. Box 6537
Cincinnati, OH 45206
(513) 421-5440
Worth Gardner,
Kathleen Panoff

CLEVELAND PLAY
HOUSE (C) (D)
Box 1989
Cleveland, OH 44106
(216) 795-7010
Josephine Abady,
Dean Gladden

GREAT LAKES THEATER
FESTIVAL (B)
1501 Euclid Ave., Suite 250
Cleveland, OH 44115
(216) 241-5490
Gerald Freedman,
Mary Bill

PENNSYLVANIA

PENNSYLVANIA STAGE
CO. (C)
J. I. Rodale Theater
837 Linden St.
Allentown, PA 18101
(215) 434-6110
Peter Wrenn-Meleck,
Rosalie Schreiber

GRETNA PRODUCTIONS,
INC. (D)
P.O. Box 578
Mt. Gretna, PA 17064
(717) 964-3627
Paul Giovanni,
Trish Rasmus

PEOPLE'S LIGHT &
THEATRE CO. (D)
39 Conestoga Rd.
Malvern, PA 19355
(215) 647-1900
Danny Fruchter,
Gregory T. Rowe

PHILADELPHIA
FESTIVAL THEATRE
FOR NEW PLAYS (D)
3900 Chestnut St.
Philadelphia, PA 10104-3105
(212) 222-5000
Carol Rocamora,
Grace Grillet

PHILADELPHIA DRAMA
GUILD (B +)
112 St. 16th St., Suite 802
Philadelphia, PA 19102
(215) 563-7530
Gregory Poggi,
Kathleen Nolan

WALNUT STREET
THEATRE (A) (D)
9th & Walnut Sts.
Philadelphia, PA 19107
(215) 574-3550
Bernard Havard,
Lynn Fitzpatrick

PITTSBURGH PUBLIC
THEATRE (C)
Allegheny Sq.
Pittsburgh, PA 15212-5362
(412) 323-8200
William Gardner,
Dan Fallon

RHODE ISLAND
TRINITY SQ.
REPERTORY CO. (C) (B)
201 Washington St.
Providence, RI 02903
(401) 521-1100
Adrian Hall,
E. Timothy Langan

TENNESSEE
CLARENCE BROWN
THEATRE (D)
P.O. Box 8450
Knoxville, TN 37996
(615) 974-3447
Thomas P. Cooke,
Kevin Coleman

TENNESSEE REP. (D)
427 Chestnut St.
Nashville, TN 37203
(615) 244-4878
Mac Pirkle,
Brian Laczko

TEXAS
PARAMOUNT THEATRE
(A)
P.O. Box 1205
Austin, TX 78767
(512) 474-2901
Linda Hansen

DALLAS THEATRE
CENTER (C) (C) (D)
3636 Turtle Creek Blvd.
Dallas, TX 75219
(214) 526-5671
Adrian Hall,
Peter Donnelly

PLAZA THEATRE (C)
2914 Greenville Ave.
Dallas, TX 75206
(214) 823-3670
Lou Moore

THEATRE THREE (D)
2800 Routh St.
Dallas, TX 75201
(214) 651-7225
Jac Alder,
Peggy Kincade

ALLEY THEATRE (B) (C)
615 Texas Ave.
Houston, TX 77002
(713) 228-9341
Jim Bernhard,
Chris Kawolsky

UTAH
PIONEER MEMORIAL
THEATRE (B)
University of Utah
Salt Lake City, UT 84112
(810) 581-6206
Charles Morey

VIRGINIA
BARTER THEATRE (D)
Box 867
Abingdon, VA 24210
(703) 628-2281
Rex Partington

VIRGINIA STAGE
COMPANY (D)
P.O. Box 3770
254 Granby St.
Norfolk, VA 23514
(804) 627-6988
Charles Towers,
Dan Martin

THEATREVIRGINIA (C)
Boulevard & Grove Aves.
Richmond, VA 23221
(804) 257-0840
Terry Burgler

WASHINGTON
A CONTEMPORARY
THEATRE (C)
Box 19400
100 W. Roy St.
Seattle, WA 98119
(206) 285-3220
Jeff Steitzer,
Phil Schermer

INTIMAN THEATRE CO.
(D)
P.O. Box 19645
Seattle, WA 98109
(206) 624-4541
Elizabeth Huddle,
Peter Davis

SEATTLE REPERTORY
THEATRE (B +) (D)
Bagley Wright Theater
155 Mercer St.
Seattle, WA 98109
(206) 447-2210
Daniel Sullivan,
Ben Moore

WISCONSIN
MILWAUKEE
REPERTORY THEATRE
COMPANY (C) (D) (D)
108 E. Wells Street
Milwaukee, WI 53202
(414) 224-1761
John Dillon,
Sara O'Connor

Dinner Theaters

by Ronn Mullen

Down through the seasons dinner theaters have provided a source of income to members of the entertainment industry. Although dinner theater has had its ups and downs, it is a form of entertainment that has been making a comeback lately. And even though types of productions in favor may change from time to time, the basic concept remains intact, and dinner theaters continue to present revues, musicals, comedies, drama, and original shows all across the nation.

Without question, it is the big, brassy, Broadway musicals that currently get preferred billing at most dinner theaters. Producers have found that today's audiences are not interested in paying to see an intimate New York apartment comedy. There are of course, exceptions, but the trend continuing for several years now, has been that the bigger and bolder the show, the greater the likelihood that dinner theaters will want to do it. For example, in 1988 more theaters performed the saga of Peggy Sawyer in *42nd Street* than any other show. The dancing, the glitter, and the glamour of the hit Broadway show is as popular in the Midwest, South, and Far West as it was on the Great White Way. *Singin' in the Rain* ran a close second to *42nd Street* and *The Best Little Whorehouse in Texas* is still a hardy staple on the dinner theater circuit. The older shows are popular, too. The celebrated *Kiss Me, Kate*, for example, is still popular.

Smaller shows are also represented at dinner theater performances. *Little Shop of Horrors*, one of the first (if not *the* first) show to make the transition from Off Broadway to dinner theater is one of these. *Nunsense*, a small-cast musical about a group of eccentric nuns, is a very popular show among dinner theater patrons. *Nunsense* began as a cabaret show at the Duplex in Greenwich Village and has been batting around various Off-Broadway theaters for a few years and is now playing in dinner theaters all over America. Nevertheless, big shows predominate.

The list of musicals playing in dinner theaters reads like a history of the American musical comedy from *Oklahoma* onward. *Annie* is still around, as are her sisters *Gigi*, *Mame*, *Nanette*, and *Dolly*. The popularity of *Sugar Babies* has spawned such look-alike titles as *The Best of Burlesque*, which in turn has led to compilation revues of musical comedy material: *The Best of Broadway*, *The Great American Backstage Musical*, *Playing the Palace* are among such efforts designed to pack as many show-stoppers into one performance as possible.

A few adventurous theaters are willing to attempt original shows. The Gaslight Dinner Theater in Memphis, Tennessee, presented an original musical version of *It's a Wonderful Life*, during the 1987 holiday season. The Barksdale Theater at Hanover Tavern in Hanover, Vermont, makes it a policy to present the unusual and original. And several other theaters around the country bring new and different material to their audiences from time to time. But it's a gamble because dinner theater audiences like what they know and don't like to be surprised after dessert. They like to come *into* the theater humming the score.

The works of Neil Simon continue to make up the bulk of nonmusical productions in dinner theaters across the states. *The Odd Couple*, always able to attract an audience, has become perhaps even more popular since the novel idea was conceived of putting women in the leading roles. Light farces and murder mysteries make up a bulk of other production schedules, but it's not all *Natalie Needs a Nightie* and *Noises Off*. *Children of a Lesser God*, *The Glass Menagerie*, *Amadeus*, and a few other weightier entries are to be seen here and there.

AUDITIONS

Casts of dinner theater productions come from a variety of sources. Approximately 65 percent of all dinner theaters nationwide list their auditions or request photos and resumes through *Back Stage*. 75 percent of existing Equity dinner theaters hold auditions in New York, Chicago, or Los Angeles. Many performers are hired as a result of these auditions. But many dinner theaters hire locally also. At least 85 percent of all dinner theaters (AEA and non-Equity) use some local talent although AEA contracts limit the number of non-Equity performers that can be used in large-cast shows. A small percentage of dinner theaters also hire performers through the twice-yearly NDTA (National Dinner Theater Association) and/or SETC (South-eastern Theater Conference) auditions. Some cast members are also acquired through agent submissions.

HOW LONG WILL A SHOW RUN?

The length of time that dinner theater productions run varies greatly. Eight weeks appears to be the average run of a production, even though some shows run only two weeks. But some shows run longer. The Chanhassen Dinner Theater complex in Chanhassen, Minnesota, runs shows from 24 to 36 weeks in any one of its four theaters. This company also has one of the longest running shows going—a production of *I Do, I Do* that has been running for 17 *years* with the *same cast*. Maynard Sloate's Sahara Dinner Theater in Las Vegas runs shows anywhere from three months to a year. One of this dinner theater's offerings was the mega-hit musical, *42nd Street*, which was practically guaranteed a successful run in this city known for its attraction to glitter.

Richard Akins Productions extends the runs of shows by packaging the productions and moving them from one theater to another, as from the Genetti to the Peddler's Village Dinner Theater in Pennsylvania. The average run at each theater is from four to eight weeks, thus giving actors from eight to 16 weeks employment in one show.

The practice of moving shows from theater to theater was once more widespread than it is today, with production packagers serving from four to eight independently owned theaters. A show was cast and rehearsed in New York by the packager and then sent to various theaters on the circuit. In recent years, theaters have chosen to mount their own productions.

DINNER THEATER—A PROFESSIONAL ENTERPRISE

Richard Akins, chairman of the National Dinner Theater Association and producer for the Genetti and Peddler's Village Dinner Theaters, and his partner David Zarnecki, are emphatic about what makes success happen and what leads to failure in dinner theaters. Their operation is a full-scale, full-time, multi-faceted enterprise that takes the expertise of a four-star restaurateur, a top-line entrepreneur, and a showman with pizzazz and foresight. And dinner theater plays and musicals constitute only one part of the Akins/Zarnecki endeavor. Star attractions in concert performance forms a major part of their enterprise. Carol Channing, the Smothers Brothers, the Lettermen, Phyllis Diller, and Doc Severinson and his Orchestra are some of the top names that they have presented, not only in their dinner theaters, but in major concert halls, such as the 15,000-seat Symphony Hall in Allentown, Pa.

"Dinner theater audiences come out," Akins says, "not only because of the type of shows that are offered—mostly glitzy musicals—but also because of star names. You have to remember that when the lights go down after a good dinner and a few drinks, what you basically have is a nightclub. Producers can't get by on a season of retreads—the 20th production of *Annie* for instance—unless you are also offering as part of your season names like Phyllis Diller. Sure, you can get away with the 20th production of *Annie,* but you'd better have something else to offer as well. You have to remember that it is a multi-use entertainment facility that you have at your disposal. And you'd better have the imagination to use it effectively."

The quality of shows that are offered in dinner theaters, both Akins and Zarnecki feel, can compare favorably to National Companies and any other professional venue you'd care to name. "Reva Rice," Akins points out, "who has since starred on Broadway in *Starlight Express,* headlined in our production of *Ain't Misbehavin'.* She was terrific then, and she's terrific now."

Fine talent is essential to dinner theater productions just as it's essential to any other type of professional entertainment. Audiences who attend dinner theater performances are mainly repeat customers and they are growing in sophistication. "You can't get by with doing *Mame* with a cast of eight on a unit set," Akins points out. "Not that you don't see that now and again . . . but you won't be seeing it again. That theater will close."

"What we have been doing, is touring our better shows," Atkins continues. "After we have mounted a first-class *La Cage aux Folles* or *Pump Boys and Dinettes* there is no reason we can't tour the show to 15,000-seat houses or to other dinner theaters across the country. Dennis Hitchcock, out in Rock Island, Illinois at Circa 21 Dinner Theater, recently played the National Touring Company of *Pump Boys.* That's the quality dinner theater audiences are expecting."

Both of the theaters to which Richard Akins Productions supplies shows are non-Equity. On the controversy over Equity and non-Equity theaters, Akins says, "We have no problem finding highly talented performers who are non-Equity. With the professional quality of the talent pool in New York, Chicago, Atlanta and Los Angeles, there is no shortage of talent." Akins points out that you can have stars in non-Equity houses by presenting them in concert evenings. He feels that there need not be a loss of audience when a theater goes from an Equity to a non-Equity house. "The Derby Dinner Theater in Indiana went non-Equity a couple of years ago," Akins said. "There has certainly been no loss of audience interest there, nor a loss of quality. The audience doesn't care if the actors belong to the union or not. They come to see the show."

Akins also talks of the right-to-work laws which exist in many states. "If an Equity actor wants to work in a non-Equity show in, say, Florida, he can, providing there is no work for him in an Equity theater—which, of course, is frequently the case. The union cannot penalize the actor for seeking work outside the union when union work is not available."

COST SHARING AND QUALITY

"Another innovation we are pursuing is co-producing, sharing the production costs with more than one theater and playing the show in more than one venue," Akins continues. "Say I'm producing *La Cage* in Philadelphia. There's no reason that same production can't play a theater in Detroit or St. Louis; we're not competing for the same audience."

Akins and Zarnecki are also adamant on finding the best directors and choreographers for their shows. "You might think of the dinner theater director as being the local high school English teacher handling a cast of New York actors," Atkins says. "That's not the case. We always look for the best directors and choreographers as well. The audience expects the show to have that New York look. You can't get that with the local high school English teacher."

Asked what he felt contributed mostly to the success of some dinner theaters and the demise of others, Akins was emphatic: "Cream rises. Quality work will triumph; that of lesser quality will falter and fall by the wayside. You have to keep your audience happy and be willing to branch out into other venues."

ORIGINAL WORKS

Most producers are afraid of trying new works and would rather keep doing *Everybody Loves Opal* and the proverbial 20th production of *Annie*. Akins and Zarnecki do not feel that such caution is warranted. "Dinner theater," says Akins, "is the ideal place for new work. I'd love to get into the position of commissioning original works. We tried a show no one had ever heard of and it broke our box office records." Which show was that? *Love, Sex and the I.R.S.*

In speaking about those members of the audience who only want to see the old standards, Akins says, "Luckily, we have our subscribers who have grown to trust us and there are the 'Group Sales' who buy the date rather than the show," Akins says. "They know they are going to see a good show and that the food will be good from past experience and they are willing to trust us. What you have to do is put the show on, make it great and hope for the best. Quality will win out."

EXPANSION AND GROWTH

While the doom-sayers are predicting the final curtain for dinner theaters, there are some pockets of growth and expansion that belie the rumor. For example, F. Scott Black's Towson Towne Musical Theater has been in operation going on ten years. Now this organization is also producing shows for the Harborlights Dinner Theater in the Fells Point section of Baltimore. Black told *Back Stage* that he is trying to schedule new shows along with old favorites. Each of the two theaters has its own unique personality. Towson Towne has followed the classic dinner theater format of serving food buffet-style. But at Harborlights, they are experimenting with uniformed waiters and candlelight. This seems to be part of a trend on the dinner theater circuit. Some theaters have converted entirely to waiter service, while others try it on some nights and retain the traditional buffet line for the remaining nights of the week.

THE CURRENT STATE OF THE ART

Dinner theaters are closing left and right. New theaters are opening north and south. Existing theaters are expanding and opening sister theaters. Equity theaters are going non-Equity. Dinner theaters are presenting concerts and special events in addition to plays and musicals; they are trading and sharing productions. It looks like everybody is doing the same show at the same time. There are 40 productions of *42nd Street* on the boards and everybody else is doing Neil Simon. Yet at the same time, a raft of original comedies and musicals are headed up for the summer season. As is apparent it's pretty hard to point to just what is happening in dinner theater right now. But time, that great teacher, will tell.

Equity Dinner Theaters

How to read this listing: The first line indicates the dinner theater to whom to direct mail. The owner or producer is then listed followed by the mailing address and phone number(s). The final line gives the Actors' Equity contract under which the theater operates. 1 = 0–199 seats; 2 = 200–329 seats; 3 = 330–449; 4 = 450–649; 5 = 650–1200; followed by the number of seats in the theater (i.e. 3/399 would indicate that the theater operates under an Actors' Equity Association Category 3 Dinner Theater contract and has 399 seats). The designation ADTI or NDTA indicates membership in one of the two national dinner theater organizations: American Dinner Theatre Institute (ADTI) (almost exclusively Equity); or National Dinner Theatre Institute (NDTA) (exclusively non-Equity).

For information regarding the American Dinner Theatre Institute, contact Joshua Cockey, Executive Director, Box 367, Cockeysville, Maryland 21030, (301) 771-0367.

For information on the National Dinner Theatre Association, contact Richard Akins, Chairman, 58 N. Ambler St., Quakertown, Pennsylvania 18951, (215) 538-3206.

CALIFORNIA

THE GRAND DINNER THEATRE
Grand Hotel
One Hotel Way
Anaheim, CA 92802
(714) 772-7710; 772-3220
Attn: Frank Wyka
3/420 seats; ADTI

HARLEQUIN DINNER PLAYHOUSE
3503 South Harbor Blvd.
Santa Ana, CA 92704
(714) 979-7550
Attn: Al & Barbara Hampton
4/515 seats

LAWRENCE WELK VILLAGE THEATRE
8975 Lawrence Welk Dr.
Escondido, CA 92026
Attn: Robert M. Dias
2/300 seats; ADTI

COLORADO

COUNTRY DINNER PLAYHOUSE
6875 So. Clinton
Englewood, CO 80110
(303) 771-1410; 771-9311
Attn: Bill McHale, prod'r.
4/470 seats; ADTI
Address all correspondence to:
P.O. Box 3167
Englewood, CO 80155

CONNECTICUT

COACHLIGHT DINNER THEATRE
266 Main St.
East Windsor, CT 06088
(203) 623-8227; 623-2021
Attn: Janis Belkin
4/599 seats; ADTI

DARIEN DINNER THEATRE
65 Tokeneke Rd.
Darien, CT 06820
(203) 655-6812; 838-8411
Attn: Jane Bergere
3/449 seats; ADTI

FLORIDA

ALHAMBRA DINNER THEATRE
12000 Beach Blvd.
Jacksonville, FL 32216
(904) 641-1212
Attn: Tod Booth, exec. prod'r
3/398 seats; ADTI

BURT REYNOLDS DINNER THEATRE
1001 E. Indiantown Rd.
Jupiter, Fl 33458
(407) 747-5261; 746-5566
Attn: Karen Poindexter, prod'r
4/449 seats; ADTI

GOLDEN APPLE DINNER THEATRE
25 N. Pineapple Ave.
Sarasota, FL 33577
(813) 366-2646; 366-5454
(B.O.)
Attn: Robert E. Turoff
2/279 seats; ADTI

THE HIRSCHFELD
THEATRE
The Castle Hotel & Resort
5445 Collins Ave.
Miami Beach, FL 33140
(305) 866-0014
Attn: Karen Poindexter
5/900 seats; ADTI

MARK II DINNER
THEATRE
3376 Edgewater Dr.
Orlando, FL 32804-3797
(407) 843-6275
Attn: Mark Howard
3/320 seats; ADTI/NDTA

ROYAL PALM DINNER
THEATRE
303 Golf View Dr./Royal
Palm Plaza
Boca Raton, FL 33432
(407) 392-3755
2/250 seats; ADTI
Attn: Jan McArt

SHOWBOAT DINNER
THEATRE
3405 Ulmerton Rd.
P.O. Box 519
Clearwater, FL 33520
(813) 576-3818; 223-2545
Attn: Maurice Shinners
4/428 seats; ADTI

ILLINOIS

CANDLELIGHT DINNER
PLAYHOUSE
5620 S. Harlem Ave.
Summit, IL 60501
(312) 735-7400; 496-3000
Attn: William Pulinsi
4/566 seats; ADTI

MARIOTT'S
LINCOLNSHIRE
THEATRE
101 Half Day Rd.
Lincolnshire, IL 60015
Attn: Kary M. Walker
5/862 seats; ADTI

DRURY LANE
OAKBROOK THEATRE
100 Drury Lane
Oakbrook Terrace, IL 60181
(312) 530-8300
Attn: Tony De Santis
5/975 seats; ADTI

DRURY LANE SOUTH
2500 W. Drury Lane
Evergreen Park, IL 60642
(312) 779-4000
Attn: John Lazzara
5/821 seats

INDIANA

BEEF 'N' BOARDS
DINNER THEATRE
9301 N. Michigan Road
Indianapolis, IN 46268
(317) 872-9664
Attn: Doug Stark/Robt. Zehn
3/449 seats; ADTI/NDTA

MINNESOTA

CHANHASSEN DINNER
THEATRE
PO Box 99
Chanhassen, MN 55317
(612) 934-1500; 934-1525
Attn: Richard Bloomberg
4/598 seats; ADTI

CHANHASSEN
PLAYHOUSE DINNER
THEATRE
Chanhassen, MN 55317
(612) 934-1500; 934-1525
Attn: Richard Bloomberg
2/135 seats; ADTI

FIRESIDE DINNER
THEATRE
51 West 78 St.
Chanhassen, MN 55317
(612) 934-1500
Attn: Richard Bloomberg
2/262 seats; ADTI
All correspondence to:
P.O. Box 99
Chanhassen, MN 55317

MISSOURI

TIFFANY'S ATTIC
DINNER THEATRE
5208 Main St.
Kansas City, MO 64112
(816) 361-2661; 561-7923
Attn: Dennis Hennessy
3/332 seats; ADTI

WALDORF ASTORIA
DINNER PLAYHOUSE
7428 Washington
Kansas City, MO 64112
(816) 561-7921; 561-1704
Attn: Dennis Hennessy
3/375 seats; ADTI
All correspondence to:
Waldorf Astoria Dinner
Playhouse, Inc.
5028 Main St.
Kansas City, MO 64112
(816) 361-2661
3/375 seats

NEBRASKA

FIREHOUSE DINNER
THEATRE
514 South 11th St.
Omaha, NE 68102
(402) 346-6009; 346-8833
Attn: Richard Mueller
2/289 seats; ADTI/NDTA

NEW YORK

AN EVENING DINNER
THEATRE
11 Clearbrook Rd.
Elmsford, NY 10523
(914) 592-2268; 592-2222
Attn: Wm. Stutler/Robt.
Funking
3/421 seats; ADTI

LAKE GEORGE DINNER
THEATRE
P.O. Box 266
Lake George, NY 12845
(518) 668-1258
Attn: David Eastwood
2/150 seats; ADTI

OHIO

CAROUSEL DINNER
THEATRE
1275 E. Waterloo Rd.
Akron, OH 44306
(216) 724-9855
Attn: Scott Griffith
5/1200 seats; ADTI
All correspondence to:
P.O. Box 7530
Akron, OH 44306

WESTGATE DINNER
THEATRE
3301 W. Central Ave.
P.O. Box 2988
Toledo, OH 43606
(419) 537-1881
Attn: Ken Shaw
2/320 seats

TEXAS

COUNTRY SQUIRE
DINNER THEATRE
135 Sunset Market Town
Amarillo, TX 79120
(806) 358-7486
Attn: Peter Fox/Della Ray
3/350 seats

DINNER THEATRE ASSOCIATIONS

AMERICAN DINNER
THEATRE INSTITUTE
Joshua Cockey, Executive
Director
Box 367
Cockeysville, MD 21030
(301) 771-0367

NATIONAL DINNER
THEATRE ASSOCIATION
Richard Akins, Chairman
58 N. Ambler St.
Quakertown, PA 18951
(212) 538-3206

Non-Equity Dinner Theaters

ALABAMA

BLUE MOON DINNER
THEATRE
1447 Montgomery, HWY.
Birmingham, AL 35216
(205) 823-3000
*Attn: Judith Peacock/
Bob King
382 seats: NDTA*

ARKANSAS

MURRY'S DINNER
THEATRE
6323 Asher Ave.
Little Rock, AK 72204
(501) 562-3131
*Attn: Ike Murry
304 seats; ADTI/NDTA*

CALIFORNIA

FIRELITE DINNER
THEATRE
4350 Transport St.
Ventura, CA 93003
(805) 656-3922
*Attn: Kathryn Taylor
125 seats; ADTI*

ROGER ROCKA'S MUSIC
HALL
1266 North Wishon
Fresno, CA 93728
(209) 266-9493
*Attn: Roger Rocka
275 seats; ADTI*

HERITAGE SQUARE
MUSIC HALL
#5 Heritage Sq.
Golden, CO 80401
(303) 279-7800
*Attn: Woody Wirth
362 seats*

DELAWARE

CANDLELIGHT MUSIC
DINNER THEATRE
2208 Miller Road
Ardentown, DE 19810
(302) 475-2313
*Attn: John O'Toole
185 seats
All correspondence to:*
P.O. Box 7301
Wilmington, DE 19803

FLORIDA

COUNTRY DINNER
PLAYHOUSE
7951 Gateway Mall
9th St. N.
St. Petersburg, FL 33702
(813) 577-5515
*Attn: David Gardner
335 seats; NDTA*

MARCO POLO DINNER
THEATRE
19201 Collins Ave.
N. Miami Beach, FL 33160
(305) 932-2233

NAPLES DINNER
THEATRE
1025 Piper Blvd.
Naples, FL 33942
(813) 597-6031
*Attn: Jules Fiske/Jim Fargo
350 seats; NDTA*

ILLINOIS

CIRCA '21 DINNER
PLAYHOUSE
PO Box 3784-1828 Third
Ave.
Rock Island, IL 61201
(309) 785-2667
*Attn: Dennis Hitchcock
336 seats; NDTA*

CONKLIN PLAYERS
DINNER THEATRE
PO Box 301
Conklin Court
Goodfield, IL 61742
(309) 965-2545
Attn: Chaunce Conklin
In Illinois 1-800-322-2304
260 seats; ADTI/NDTA

SUNSHINE DINNER
THEATRE
115 West Kirby Ave.
Champaign, IL 61820
(217) 359-4503
*Attn: Arthur L. Barnes
200 seats; NDTA*

INDIANA

DERBY DINNER
THEATRE
525 Marriott Dr.
Clarksville, IN 47130
(812) 288-2634
*Attn: Bekki Jo Schneider
574 seats; NDTA*

IOWA

INGERSOLL DINNER
THEATRE
3711 Ingersoll Ave.
Des Moines, IA 50312
(office) (515) 274-4686
*Attn: Charles Carnes
270 seats; ADTI/NDTA*

KANSAS

CROWN UPTOWN
DINNER THEATRE
3207 E. Douglas
Wichita, KS 67218
(316) 681-1566
*Attn: Karen & Ted Morris
550 seats; NDTA*

MARYLAND

BURN BRAE DINNER
THEATRE
Rt. 29
Burtonville, MD 20866
(301) 384-5800
Attn: John Kinnamon
350 seats; NDTA

HARBORLIGHTS DINNER
THEATRE
511 So. Broadway
Baltimore, MD 21231
(301) 522-4126
Attn: F. Scott Black
196 seats; ADTI

HARLEQUIN DINNER
THEATRE
1330 E. Gude Dr.
Rockville, MD 20850
(301) 340-6813
Attn: Nicholas Howey/
Kenneth Gentry
384 seats; NDTA

PETRUCCI'S DINNER
THEATRE
312 Main St.
Laurel, MD 20707
(301) 725-5226
Attn: C. David Petrucci

TOWSON TOWNE
MUSICAL DINNER
THEATRE
7800 York Rd.
Towson, MD 21204
(301) 321-6595
Attn: F. Scott Black
250 seats

MICHIGAN

CORNWELL'S
TURKEYVILLE DINNER
THEATRE
18935 15½ mile Rd.
Marshall, MI 49068
(616) 781-7933; 781-4315
Attn: David M. Pritchard
150 seats; ADTI/NDTA
All correspondence to:
Pritchard Productions
PO Box 734
Marshall, MI 49127

SCHULER'S
STEVENSVILLE DINNER
THEATRE
5000 Red Arrow Hwy.
Stevensville, MI 49127
(616) 781-7933
Attn: David M. Pritchard
175 seats; ADTI/NDTA
All correspondence to:
Pritchard Productions
PO Box 734
Marshall, MI 49127

MISSOURI

GOLDENROD
SHOWBOAT
700 No. L. K. Sullivan
Blvd.
St. Louis, MO 63102
(314) 621-3311
Attn: Frank Pierson
400 seats; ADTI/NDTA

NEBRASKA

UPSTAIRS DINNER
THEATRE
221 S. 19th St.
Omaha, NE 68102
(402) 344-3858
Attn: Anne Ausdemore
200 seats; NDTA

NEW JERSEY

NEIL'S NEW YORKER
DINNER THEATRE
Route 46
Mountain Lakes, NJ 07046
(201) 334-0010
Attn: Jack Bell
375 seats; NDTA

NEW YORK

ISLAND SQUIRE DINNER
THEATRE
PO Box 428
Middle Island, NY 11953
(516) 732-2240
Attn: John Wyle
150 seats

NORTH CAROLINA

THE BARN
120 Stage Coach Trail
Greensboro, NC 27409
(919) 292-2211
Attn: Thomas F. Hennis, Jr.
322–336 seats; NDTA

OHIO

LA COMEDIA DINNER
THEATRE
PO Box 204
Springboro, OH 45066
(513) 746-3114
Attn: Ed Flesch
622 seats; NDTA

PENNSYLVANIA

ALLENBERRY
PLAYHOUSE
PO Box 7, Rte. 174
Boiling Springs, PA 17007
(717) 258-6120
Attn: John Heinze
NDTA

DUTCH APPLE DINNER
THEATRE
510 Centerville Rd.
Lancaster, PA 17601
(717) 898-1900
Attn: Prather Productions
350 seats; ADTI/NDTA

GENETTI DINNER
PLAYHOUSE
Route 309
Hazelton, PA 18201
(717) 455-3691
Attn: Richard Akins
Productions
270 seats; NDTA

HUNTINGDON VALLEY
DINNER THEATRE
2633 Philmont Ave.
Huntingdon Valley, PA
19006
(215) 947-6000

PEDDLER'S VILLAGE
DINNER THEATRE
Route 263
Lahaska, PA 18931
(215) 794-3460
200 seats; NDTA

VIRGINIA

BARN DINNER THEATRE
Salem, VA
(703) 387-2276
Attn: Mary Gilchrift

BARKSDALE DINNER
THEATRE
PO Box 7
Hanover, VA 23069
(804) 537-5333
Attn: Nancy Kilgore
199 seats

SWIFT CREEK MILL
PLAYHOUSE
PO Box 41
Colonial Heights, VA 23834
(804) 748-5203
Attn: Wamer J. Callahan
240 seats

TIDEWATER DINNER
THEATRE
6270 Northampton Blvd.
Norfolk, VA 23502
(804) 461-2933
Attn: Maureen J. Sigmund
299 seats; ADTI/NDTA

WISCONSIN

FANNY HILL SUPPER
CLUB & DINNER
THEATRE
Route 5
Eau Claire, WI 54701
(715) 836-8184

FIRESIDE PLAYHOUSE
1131 Janesville Ave.
Ft. Atkinson, WI 53538
(414) 563-9505
Attn: E. Flesch
488 seats; NDTA

NORTHERN LIGHTS
PLAYHOUSE and
PINEWOOD DINNER
THEATRE
PO Box 256
Hazelhurst, WI 54531
(715) 356-7173
Attn: Michael D. Cupp
NDTA

Theater for Young Audiences

by Joseph J. Schwartz

Theater for Young Audiences offers great opportunities to actors searching for experience, credits, and gainful employment. With more than 50 producers regularly mounting Equity children's shows each season (and dozens of non-union producers providing similar opportunities), performers looking to start a professional career would do well to take a closer look at acting for the younger set.

A GATEWAY TO EQUITY

There are a great many more chances for a non-union actor to get into Equity through a TYA (Theater for Young Audiences) contract than any other way. At least that's how Peter Harris, Equity's business representative for TYA, sees it. Harris maintains that producers are often unable to find actors willing to take on the rigors of touring with a TYA contract, which can include long periods of time away from New York, long hours of traveling and multi-performance days. Therefore, they frequently open TYA auditions to non-union performers, who subsequently become Equity members.

THE TYA CONTRACT

The TYA contract guarantees actors a minimum wage on either a weekly or per performance basis. In the weekly contract, which guarantees a performer a minimum of two week's work, actors must be paid no less than $251 per week. Assistant stage managers are paid the same amount but receive an additional $11 if they are also required to act. A first or second assistant stage manager who also acts is guaranteed no less than $267 for a week's work, while a stage manager must be paid $328 for the same length of time and may not act or understudy. A per-performance TYA contract guarantees an actor a minimum of $40.25 per show. The wage is scaled accordingly for the various stage managerial assignations.

The TYA workday cannot exceed 10 hours and includes an hour for lunch. Rehearsing, performing, and traveling are all considered as part of the 10-hour workday and actors are guaranteed a 12-hour rest period between days. Performances are limited to 12 a week and must last no more than 90 minutes, including any live, educational demonstrations given by performers after a show. Additional compensation of $17.75 per show must be paid after nine performances in any given week, and a $29.25 per night per diem must be paid to performers traveling away from the theater's home base. Overtime is provided at $3.75 per half hour during the workday and $9.50 per hour during the rest period.

To some in the field, the guarantees provided by the TYA contract may not seem overly attractive, but Barbara Colton, who was formerly first vice president for Equity and who was also TYA Committee Chair, recalls what children's theater was like before an Equity contract existed. Colton worked the children's theater circuit in

1961, and remembers working a three-performance day and being paid on a sliding scale: $7 for the first show, $5 for the second, and $3 for the third. "Today the Equity producer can only do a three-performance day twice a week and this must be non-consecutive," she says. "A standard weekly contract with a weekly guarantee and a per diem was absolutely unheard of before 1969. Frequently the actors had to maintain their own costumes, there was no rehearsal salary and you were paid by the performance."

This is not to say that an age of enlightenment has taken over the entire theater establishment. Horror stories still abound of non-union children's theater companies that require actors to do manual labor, load-ins, set and prop maintenance, costume repair, and assorted duties in addition to traveling and acting. But such stories are in the minority, and most performers' experiences of non-union children's theater are positive.

WHY ACTORS SHY AWAY FROM CHILDREN'S THEATER

It may be that some actors shy away from children's theater because they are uncomfortable performing for children, but many theater professionals feel that the reasons have more to do with economic and professional considerations.

"Agents will not come to see actors in children's shows," says John Ahearn of the Gingerbread Players. He maintains that since actors want to advance their careers they stay away from children's productions because of the lack of the critical spotlight. "Actors aren't really investigating children's theater because agents feel the productions are not as good as other shows. But they *are* as good."

"It's difficult to get actors to leave New York," explains Charles Hull, producer of the 28-year-old Theaterworks/USA, one of the nation's oldest professional children's theater companies. "Actors feel that if they are away from New York they will miss something," says Hull. That "something" Hull refers to may be an important audition, a showcase or a part in a Broadway play.

Some actors who object to performing in children's theater seem to attach a cultural stigma to the simple act of performing in a children's show. They hold the misconception that what's being done on stage in children's theater is not really legitimate theater, but some kind of simplified bastard version. "I wonder about that," muses actress Amy Butler, an eight-year veteran of the children's theater circuit. "I know people who compromise what they are doing all the time, and sometimes they feel better doing a showcase or a 'scene night' for free rather than being paid to do a children's show. I'd rather get paid."

Cultural stigma notwithstanding, many of the country's top performers got their start performing for the younger set, with many of them supporting themselves through these performances for many years. Among the well-known performers who have appeared in children's theater are Henry Winkler, John Travolta, and F. Murray Abraham. In addition, there are numerous examples of established stars coming back to children's theater to do an occasional show or benefit. Elaine Stritch and Richard Kiley are cases in point.

A LIMITED GATE

Money is, of course, at the heart of mounting any successful theatrical production and TYA is no exception. According to Hull, whose Theaterworks/USA company works in agreement with the Equity TYA contract, his cost in mounting a production is approximately $30,000. This does not include the costs incurred while running or maintaining the production. And even though other companies may have fewer costs, one of the common complaints among children's theatrical producers is that the money one can charge is very limited. "There is a very limited gate," says Judith Martin, founder and artistic director of the Paper Bag Players, a non-union company that has been producing shows for 30 years. "The money we take in from ticket sales never meets our expenses. We have to be constantly fundraising."

Gingerbread's Ahearn agrees. "The Labor, the artwork, costumes, scenery, salaries, rent have all gone up. And we always, always have to consider how much organizations are funded to bring in these shows."

The funding that Ahearn refers to are all the budget appropriations, state art council grants, parent/teacher organization donations and educational cultural monies that usually pay for children's theater when it tours to public and private schools around the country. "In children's theater you can't make a lot of money because people will only pay so much for a seat for a child," Ahearn says.

In the absence of high monetary reward, one can only think that producers who go into mounting children's shows have ulterior motives. "It can be very exhilarating," says Martin. "We feel we make a very interesting kind of theater. It's where our talents lie and it's a very artistically demanding situation," she adds. Charles Hull says that "It's fun." And finally Ahearn cites the fact simply that there's a great feeling in doing quality work.

Equity Theater for Young Audiences Companies

The following is a list of TYA companies in the Eastern, Midwestern, and Western regions of the United States. They are listed alphabetically in their appropriate regions, followed by an address, phone number, and the name of the artistic and/or producing director. *Indicates companies which are not currently active on TYA contract.

Producers League of TYA

ASOLO STATE
THEATRE, INC.
P.O. Box Drawer E.
Sarasota, Florida 34230
(813) 355-7115
Don Creason,
Lindia M. DiGabriele

FANFARE THEATRE
ENSEMBLE
100 E. 4th St.
New York, NY 10003
(212) 674-8181
Joan Shepard

GINGERBREAD PLAYERS
& JACK
35-06 88th St.
Jackson Heights, NY 11372
(718) 424-2443
John Ahearn

MAXIMILLION
PRODUCTIONS
98 Riverside Drive, #7H
(212) 874-3121
Max Traktman,
Peggy Traktman

THEATREWORKS, USA
890 Broadway, 7th fl.
New York, NY 10003
(212) 677-5959
Charles Hull,
Jay Harnick

TRAVELLING
PLAYHOUSE
104 Northampton Drive
White Plains, NY 10603
(914) 946-5289
Kay Rockefeller,
Ken Rockefeller

Independent Producers

EASTERN STATES

ALLIANCE THEATRE
Robert W. Woodruff Arts
Ctr.
1280 Peachtree St. NE
Atlanta, GA 30309
(404) 898-1132
Edith H. Love,
Wm. B. Duncan

AMERICAN STAGE (TYA)
P.O. Box 1560
211 3rd St. South
St. Petersburg, FL 33731
(813) 823-1600
John Berglund

*BARTER THEATRE
Box 867
Abingdon, VA 24210
(703) 628-2281
Rex Partington

CARPENTER CENTER
FOR THE PERFORMING
ARTS
525 East Grace St.
Richmond, VA 23219
(804) 782-3930
Sue Bahen,
Bob Foreman

*CITY KIDS
FOUNDATION INC.
99 Hudson St.
New York, NY 10013
(212) 219-4550
Laurie Meadoff

COCONUT GROVE
PLAYHOUSE
Attn: Education Dept.
3500 Main Highway
Miami, FL 33133
(305) 442-2662
Arnold Mittleman,
Judith Delgado

CREATIVE THEATRE
FOR CHILDREN, INC.
30 North Van Brunt St.
Englewood, NJ 07631
(201) 568-4446; 568-5448
Adlynn Gordon

CYGNET PRODUCTIONS,
INC.
1261 Broadway, #505
New York, NY 10001
(212) 725-1375
Sterling Swann

DEAR KNOWS LTD.
236 a W. 19th St., Suite 149
New York, NY 10011
(212) 921-2800
Ken LaZebnik

*DELAWARE THEATRE
COMPANY
P.O. Box 516
Wilmington, DE 19899
(302) 594-1104
Dennis Luzak

*DFB PRODUCTIONS,
INC.
177 E. 79th St.
New York, NY 10022
(212) 794-9311
Dr. Frederick Bernstein

EMPIRE STATE
INSTITUTE FOR THE
PERFORMING ARTS
(ESIPA)
Empire State Plaza
Albany, NY 12223
(518) 443-5222
Patricia B. Snyder

FLOATING HOSPITAL
Children's Theatre
275 Madison Ave.
New York, NY 10016
(212) 685-0193
Madeline Burgess

FOUNDATION THEATRE
Burlington County College
Pemberton, NJ 08068
(609) 894-9311 (ext. 423)
Julie Ellen Prusinowski

GEORGIA
SHAKESPEARE
FESTIVAL
4484 Peachtree Rd. NE
Atlanta, GA. 30319-2797
(404) 261-1441 (Ext. 343)
Lane Anderson

HIPPODROME STATE
THEATRE (TYA)
25 SE 2nd Place
Gainesville, FL 32601
(904) 375-6170
Margaret Bachus

HOSPITAL AUDIENCES
INC.
220 W. 42nd St.
New York, NY 10036
(212) 575-7666
Max Daniels

*JEWISH THEATRE FOR
YOUNG AUDIENCES
c/o Dave De Christopher
374 Richmond Terrace, #1F
Staten Island, NY 10301
(718) 448-7248
Joyce Klein

*JOHN F. KENNEDY
CENTER FOR THE
PERFORMING ARTS
Kennedy Center
Washington, DC 20566
(202) 254-7190
Carole C. Sullivan

LINCOLN CENTER
INSTITUTE
140 W. 65th St.
New York, NY 10023
(212) 877-1800
*June Dunbar,
Mark Schubert*

*MAINSTAGE
PRODUCTIONS, LTD.
35 W. 92nd St.
New York, NY 10025
(212) 864-5217
Harve Brosten

*MOONSTONE, INC.
349 W. 85th St., #32
New York, NY 10024
(212) 724-1649
Thelma Carter

NORTH CAROLINA
SHAKESPEARE
FESTIVAL
305 North Main St.
High Point, NC 27260
(919) 841-6273
Pedro Silva

PUSHCART PLAYERS
197 Bloomfield Ave.
Verona, NJ 07044
(201) 857-1115
*Ruth Fost,
Carole Wechter*

SCHOOLTIME THEATRE,
INC.
Rd. 2, Box 289
Irwin, PA 15642
(412) 744-3345
Merle Smith Kuznik

SHAKESPEARE AND
COMPANY
The Mount
Lenox, MA 02140
(413) 637-1197
*Dennis Krausnick,
Deborah Sims*

SHAKESPEARE FOR
SCHOOLS CO.
41 Madeline Ave.
Clifton, NJ 07011
(201) 546-0624
Janet Villas

SHAKESPEARE TO GO
215 E. 80th St.
New York, NY 10021
(212) 737-6608
Caroline Cornell

STAGE ONE:
Louisville Children's Theater
425 West Market St.
Louisville, KY 40202
(502) 589-5946
Moses Goldberg

*STARLITE
30-60 29th St.
Astoria, NY 11102
(718) 828-3176
Karen Kenny

STREET THEATRE
TOURING COMPANY
228 Fisher Ave., Rm. 226
White Plains, NY 10606
(914) 761-3307
Gary Smith

THEATRE FOR A NEW
AUDIENCE
26 Grove St., #6G
New York, NY 10014
(212) 505-8345
Jeffrey Horowitz

*THUNDERBIRD LTD.,
INC.
(Totem Pole Playhouse)
9555 Golf Course Rd.
Fayetteville, PA 17222
(717) 352-2164
Carl Schurr

VEE CORPORATION
(SESAME/MUPPETS)
Lumber Exchange Bldg.
10 South Fifth St.
Minneapolis, MN 55401
(612) 375-9670
Vincent E. Egan, Pauline Knight

WOODEN O, INC.
600 W. 58th St.
New York, NY 10019
(212) 874-6147
Gayther Myers

YATES MUSICAL
THEATER FOR
CHILDREN
19 Morse Ave.
East Orange, NJ 07017
(201) 677-0936
William Yates, Sr.

MIDWEST STATES

DRURY LANE SOUTH
PRODUCTIONS
J.R.J. THEATRICALS,
LTD.
2500 West Drury Lane
Evergreen Park, IL 60642
(312) 422-8000
John R. Lazzara

DRURY LANE AT
OAKBROOK CHILDREN'S
THEATRE
100 Drury Lane
Oak Brook Terrace, IL
60181
(312) 530-8300
Anthony DeSantis

LORELEI PRODUCTION/
ON STAGE
P.O. Box 25365
Chicago, IL 60625
(312) 275-6836
Bob Boburka, Michelle Vacca

M & W PRODUCTIONS,
INC.
925 East Wells, #416
Milwaukee, WI 53203-0910
(414) 272-7701
Tom Marks, Michael Wilson

MARRIOTT
LINCOLNSHIRE
101 Half Day Rd.
Lincolnshire, IL 60015
(312) 643-0200
Kary Walker

MUNY/STUDENT
THEATRE PROJECT
4219 Laclede
St. Louis, MO 63108
(314) 531-1301
Kathryn White

MUSIC THEATRE
WORKSHOP
1730 West Catalpa
Chicago, IL 60640
(312) 561-7100
(Weekly)
Elbrey Harrell

OLD LOG CHILDREN'S
THEATRE
Old Log Theater, Box 250
Excelsior, MN 55331
(612) 474-5951
Don Stolz

REPERTORY THEATRE
OF ST. LOUIS
Imaginary Theater
Company
P.O. Box 28030
St. Louis, MO 63119
(314) 968-7342
Stephen Woolf

SEEM TO BE PLAYERS
P.O. Box 1601
Lawrence, KA 66044
(913) 842-6622
Rick Averill

THEATRE FOR YOUNG
AMERICA
7204 West 80th St.
Overland Park, KA 66204
(913) 648-4600
Gene Mackey

WESTERN STATES

A CONTEMPORARY
THEATRE
100 West Roy St.
Seattle, WA 98119
(206) 285-3220
Philip Schermer

AMERICAN LIVING
HISTORY THEATRE
P.O. Box 2677
Hollywood, CA 90028
(213) 876-2202
Jay W. Malinowski

BILINGUAL
FOUNDATION OF THE
ARTS
421 N. Ave. 19
Los Angeles, CA 90032
(213) 255-4044
Carmen Zapata

CASA MANANA
PLAYHOUSE
P.O. Box 9054
Ft. Worth, TX 76107
(817) 332-9313
Charles Ballinger, Bud Franks

DENVER CENTER
THEATRE COMPANY
1050 13 St.
Denver, CO 80204
(303) 893-4200
Sarah Lawless

FANTASY THEATRE
P.O. Box 19206
Sacramento, CA 95816
(916) 442-5635
Timothy Busfield

LA JOLLA PLAYHOUSE
P.O. Box 12039
La Jolla, CA 92037
(619) 534-6760
Alan Levey

*OLD GLOBE THEATRE
Balboa Park
P.O. Box 2171
San Diego, CA 92112
(619) 231-1941
Tom Hall, Noel Craig

SEATTLE CHILDREN'S
THEATRE
305 Harrison St.
Seattle, WA 98109
(206) 443-0807
Linda Hartsell

SEATTLE REPERTORY
Seattle Center
155 Mercer Street
Seattle, WA 98109
(206) 443-2210
Benjamin Moore

SOUTH COAST
REPERTORY
655 Town Center Drive
P.O. Box 2197
Costa Mesa, CA 92626-1197
(714) 957-2602
Paula Tomei

THEATRE WEST
3333 Cahuenga Blvd. W
Los Angeles, CA 90068
(213) 851-4839
Nadine Kalmes

P. WEINSTOCK
PRODUCTIONS
423 S. LeDoux Rd., #3
Los Angeles, CA 90048
(213) 278-8679
Phil Weinstock

PART SIX

Off the Main Stage

Theme Parks

by Thomas Walsh

In terms of sheer quantity of people, theme parks probably offer the best exposure anywhere for the performing artist. Some ten million persons pass through the gates of a good-sized, year-round theme park. This averages out to over 27,000 audience members a day. Such numbers add up to an equation that spells out opportunities for intense, varied experience, and career advancement.

Only a handful of the better-known theme parks are open 365 days a year. Most, however, are seasonal operations, generally presenting daily shows from early spring through Labor Day. Nevertheless, audiences at all theme parks are huge. A show may run for 30 seconds, or it can last 20 minutes, an hour, or even all day long. Salaries vary greatly but are generally considered fair, and perks at the theme park are always good. Housing and transportation may be provided. Training, workshops, and internships are usually available and college credits can sometimes be obtained. Additionally, as employees of the theme parks, theater personnel frequently receive unlimited access to the park's multitude of attractions (rides, games, and other shows, etc.). The benefits of working three months, or even a year, in the gorgeous and invigorating outdoor environment that is the setting for most theme parks cannot be overstated. If you compare the pleasures of pushing the sets around at a rep house to the prospect of a summer in Anaheim or an autumn in Orlando, you will probably agree.

The following listings contain information about theme parks nationwide. Nearly all theme parks issue open calls prior to each season for performers, as well as audio engineers, lighting technicians, costumers, dressers, stagehands, and many more. The packages offered to technical personnel are as attractive as they are for performing artists.

ALLAN ALBERT, INC.

The New York-based Albert company serves as a clearing house and central casting headquarters for two large East Coast parks: Hersheypark in Hershey, PA, and Action Park in Vernon Valley, NJ. This company has been expanding its borders, and has recently presented the first theme park shows in China before an audience of nearly 50,000 people. Further territorial treks by the Albert company are in the works.

Action Park

One of America's largest water parks, located just an hour and a quarter from midtown Manhattan, is a neighbor of the Vernon Valley/Great Gorge ski areas and has been offering theatrical productions since 1981. Its season runs from approximately June 1 to Sept. 5, and presents various showcases that feature a wide variety of entertainers.

Applicants must be at least 17 years old or be high school graduates, and the management prefers that prospective employees be under 25 years of age. On the technical end, stage managers, seamstresses, and a company manager are hired.

Action Park residual benefits are excellent: luxury condominiums with all amenities are available (adjacent to the park) for about $35 to $45 per week, and employees have access to the parks at all times, including pools and water rides. The weekly pay begins around $250, plus bonuses.

Hersheypark

"Chocolatetown, U.S.A." is the home base for Hersheypark, which is a pretty fair attraction in itself—and upwards of 30,000 people flock to this park daily. Hersheypark, which has featured live productions for the past 15 seasons, is approximately three hours from New York City by car and has been in existence for 50 years.

Criteria for performers are the same as for Action Park. Additionally, singers must dance and move well, and dancers must be proficient in jazz and tap. Technicians required are stage managers, seamstresses, and sound and lighting technicians.

All applicants are offered a salary package ranging from approximately $285 to $300 weekly, plus bonuses. Employees are provided housing at a subsidized rate (about $45 per week), have free access to park facilities at all times, and may use the employee cafeteria. A limited number of guest passes are available.

THE BUSCH ENTERTAINMENT CORPORATION

The Busch Entertainment Corporation, a subsidiary of Anheuser-Busch Companies, Inc., is at the helm of four U.S. theme parks: Busch Gardens—The Dark Continent, in Tampa, FL; Busch Gardens—The Old Country, in Williamsburg, VA; Sesame Place, a "play park" for younger folks (and their parents), in Langhorne, PA; and Adventure Island, a water park in Tampa, which is adjacent to The Dark Continent.

Only two of the Busch Gardens theme parks will be reviewed here, The Dark Continent and The Old Country. Sesame Place is a relatively new theme park (1983) and hires fewer performers than the two parks that are listed. The other park, Adventure Island, is a water park that does not hire stage performers or strolling entertainers. Addresses for these latter two parks are included in the list at the end of this chapter.

The Anheuser-Busch parks function as a leading "farm system for the high-powered reaches of Broadway, television, stage, and motion pictures," says entertainment director Joseph G. Peczi. "Almost every year, one of our performers hits the big time. In 1987 it was Michael Maguire, who won a Tony Award for his role in Broadway's *Les Miserables.*"

Two of the Busch Gardens venues, The Dark Continent and the Old Country, conduct annual safaris to track down singers, dancers, actors, actresses, variety artists, technicians, and stage managers. Busch Gardens theme parks feature Broadway-style variety revues, country and contemporary song-and-dance productions, German and Italian shows, and strolling bands.

Applicants for auditions must be at least 18 years of age and must be available for full-time seasonal employment. A detailed resume is a must. Audition requirements are as follows: Singers are required to perform an up-tempo song and a ballad (bring your own sheet music), and must dance a choreographed piece; dancers must dance and perform a vocal selection; actors must present a comic monologue—improvs and dialects are important; variety artists are required to come up with some type of patter; and musicians must also present vocal material. Auditioners should limit their presentations to two minutes and be prepared to present additional material upon request.

Performers have access to free classes in dance, vocal instruction, and instrumental training, and can participate in choral, band, jazz, and dance concerts.

Busch Gardens—The Dark Continent

The Dark Continent is a 300-acre representation of yesteryear Africa. It is one of the most popular attractions on Florida's west coast. A year-round showplace, The Dark Continent offers three- and six-month contracts to performers, renewable up to one year.

Among Dark Continent's attractions are animal shows, strolling performers, Broadway-style shows, thrill rides, exhibits, shops, and games.

The Dark Continent hires singer/dancers, musicians, actors, technicians, and belly dancers. Wages start at $6.50 to $8.00 per hour. Perks include 22½ vacation hours after six months of employment, overtime pay for special functions, a full medical plan, and two cases of beer per month (Anheuser-Busch, of course).

Busch Gardens—The Old Country

A 360-acre family entertainment park three miles east of historic Williamsburg, VA, The Old Country consists of eight authentic European hamlets ranging from Oktoberfest (Germany) to Banbury Cross (England). From April to October, the park's strolling performers, magicians, musicians, and storytellers play host to approximately two million visitors.

The park has introduced an all-new ice show, *Hot Ice*, featuring Olympic-style ice skating and dancing. Other entertainment includes the musical show *Journey into Music*, which takes audiences through five nostalgic destinations while recreating the musical spirit of the past, and the production *Enchanted Laboratory*, a computer-animated show featuring special effects and "audio-animatronic" characters which interact in precision timing with a human performer.

Salaries range from approximately $254 to $385 weekly, and benefits include free classes and seminars in dance, music, and drama.

The Old Country presents up to 17 hours of live entertainment in 84 to 100 shows daily. Nationwide auditions begin in the fall and are usually completed by mid-December.

CEDAR POINT/THE AMAZEMENT PARK

Over 700 performances are staged annually at Cedar Point, and after nearly 120 years of entertaining America's Midwest, the 364-acre, four-theater park can list many alumni who have graduated to Broadway, television, films, major theaters, and concert halls nationwide.

Positions are available for musicians (everything from banjo and bass to trumpet and tuba), singers, singer/dancers, singer/musicians, MCs, speciality acts, and about 20 technicians.

The Cedar Point season runs from early May through Labor Day, with some acts held over for bonus weekends in September. Salaries range from approximately $235 to $295 weekly; most positions also offer bonuses by the week. Musicians must be members in good standing of the American Federation of Musicians and the minimum age for all live-show employees is 18. Benefits include low-cost housing, free workshops, movies, dances, and beach and ride privileges.

WALT DISNEY COMPANY

For the theatrically trained individual seeking big-time exposure and experience, the Disney empire holds some of the most powerful cards in the deck. Applicants may submit resumes throughout the year for any and all positions. Disney's yearly talent search is so vast that company representatives are reluctant to release even a rough estimate of the number of people they hire. Suffice it to say that the annual lineups of professional singers, dancers, musical-theater performers, and orchestra members interning in the Disney Company is vast. Applicants are generally selected in the fall.

Walt Disney World

This Disney facility offers productions such as *Broadway at the Top*, *Hoop-Dee-Doo Revue*, and *Fantasy Follies*, featuring old-time vaudeville, contemporary Broadway, country/western, pop, and jazz styles.

Auditions are open to union and non-union performers. Employment begins in May or June. Hopefuls must attend a preliminary call to be considered for callbacks. Those who are called back will receive written or phone notification. The All American College Band and Orchestra also audition here. They seek musicians who have a flair for jazz and popular music.

Disney World benefits are quite broad, beginning with a base pay for chorus and principal performers of $298 to $432 per week. One-year contracts and summer employment are available; full-timers generally work a five-day, 40-hour week and are compensated for overtime. Other incentives include relocation assistance, health and dental benefits, paid vacations and sick days, and rehearsals at full salary.

Disney World does not interview technicians, stage managers, or variety acts, but resumes are accepted year-round.

Epcot Institute of Entertainment Arts

"There is no other program like this anywhere," trumpets the Epcot literature, "a chance for the most promising dancers, singers, and instrumentalists to develop their talents." Indeed, the institute's incentive for newcomers is attractive—an opportunity to become part of a school in which the classroom is the largest entertainment showcase in the world.

Epcot offers an internship to performers seeking intense training and experience in virtually every area of the entertainment field. Interns attend classes, workshops, and seminars with acclaimed professionals and Disney Entertainment staff members. Benefits to interns include housing and utilities (two interns per two-bedroom furnished apartment), a weekly stipend of approximately $212, workshops and master classes, extensive talent and career coaching, and significant show experience in a variety of formats.

Auditioners must be at least 18 years old and must bring a current picture, resume, and letter of recommendation; a four-month commitment is required. Audition guidelines for singers and dancers are identical to those for Disney World. For instrumentalists, popular music, show band, and jazz experience are preferred.

The Epcot Institute is continually seeking interested professionals for special events and industrials, and replacements for stage shows. Interested individuals are encouraged to send pictures and resumes. All inquiries will be placed on the audition mailing list.

Disneyland

Disneyland has been operating at Anaheim since 1955. Open 365 days a year, Disneyland's live-entertainment lineups change on an almost constant basis, and talent is recruited nationwide.

New concepts for performers are dreamed up continually at Disneyland, and the entertainment staff chooses the formats and meets the talent needs in shifting patterns. Musical performers dominate Disneyland's roving-entertainment scenario, but all shapes and sizes of talent are sought and staged. The Disneyland Band, a 16- to 17-member ensemble, is among the constants on the park's musical roster; performers are scattered throughout the seven lands of the 76.6-acre Disneyland property.

DOLLYWOOD

Dollywood is a corporation partially owned and controlled by country music/film/ television star Dolly Parton. Formerly known as Silver Dollar City, this theme park corporation rechristened itself as Dollywood in May of 1986, undoubtedly boosting future attendance beyond the already formidable 1 million figure it had reached previously. Dollywood runs productions from the last weekend in April to the last weekend in October.

Singers, roving groups, individual performers, and several musical groups entertain throughout the park daily. In April of 1988, a 2,000-seat, $3 million state-of-the-art theater was unveiled. Gospel, country, and bluegrass music are the main fare at this theater. Performers are paid for a six-day work week. Pay is approximately $240 to $500 and incentive bonuses and profit-sharing are offered.

HARCOURT BRACE JOVANOVICH, INC.

The Harcourt Brace Jovanovich publishing empire has a flock of six entertainment parks. These parks lean to the nautical side, theme-wise—four of the parks are "sea worlds." As would be expected, with such a heavy emphasis on nautical themes, Harcourt Brace Jovanovich hires many specialty performers, such as divers, swimmers, water skiers, and so on. Even so, they still use a fair number of singers, dancers, and actors, although hiring is generally done locally. For information about auditions, contact the theme park in which you are interested. The Harcourt Brace Jovanovich theme parks are: Boardwalk and Baseball, Orlando, FL; Cypress Gardens, Cypress Gardens, FL; Sea World of Florida, Orlando, FL; Sea World of San Diego, San Diego, CA; Sea World of Ohio, Aurora, OH; and Sea World of Texas, San Antonio, TX. Corporate headquarters for HBJ is located at: Harcourt Brace Jovanovich Building, Orlando, FL 32887.

KINGS PRODUCTIONS

The Kings Entertainment Company of Cincinnati is one of the largest producers of live shows for theme parks in North America. It produces shows for the following theme parks: Kings Dominion in Richmond, VA, Carowinds in Charlotte, NC, Great America in Santa Clara, CA, Kings Island in Cincinnati, OH, and Wonderland in Toronto, Ontario. Shows at Kings Productions sites usually run from March to December and generally are staged from 15 to 30 minutes, five to six times a day.

"Kings" hires over 700 theatrical people for its five theme parks. Actors, singers, dancers, instrumentalists, specialty acts, technicians, backstage personnel, hosts, hostesses, escorts, and others are auditioned during nationwide casting tours throughout the United States and Canada. Applicants must be at least 16 at the time of employment. The weekly pay scale is approximately $230 to $260 for singers, dancers, variety acts, and instrumentalists, $195 to $230 for technicians, and $150 to $210 for "walkabouts," hosts, hostesses, and escorts. Housing and transportation are not provided.

Kings Productions sponsors free seminars by leading show-business people, industrial shows for corporate clients, and a tour of the Orient and Europe in conjunction with the U.S. Department of Defense.

OPRYLAND

Over a dozen live musical productions go up at this park. Covering the full spectrum of American music, the multiple scenarios spotlight ballet, jazz, tap, gymnastics, and every conceivable musical motif. Singers, dancers, musicians, specialty acts, and technicians are recruited for shows that are witnessed by an audience of more than two million people.

Rehearsals begin in February and productions start in late March and run through early November. The pay scale runs from around $225 (audio engineers) to $533 (conductor/pianists) for a six-day work week. Rehearsal pay is hourly, and returning employees receive a salary advantage.

Opryland's 25-city audition tour starts in the fall and usually concludes in Nashville around early January.

SHOW BIZ INTERNATIONAL, INC.

Show Biz International, Inc. is an independent production company with long experience in coordinating family-style entertainment for theme parks. This Indiana-based group is at the forefront of four theme parks in the U.S. and Canada: Canobie Lake in Salem, NH, Darien Lake in Darien Center, NY, Holiday World in Santa Claus, IN, and Playland in Vancouver, BC.

The company hires approximately 400 seasonal employees, including directors, producers, writers, artists, choreographers, arrangers, costumers, designers, magicians, singers, dancers, musicians, and technicians, for a general package of musical extravaganzas, patriotic salutes, and Broadway-style blockbusters.

All those hired are under contract with their respective parks. Length of season is set by each site, opening as early as mid-April and as late as mid-June and extending past Labor Day, with some additional weekend work in October.

Salary at Show Biz International is from about $190 to around $400 a week; performers appear four to six times a day during a season that runs from mid-April through Labor Day, with some additional weekends in October.

SIX FLAGS

As one of the country's top five employers of young people, the Six Flags Corporation annually plays host to more than 16 million visitors nationwide. This company has been showcasing live productions since 1961. Six Flags operates seven theme parks featuring musical revues and family-oriented shows. The theme parks are: Astroworld in Houston, TX, Six Flags Great Adventure in Jackson, NJ, Six Flags Great America in Gurnee, IL, Six Flags Magic Mountain in Los Angeles, CA, Six Flags Over Georgia in Atlanta, GA, Six Flags Over Mid-America in Eureka, MO, and Six Flags Over Texas in Arlington, TX.

The Six Flags Corporation primarily hires singers and dancers, but also hires street entertainers, variety acts, musicians, off-beat vocalists, such as barbershop quartets, etc., and bands specializing in country-western, bluegrass, and ragtime. Pay rates average from $5.00 to $6.00 per hour. Seasons vary from park to park, though most performers are asked to work five-day work weeks during daily summertime operation and on weekends in the spring and fall.

WORLDS OF FUN

This theme park has hosted more than 18 million visitors since its inception in 1973. Worlds of Fun is geared to musical-theater and conducts auditions for singers and dancers in February. Rehearsals begin in mid-March for a season that runs from April through October. Salaries hover around $200 a week, and bonuses can run up to $700 for the season.

Theme Parks and Show Producers

The following is a list of theme parks and theme park show producers. They are listed alphabetically by the name of the park or production company. The names given are, in most cases, the entertainment coordinators at the parks.

ACTION PARK
P.O. Box 848
McAsee, NJ 07428

ALLAN ALBERT, INC.
561 Broadway
Suite 10C
New York, NY 10012
(212) 966-8881

ASTROWORLD
9001 Kirby Dr.
Houston, TX 77054
(713) 799-8404
Att: Michael Svatek

BOARDWALK AND
BASEBALL
P.O. Box 800
Orlando, FL 32802
(305) 648-5151, ext. 7222
Att: Bob LaPratt

BUSCH GARDENS—
THE DARK CONTINENT
P.O. Box 9158
Tampa, FL 33674-9158
(813) 988-5171
Att: Doug Braconnier

BUSCH GARDENS—
THE OLD COUNTRY
P.O. Drawer F.C.
Williamsburg, VA 23186
(804) 253-3300
Att: Linda Cuddihy

CEDAR POINT/THE
AMAZEMENT PARK
C.N. 5006
Sandusky, OH 44870
(419) 626-0830
Att: Gary Lensenmayer

CYPRESS GARDENS
P.O. Box 1
Cypress Gardens, FL 33884
(305) 351-5901
Att: Steven DeWoody

DISNEYLAND
1313 Harbor Blvd.
Anaheim, CA 92803
(714) 490-3125;
(714) 999-4000
Att: Dave Goodman

WALT DISNEY WORLD
P.O. Box 10,000
Lake Buena Vista, FL
32830
(305) 345-5745
Att: Larry Smith

WALT DISNEY WORLD/
EPCOT INSTITUTE
Auditions '89
P.O. Box 10,000
Lake Buena Vista, FL 32830
(305) 345-5755
Att: Bob Radock

DOLLYWOOD
700 Dollywood La.
Pigeon Forge, TN
37863-4101
(615) 428-9433
Att: Michael Padgett

HERSHEYPARK
100 West Hersheypark Dr.
Hershey, PA 17033
(717) 534-3349
Att: Bonnie Bosso

KINGS PRODUCTIONS
1932 Highland Ave.
Cincinnati, OH 45219
(513) 241-8989
Att: Dan Schultz

OPRYLAND
2802 Opryland Dr.
Nashville, TN 37214
(615) 871-6656
Att: Susan Bablove

SEA WORLD OF
FLORIDA
6277 Sea Harbor Dr.
Orlando, FL 32887
(305) 345-5168
Att: Entertainment Dept.

SEA WORLD OF OHIO
1100 Sea World Dr.
P.O. Box 237
Aurora, OH 44202
(216) 562-8101
Att: Entertainment Office

SEA WORLD OF
SAN DIEGO
1720 S. Shores Rd.,
Mission Bay
San Diego, CA 92109
(619) 222-6363
Att: Entertainment Dept.

SEA WORLD OF TEXAS
2548 Boardwalk
San Antonio, TX 78217
(512) 523-3000
Att: Henry Hartman

SESAME PLACE
100 Sesame Rd.
Langhorne, PA 19067
(215) 752-7070
Att: Greg Hartley

SHOW BIZ
INTERNATIONAL, INC.
5142 Old Boonville Highway
Evansville, IN 47715
(812) 473-0880
Att: Maria A. Rivers

SIX FLAGS
CORPORATION
SHOW PRODUCTIONS
1168 113th St.
Grand Prairie, TX 75050
(214) 988-8332

SIX FLAGS GREAT
ADVENTURE
P.O. Box 120
Jackson, NJ 08527
(201) 928-2200
Att: Show Operations

SIX FLAGS GREAT
AMERICA
P.O. Box 1776
Gurnee, IL 60031
(312) 249-1776, Ext. 4650
Att: David Carter

SIX FLAGS MAGIC
MOUNTAIN
P.O. Box 5500
Valencia, CA 91355
(805) 255-4858
Att: Show Operations

SIX FLAGS OVER
GEORGIA
P.O. Box 43187
Atlanta, GA 30378
(404) 948-9290
Att: Show Operations

SIX FLAGS OVER
MID-AMERICA
P.O. Box 666
Eureka, MO 63025
(314) 938-5300
Att: Show Operations

SIX FLAGS OVER TEXAS
P.O. Box 191
Arlington, TX 76004
(817) 640-8900
Att: Show Operations

WORLDS OF FUN
4545 Worlds of Fun Ave.
Kansas City, MO 64161
(816) 454-4545
Att: Gary Noble

Cruise Lines

by John Allen

Performers who are adventurous and who like to travel during the summer months might consider the possibility of working on a cruise ship. Cruise ship work offers many attractive features, such as travel to exotic ports of call in the Caribbean or South America, dancing and dining under the stars, a light work schedule, free time to explore new locations, sunbathing—in short, a pampered life on the high seas.

THE SHOWS

Cruise ships usually feature one of two kinds of shows—musical revues or Las Vegas-style revues. The better cruise lines, however, may run both types of shows on a single voyage. Within these contexts, two to four different shows may be offered (depending on the length of the cruise), each of which will be performed once during the cruise. Performers generally work two shows per evening (an early and a late show) three or four nights per week.

The musical revues on ships generally run 45 to 60 minutes and use from four to ten performers. They contain little substance but are well-produced with a lot of flash, and spectacular costumes. Glitz is very important on all ships.

Las Vegas-style revues consist of self-contained acts: always a comedian and a magician, and usually one or two other novelty acts. Between these acts showgirls make an appearance in exotic, skimpy costumes.

PAY

Pay on ships varies widely depending on the line. For showgirls and those in musical revues it can be as low as $200 per week or as high as $400 per week. Room and board are always free, but the quality of the rooms vary depending on whether you are put up in passenger or crew quarters. For single acts the pay ranges from $300 per week (per person) up to $1,000 per week or more, depending on the line, your experience, and your name. Performers are usually paid through the production company or agent who hired them, not the shipping line itself.

PERFORMANCE SPACE

Performance spaces on ships are generally less than ideal. In this sense, ships have one thing in common with New York City—there is not enough space. Performance space aboard ship often serves a number of different functions—that of ballroom, meeting room, game room, and so forth.

The room's design (or lack of it) will dictate much about the blocking of a show. Stages are usually set at floor level and the seats are not raked. Audiences are seated in the round and often are able to see performers from the waist up only. Sightlines are often so bad that shows may actually be seen well by only a few members of the audience, although they are usually enjoyed by all nevertheless.

DRESSING ROOMS

The best cruise lines provide adequate dressing rooms, but on many ships dressing room space is hardly satisfactory. Many ships have no dressing rooms whatsoever. In this case costume changes must be done in partial view of the passengers. Cramped, tiny spaces are the norm, with no running water or separate dressing areas for men and women.

On many ships performers must make up in their cabins. In such instances, the dressing room is used only for changes; even so, it is usually too small to comfortably accommodate everyone.

CRUISE STAFF HIERARCHY AND EXTRA DUTIES

Most performers aboard ship are hired as members of the cruise staff. As such, you, the performer, will be given duties that are not directly connected to your function as an entertainer. (The exception to this is those performers who are hired as an act. Because of their investments in costumes, material, charts for the band, and so on, they are not given other duties.)

The Cruise Director will be your immediate boss and will be in charge of distributing cruise staff duties. The cruise director deals with problems and conflicts among the staff and will also host many of the games and activities at which you will help. Additionally, the Cruise Director is assisted by a Social Hostess (or two) and a number of Assistant Cruise Directors. You will find yourself assisting all of these people during your cruise staff duties.

CRUISE STAFF DUTIES

The cruise staff is technically on call 24 hours a day, although obviously such demands will not be made upon your time. Most ships have some sort of equitable distribution of extra-duty activities so that even *heavy* schedules will require no more than three hours of extra work per day. This may cut into your sunbathing time, but it certainly cannot compare with the work required in most non-Equity stock situations.

So, what are these dreaded duties? Let's see, there's *library*. Yes, you may have to spend 30 minutes twice a day in a room with books in it and check them out to the two or three passengers who might want to do a little reading. Or there is *bingo*. No, you probably won't call the game, but you may have to walk among the crowd and call out the winning card. And then there is *horseracing*, (ship style) where you might have to move wooden horses along a track.

Each ship has its own stash of standard and original games which you will probably have to help with. None of them are taxing or difficult and if you let yourself go you will probably enjoy them.

SOCIALIZING

As in many summer stock situations you may be expected to do a certain amount of socializing. On a ship you are always in the public eye and are seen as a representative of the ship. As such you will be required to be dressed properly at all times, to be helpful and courteous to the passengers, and to be ready to sit and chat with them whenever they want to.

EMBARKATION/DISEMBARKATION

There are two cruise staff duties which are definitely no fun. They are disembarkation and embarkation. Anytime that people must wait in lines they will be unhappy, and the lines are slow and long when the passengers are boarding at the start of the cruise and when they leave the ship at the end of the cruise. Additionally, when disembarking there are customs, rules and officials to deal with, which means more lines, more waiting, and more dissatisfaction.

At these times you may be required to direct the passengers, keep the peace, answer questions, and you will be expected to be courteous and pleasant, no matter what the circumstances.

SEASICKNESS

If you suffer from motion sickness when in a car or airplane, be sure to take some Dramamine with you. If this remedy helps you on land, it may do the trick on water, too. Just be sure to take it *before* the ship starts rocking!

Most passengers get used to the motion of the ship in just one or two crossings. Some people, however, experience chronic sea-sickness. For them, any rough crossing can be miserable, Dramamine or not.

OTHER CULTURES

Most cruise ships are owned and operated by foreign companies. This means that on almost every ship the vast majority of the crew are not Americans, even though most of the passengers are, and that most of the crew speak little, if any, English. Be prepared to be in a minority and to encounter some trouble in communicating. On some ships, crew members whose English improves are promoted to positions where they are more in contact with English-speaking passengers.

On many ships there is an unofficial caste system. Almost all of the cabin stewards, cocktail waiters and waitresses are from third world countries. They work 14 to 16 hours per day and are paid an unconscionably small amount. The restaurant employees come mostly from western countries. They are paid better but work just as hard. Casino workers, on the other hand, receive good pay, and work reasonable hours. A high percentage of Americans are frequently employed as casino workers.

The cruise staff and entertainers are usually mostly British or American (with the exception of the bands, which come from various countries), receive good pay, and have a light work schedule. Exceptions among the cruise staff are the Cruise Director, Assistant Cruise Directors, and Social Hostesses, who are paid well but earn it the hard way, sometimes working as much as 14 hours in a day. Some vessels are staffed almost entirely from the country of origin, so there is less disparity in pay and more cohesion among the crew. These ships are generally more organized and easier to work on. Of course, the exposure to different cultures can be exciting and enjoyable, as long as you remember that "your way" (or "the American Way") is not necessarily the only or the best way to do things.

WORKING ATMOSPHERE

It is the officers who set the tone for the interpersonal relations among the crew. Some officers are personable, and promote an open and congenial atmosphere where information and camaraderie are shared. Other officers, however, can be cold and arrogant. Their style is abrupt and dictatorial. They enforce a plethora of rules that have no rhyme or reason. It is hard to get accurate information from them and the lack of communication on their ships is extremely frustrating. The general tone on ships run by such officers can be unpleasant.

All ships use a fining system to enforce the rules. These rules must be followed—at sea the captain and his officers are in *charge*. Your American citizenship will not give you privileged status and will not exempt you from rules and regulations, even when some of them are petty.

About 90 percent of the ship's crew are not allowed in public areas, except to work. They live in crew quarters, eat in crew messes, and drink in the crew bar; even during leisure hours they are *not* allowed in the areas where the passengers are. Entertainers, musicians, and the cruise staff, on the other hand, are encouraged to socialize with the passengers. Officers and security personnel are always permitted access to passenger areas.

LIVING QUARTERS

Almost all crew members are housed in crew quarters. A ship is a finite space, so even passenger cabins can be small. Crew cabins are *always* small, and shared; they usually contain one or two sets of bunk beds and often do not have a bathroom—bathrooms in crew areas are dormitory style.

On many ships, however, entertainers are housed in passenger cabins. Although they too, must be shared, these cabins are still larger than the crew cabins and do have a private bathroom.

Most of the crew are only allowed to eat in the crew messes, i.e, dining rooms, of which there may be three or four. These are sometimes set up internationally; for example, there may be an Italian mess, a Greek mess, a Caribbean mess, or even a Bangladesh mess. The officers' messes are always separate from the crew's messes.

As an entertainer, however, you may have the option, or you may even be required, to eat in the passengers' restaurant, although in a section reserved for the staff. You will be able to order from the same menus as the passengers and enjoy the same service as they do which, incidentally, is generally slow! Entertainers are also permitted to eat at the buffets, teas, and so forth, which are provided regularly for the passengers. Most crew members are excluded from such activity.

Although your food and cabin are free, on some lines you are still expected to tip the waiter and cabin steward a nominal amount. Tips should be a minimum of $1 per meal to your waiter and $10 per week to your steward.

DRESS CODES

A strict dress code is enforced on every ship. On some nights formal attire is required. On these nights men are expected to wear a tux or suit. There are "informal" and "casual" occasions, too. Only when you get off the ship can you dress as you please.

SHIP HOSPITALS

Cruise ship hospitals are equipped with a doctor and one or two nurses. Soon after your arrival you will be given a cursory exam by the head nurse in order to record your medical history and to check your physical condition.

Unfortunately, cruise hospital staffs are more capable of dealing with seasickness than any real ailment and are either unwilling or unable to deal effectively with most illnesses. Salaries for doctors and nurses are below standard, so that the most highly qualified among them are not always attracted to employment on cruise ships. Diagnostic equipment aboard ship is minimal and ship hospitals carry only limited supplies. To make matters worse, nurses may be severely limited in what they are allowed to do. For example, a nurse may only be permitted to administer seasickness shots and to help people on and off the ship. All these factors add up to poor medical treatment. This situation does not bode well if you have a history of illness. If you are not in top physical condition, you should think twice before setting sail on a cruise ship.

PERKS

A great perk that some ships offer is that your friends and family can sail for about half price. The fare is paid in *cash* to the Chief Purser, which raises some thought-provoking questions. Is this transaction recorded or isn't it? Is it accounted for or not? Perhaps it does not matter. Even if you are "greasing the wheels" your friend will still be able to get on board! The person to ask about this perk is the cruise director.

Another perk that cruise ships offer entertainers is free time. Although the staff cannot sunbathe with passengers, ships do reserve a spot where the staff can sunbathe. You are also allowed in the public areas in your free time even though you are not allowed to congregate in those areas with other staff members. And, of course, your cabin can be your retreat and you can spend free time there.

SAFETY ON THE SEAS

Inevitably, the question of the safety on board these cruise ships will enter your mind. And if it doesn't before you take the job, it certainly will after you experience your first rough crossing. No matter how big and stable the ship looks (and some can seem like a small city), when the sea is rough that ship will rock—and that will make you wonder. Tragedies on cruise ships are very rare, but occasionally a mishap will occur. One summer a ship off the Miami coast was evacuated due to fire. Five years ago an Alaska-bound ship was evacuated. It is infrequent, but disaster can happen.

By far the greatest cause for concern on a ship is fire. Collisions are unlikely and the seas are well-charted so that running aground is also uncommon. But fire is a potential hazard on every ship because of factors like electricity, cooking done in restaurants, and cigarette smokers.

In case of fire, heavy metal doors acting as fire screen doors can be shut automatically from the bridge. These doors can contain a fire in a specific area. Fire screen doors are, however, difficult to open manually, because they are so heavy, and on some ships they may even lock. Nevertheless, they can usually be forced open with brute force if you find yourself on the wrong side in an emergency.

LIFE JACKETS, LIFE BOATS AND SAFETY DRILLS

All ships are required to have safety drills for crew and passengers *before* the ship reaches the open seas. (Cruises to nowhere are not required to have these drills.)

Unfortunately, no matter how well-trained the crew is, passengers rarely take these drills seriously.

International regulations and agreements dictate that ships must carry enough life jackets for every single person aboard—and there must be sufficient life boats to accommodate the entire crew and all passengers. On the surface these rules are followed. Unfortunately, compliance on paper does not guarantee a safe ship. Frequently crews are not well-trained in safety procedures. Maintenance may be poor on lifeboats and the crew may not be regularly rehearsed in their operation. There have been recent reports of engines in lifeboats breaking down; in one incident crew members had forgotten to put the plugs in a boat, and the boat began to take on water—and passengers were aboard! In these incidents no one was hurt, but the potential for tragedy was there.

The likelihood of an incident at sea is remote but be aware that it can happen. Take safety instructions and drills seriously, and make it your business to know what to do in an emergency.

AN INTERNATIONAL FAMILY

In the best of circumstances living on a ship can be a very rewarding experience. When you see a thousand new faces each week, those faces which are familiar become very important. Because of this, crew members share a closely-knit bond. Wonderful friendships can occur among people from different cultures, and you may discover that you have become a member of an international family.

In the worst of circumstances where the quarters are close, where no sense of unity exists among the crew, and where the staff is discontent, life aboard a ship can be unbearable.

As in most situations, your own attitude can make a huge difference to the outcome of your shipboard adventure. If you are a picky eater, if you hate sharing a room, if you detest dormitory-style bathrooms, then a cruise ship may not be for you. But if you are easy-going and are willing to trade a few comforts and a few hours of work each day for good pay, sun time, some socializing and free trips to the vacation wonderlands of the world, then cruise work could be perfect for you.

Cruise Lines

Entertainment Directors

Many cruise lines employ an Entertainment Director to handle entertainment bookings for its ships. The responsibilities of this position may vary from one line to another, and from one season to the next. Sometimes Entertainment Directors book talent directly; at other times they book solely through agents.

Even if you have already contacted cruise agents and producers it would probably be worthwhile to contact cruise lines you are interested in directly. Send pictures and resumes to the Entertainment Director, unless otherwise specified below. Don't send tapes or other materials unless they are requested.

ADMIRAL CRUISES
1220 Biscayne Blvd
Miami, FL 33132
(305) 374-1611
Hires novelty acts; singers. Director of Entertainment: William Yule.

AMERICAN HAWAII CRUISES
550 Kearny St.
San Francisco, CA 94108
(415) 392-9400
Submit entertainment inquiries to: Personnel Department: 604 Fort St., Honolulu HI 96813

BERMUDA STAR LINES
1086 Teaneck Rd.
Teaneck, N.J. 07666
(201) 837-0400
Variety artists, musical prod'n revues. All inquiries to Gerard Purcell & Assoc., Attn: Donald Tabler, 210 E. 51 St. New York, NY 10022

CARNIVAL CRUISE LINES
5225 N.W. 87th Ave.
Miami, FL 33178-2198
(305) 599-2600
Hires entertainer/cruise director, entertainers, musicians. Address pictures, resumes, and tapes to Tom Lacey. Musicians, contact Rob Waterfield, music supervisor.

CHANDRIS FANTASY CRUISES
900 Third Ave.
New York, NY 10022
(212) 223-3003
Entertainment Director: Fofy Lampropoulos.

COSTA CRUISES
One Biscayne Tower
Miami, FL 33131
(305) 358-7330
Entertainment hired through Caribbean Cruise Management (See Agents & Producers).

CUNARD LINE
555 Fifth Ave.
New York, NY 10017
(212) 880-7500
Hires singers, comedians, specialty acts, classical entertainers. Also uses musicians (only duos/trios), dancers (hired in Europe), piano bar performers, dance teams. Books through Garry Brown Associates or Bramson Entertainment (See Agents and Producers).

HOLLAND AMERICA LINE
300 Elliot Ave. West
Seattle, WA 98119
(206) 281-3535
Books through Bramson Entertainment Bureau.

NORWEGIAN CARIBBEAN LINE
2 Alhambra Plaza
Miami, FL 33131
(305) 447-9660
In-house production department (Jean Ann Ryan Prods.) produces revues. Also books shows produced outside and variety acts. Hires through open auditions, agents. Accepts pictures, resumes, tapes. Variety performers should contact M.A. Prod'ns.

OCEAN CRUISE LINES
1510 S.E. 17th St.
Ft. Lauderdale, FL 33316
(305) 764-3500
Bookings made only in London:
447-723-5557

PREMIER CRUISE LINES
101 George King Blvd.
Cape Canaveral, FL 32920
(407) 783-5061
Casts thru independent producers for themed musical revues. Also books cabaret artists, mainly comedians and novelty acts. Submissions of promo material accepted; send attn: Jim Flynn, Entertainment Director.

PRINCESS CRUISES
2029 Century Park East, Suite 3000
Los Angeles, CA 90067
(213) 553-1770
Cruises to Caribbean, Mexico, S. America, Alaska, Mediterranean. Hires vocalists, comedians, duos, trios, magicians. Also produces in-house revues. Send tapes (audio and VHS) and resumes to Entertainment Department.

REGENCY CRUISES
260 Madison Ave.
New York, NY 10016
(212) 972-4774
Hires production groups, dancers, comedians, novelty acts. Casting through independent producers, agents, or direct submissions. Entertainers frequently double as cruise staff. Contact: Joe McGrath, Entertainment Director.

ROYAL CARIBBEAN CRUISE LINE
903 South America Way
Miami, FL 33132
(305) 379-2601
Hires dance teams, DJs, singers, novelty acts. Robin Netscher, Entertainment Manager.

ROYAL CRUISE LINE
One Maritime Plaza, Suite 660
San Francisco, CA 94111
(415) 956-7200
Hires vocalists, cabaret performers, bands, variety acts through Bramson. (See Agents & Producers.) Also hires fully produced revues.

ROYAL VIKING LINE
750 Battery St.
San Francisco, CA 94111
(415) 398-8000
Hires variety and cabaret-type acts: comics, ventriloquists, classical artists, jugglers, vocalists, instrumentalists. Talent booked directly, as well as through agencies worldwide. Send materials to Greg Von Seeger.

SEAESCAPE, LTD
1080 Port Blvd., Port of Miami
Miami, FL 33132
(305) 377-9000
Hires singer/dancers for four different 45-minute revues. Two shows per day, six days per week. Entertainers live on ship with crew; four-month contracts. Uses in-house production department. (See Agents & Producers.) Contact: Gene Hull, Dir. of Entertainment; Robin Cahill, Mgr. of Entertainment.

SITMAR CRUISES
10100 Santa Monica Blvd.
Los Angeles, CA 90067
(213) 553-1666
Hires vocalists, comics, magicians, Broadway-type revues. Also uses classical pianists, jazz singers, strolling strings, etc. Books revues and entertainers through inquiries in writing to Bruce Krumrine, Dir. of Passenger Programs. Musicians: contact Abe Weinstein, 1500 Bay Rd. #1239, Miami, FL 33139. DJs: contact Don Blanton, 17011 Beach Blvd., #800, Huntington Beach, CA 92647.

SUN LINE CRUISES
One Rockefeller Plaza, Suite 315
New York, NY 10020
(212) 397-6400
Hires singers, dancers, dance groups, comedians, magicians. Cruises to Caribbean and Europe. Contact: Tina Smith, Entertainment Director.

Cruise Agents and Producers

Many cruise lines will hire a booking agent to put together an entertainment package for a particular cruise. Some work exclusively with one agent; others use both booking agents and their own Entertainment Director to fill their entertainment needs.

Agents and Entertainment Directors, in turn, may book revues, acts, or shows produced by an independent production company. A couple of larger cruise lines work exclusively with their own in-house producer. Most, however, rely on shows produced by independent contractors.

Performers interested in cruise work, no matter what their specialty, should introduce themselves to cruise agents *and* producers.

AUGMAR INC.
200 W. 54th St., #55
New York, NY 10019
(212) 757-7577
Augie & Margo Rodriguez produce revues thru Gerard W. Purcell & Assoc.

BRAMSON ENTERTAINMENT BUREAU
1440 Broadway
New York, NY 10018
(212) 354-9575
President: Ephraim Abramson; VP: James Abramson. Largest booking organization for cruise work. Books comedians, 'big name' entertainers, novelty acts, singers, musicians. Books shows, revues from independent producers. Books for such cruise lines as Cunard, Sitmar, Holland America, Ocean Cruise and Royal Cruise. Accepts videotapes, VHS or ¾", especially of novelty acts, comedians.

CARIBBEAN CRUISE MANAGEMENT, INC.
World Trade Center
80 S.W. 8th St., Suite 2640
Miami, FL 33131-3097
(305) 374-0990
Vice President of Entertainment: Felice Campagna. Hires entertainers for Costa Cruises.

FIESTA FANTASTICA
1637 S.W. 27th Ave.
Miami, FL 33145
(305) 854-2221
Producer: Marcelo Productions. Books individual singers and dancers for revues (no variety, specialty or solo acts) for Holland America cruise line. Holds open calls. Accepts pictures, resumes, and tapes. Send to: Marcelo Palacio, Paul McEvoy.

G&C ENTERTAINMENT
P.O. Box 1063 Ansonia Station
New York, NY 10023
(212) 874-4770
Casts for cruise line performers: singers, magicians, specialty acts.

GARRY BROWN ASSOCIATES
27 Downs Side, Cheam, Surrey
SM2 7EH England
01-643-3991/8375
Agent: Garry Brown. Books variety acts, stars, revues, other entertainment for Cunard Line. Holds showcases in New York, other major cities seeking talent. Watch Back Stage for announcements. Accepts pictures, tapes, videos (American, English, European VHS).

GERARD W. PURCELL & ASSOCIATES
210 E. 51st St.
New York, NY 10022
(212) 421-2670
Agent: Donald Tabler. Books variety acts; places cruise staff for various cruise lines. Contract is with individual cruise line. Accepts pictures and resumes. Entertainment consultants for several cruise lines.

IMPACT PRODUCTIONS
133 W. 72nd St., Suite 601
New York, NY 10023
(212) 874-0960
Producer: Joyce Flynn. Produces musical shows, revues for cruise lines and corporate events. Contract is with individual cruise line. Hires dancers and singers for both cruise work and corporate shows. Holds open calls; watch for announcements. Accepts pictures, resumes and tapes. Send attn: Joyce Flynn.

JEAN ANN RYAN PRODUCTIONS
308 S.E. 14th St.
Fort Lauderdale, FL 33316
(305) 523-6399
Producer: Jean Ann Ryan; General Manager: Joanne Maiello. Produces revues, Broadway-style productions for Norwegian Cruise Lines. Producing 42nd Street *for S.S. Norway, and* A Chorus Line *for M.S. Seaward. Cabaret and novelty acts booked. Also hires technical staff. Major audition tours twice each year; New York in autumn and January. Performers with resumes on file will be notified about auditions. Contracts for six months.*

MCL PRODUCTIONS
165 W. 46th St., Suite 1211A
New York, NY 10036
(212) 921-9488
Agents: Chip Lavely, John Arcangeli. Produces Broadway, Hollywood, Decades, *and* Baggy Pants *revues; magic shows; star packages. Shows booked by Bramson Entertainment Bureau, and directly with lines. Accepts pictures, resumes, and tapes. Holds two or three open calls per year. Contracts talent for four months.*

MILLER-REICH ENTERPRISES
1922 N.E. 149th St.
North Miami, FL 33181
(305) 949-0227
Agent: Leonard Miller. Books dancers and singers for Carnival Cruise Lines and Royal Caribbean Cruise Lines. Produces lavish Vegas-style shows as well as B'way concepts. Auditions held mostly in New York (at least six times yearly), and in London (two or three times yearly). Long-term contracts (one-year) are with Miller-Reich Enterprises. Accepts pictures, resumes, tapes, videos and C.V. Also accepts resumes from technical staff.

SEAESCAPE, LTD.
1080 Port Blvd., Port of Miami
Miami, FL 33132
(305) 377-9000
In-house production company for SeaEscape Ltd. Produces thematically constructed revues. Contracts are from 3 to 6 months. Accepts pictures, tapes, and resumes. Contact: Gene Hull, Director of Entertainment; Robin Cahill, Manager of Entertainment.

SHERIDAN VENTURES
306 W. 18th St.
New York, NY 10011
John Sheridan works as an independent producer for Chandris Cruise Lines.

PETER GREY TERHUNE PRESENTS
P.O. Box 715
Cape Canaveral, FL 32920
(407) 783-8745
Co-producers: Peter Terhune, Cathy Abram. Produces custom revues, shows for cruise lines, industrials, resorts. Average talent contract is for five months. Accepts pictures, resumes, and tapes. Auditions in NY, Nashville, Florida, colleges, and universities. Seeks singer/dancers with "wholesome" appearance. Shows booked by Bramson Entertainment or independently with cruise lines.

Summer Stock: Combined Auditions

by Jill Charles

Combined auditions are the means by which many summer stock companies fulfill their casting requirements. These auditions are held at central locations in different parts of the country, and representatives, such as managers and producers, from various theater companies gather at the audition sites to audition and interview the performers and theater personnel they are going to need during the coming season.

Listed here are 20 locations where state and regional combined auditions are held for summer stock companies throughout the country. If you don't have an Equity card yet, and you've been frustrated at not being able to get auditions, now is your chance, since the bulk of representatives attending these regional combined auditions are from non-Equity companies. Do you double as a carpenter, costumer, or lighting designer? You may be able to parlay your technical skills into a full season somewhere with an acting/tech combination that will actually leave you with money in your pocket come Labor Day. This is a good time, too, if you have honed your special skills, like singing, dancing, stage combat, or juggling, to take advantage of some unique theatrical opportunities offered by outdoor dramas and Renaissance Faires.

So, look over the list below, and start applying for audition slots. Many of these auditions are nothing but "cattle calls," true, but it's an efficient way of being seen by many companies. Combined auditions also present an excellent opportunity to test your audition technique, which is also a good reason for trying to get to more than one audition.

COMBINED AUDITION PROCEDURES

In general, this is the way combined auditions work: you write to the given address, usually several months in advance of the audition and request an application form. When you receive your application you fill it out and return it with an application fee. If your application is early enough, and you are not screened out (screening is usually based on a minimal level of experience), you will be given an audition time. At callbacks, after the audition, if the company likes your work, you will be: a) scheduled for a second audition to take place at a future date; b) offered a job then and there; or c) contacted later for another audition or with a job offer.

Director, designers, stage managers, management persons, and technicians, are usually interviewed at separate times from the performers' auditions. There are various mechanisms for doing this, but the first step is always the application, and the organization running the combined auditions will take it from there.

Many of the auditions listed here are regional auditions, run by a state or regional theater organization. Some require that you be a resident of, or attending school in the state or region holding the auditions. You may have to join the regional organization to be eligible to participate in the auditions. Many of these regional auditions are held as a part of that regions' annual conference. You should write several months in advance of the auditions, as most of them have deadlines for receiving the application of at least one month beforehand.

Audition rosters fill up quickly, so even if your application is made by the deadline date, you still are not guaranteed an audition. If you don't get an audition, sometimes you can be placed on a waiting list; or you can stand by at the audition in the hope that there will be a last minute opening.

At a typical combined audition you will encounter 30 to 50 producers and directors. With so many persons involved, and because of the strict time limitations on auditions this imposes, it is crucial to come into the situation well-prepared in all respects. The following guidelines are directed toward the special problems presented by these auditions.

1. Follow directions: Read the application carefully and fill it out correctly. Because of space and time limitations, all applications are not accepted, and incomplete applications are usually rejected automatically.

2. Research the companies: Along with your audition notification, you should receive a tentative list of the companies for whom you will be auditioning. Find out what these companies are all about and then gear your audition pieces toward those companies that you are interested in. Prepare a classical piece if you are auditioning for a Shakespearean troupe, or a song and dance routine if you are trying to get into a musical comedy company.

3. Prepare your pieces: Be well-prepared. You should know your pieces thoroughly at least two weeks before the audition. *Never* make the mistake of performing a monologue that you learned the night before—at an audition that's a guaranteed way of going up on your lines.

4. Photo/Resumes: Take a good supply of 8×10 photo/resumes to the audition. Make sure that vital statistics are up-to-date and accurate, especially your contact phone number.

5. Sheet Music: Sheet music must be in good condition and clearly marked for the accompanist. Not all accompanists can transpose music at sight, so it is especially important that your music be in the right key.

6. Dress: Dress as you would for any audition. Present yourself as a person, not as the character you are performing—wear something flattering that makes you feel good. The mistake women most often make is to wear a leotard or something revealing; the mistake men most often make is to underdress, to wear old jeans and a T-shirt.

7. Audition Introduction: The way you enter, look at the auditors, and say your name and the title and character of the piece you're doing are as important as the audition itself. Don't explain the piece; be yourself.

8. Be professional: Your manner should demonstrate confidence, competence, and a pleasant personality. Take the time to be nice to those whom you meet, from the people at the registration desk, to the timekeepers, to the gofers, to the company representatives, to your colleagues.

9. Attitude: Remember that the auditors are not your enemies. They are there to cast their seasons, and they want you to be good. Keeping this in mind will help you to approach the audition with a positive attitude.

10. Callbacks: Try to make it to any and all callbacks. If time restrictions or scheduling prevent you from attending, contact any company you are interested in and try to set up another appointment. When you are speaking with a company that has shown some interest in you, get as much exact information as you can about what they are offering. Make written notes. Combined audition weekends are chaotic events, and details of important meetings and conversations can be difficult to re-collect; written notes will prove to be an indispensable source of reference once you are back in your home environment.

Combined Audition Sites

ASSOCIATION OF KANSAS THEATRE
Auditions: *usually in late February*
Place: *rotates through different locations in the state*
Write for Application to: *Louise Hanson, Executive Director*
Association of Kansas Theater
1628 Dudley Ct.
Lawrence, KS 66044
(913) 842-3502
Deadline: pre-registration required, 2 weeks before auditions
Eligibility: open to anyone
Fee: no fee for AKT members: $15 fee for non-members
Format: 2 min. for short dramatic reading, dance combination or movement, and/or song (bring well-marked music, accompaniment provided); Performers bring 12 photo/resumes
Interviews for tech/design (bring portfolio & resume)

BAY AREA REGIONAL AUDITIONS
(San Francisco & Bay Area companies)
Auditions: *preliminary auditions in February, final auditions in March*
Place: *Bay Area theater*
Write for Application to: Theater Bay Area
2940 16th St., Suite #102
San Francisco, CA 94103
(415) 621-0427
Eligibility: for Bay Area actors only.

GREAT LAKES THEATER CONFERENCE (GLTC)
(Companies in 5 member states: IL, WI, IN, OH, MI)
Auditions: *sometime in March*
Place: *varies*
Write for Application to: Great Lakes Theater Conference
Barbara Evans, Auditions Coordinator
Hanover College, Box 2
Hanover, IN 47243
Eligibility: Applicant must participate in one of the statewide auditions at one of the 5 member states listed above. A maximum of 125 applicants are selected after screening at these state auditions.
Fee: $5 eligibility fee payable at state auditions $15 audition fee payable at GLTC.
Format: 2 monologues, song (optional), maximum of 4 minutes; Performers only, no technician interviews.

ILLINOIS THEATER ASSOCIATION
Auditions: *early March*
Place: *Chicago location*
Write for Application to: *Mr. Wallace Smith, Executive Director*
Illinois Theater Association
1225 West Belmont
Chicago, IL 60657
(312) 929-7288
Applicants who pass the audition are eligible for GLTC Auditions (see above) if desired.

INDIANA THEATER ASSOCIATION
Auditions: *Early February*
Place: *rotates through Indiana colleges*
Write for Application to: *Barbara Evans, Executive Director*
Hanover College, P.O. Box 2
Hanover, IN 47243
Deadline: usually in January
Eligibility: Applicant must be a member of a professional union, or be recommended by a professional director. Applicants under 17 years of age must attend a screening.
Fee: $15 for state residents; $20 for out-of-state.
Format: singing or non-singing: 2 minute limit, interviews for tech/design/management
Applicants who pass the audition are eligible for GLTC Auditions (see above) if desired.

LEAGUE OF RESIDENT THEATER (LORT) LOTTERY AUDITIONS
These are Eligible Performer auditions which are held twice a year in New York City for the fall/winter and spring/summer seasons. Contact AEA at 165 West 46th St., NYC 10036. Since there are more applicants than available audition slots, selection is made by lottery. There are also interviews for Stage Managers. LORT theaters are required to attend by Equity.

MICHIGAN THEATER ASSOCIATION
Statewide Professional Theater Auditions
Auditions: *late February*
Place: *rotates throughout the state*
Write for Application to: Michigan Theater Association
Box 734
Marshall, MI 49068
(616) 781-7933
Application Deadline: early February
Eligibility: at least 20 years of age or college sophomore.
Fee: $30 plus additional $5 (non-refundable) for adjudication into Great Lakes Theater Conference GLTC
Format: Each audition will be limited to 2 min. and will include two contrasting monologues. Applicant may add 16 bars of song after time limit; optional dance auditions; tech interviews arranged.
Applicants who pass the audition are eligible for GLTC auditions (see above).

MID-AMERICA THEATER CONFERENCE AUDITIONS
(Includes MN, IA, MO, ND, SD, NE, KS)
Auditions: *mid-March*
Place: *Auditions are held in the states listed above.*
Write for Application to: *Kennis Wessel, Coordinator*
Dept. of Theater & Media
317 Murphy Hall
University of Kansas
Lawrence, KS 60045
Application Deadline: Early February (If audition slots are available after the cut-off date, later applicants will receive time slots on a first-come, first-served basis.)
Eligibility: no residency requirement
Fee: $5 audition fee if member of MATC if non-member, $18.50 for students, $35 for non-students.
Format: 2 minutes, with or without song; pianist provided. Bring music in the correct key. Singing/dancing auditions are held at the end of each day.

MIDWEST THEATER AUDITIONS
(Sponsor: Conservatory of Theater Arts, Webster University: 60 companies)
Auditions: *mid-February, 3 days.*
Place: *Loretto-Hilton Theater, Webster University, St. Louis, MO.*
Write for Application to: *Peter Sargent, Coordinator*
                              Midwest Theater Auditions
                              Webster University
                              470 E. Lockwood
                              St. Louis, MO 63119
Application Deadline: early January
Eligibility: No residency requirements
Non-Equity application form signed by an instructor or director; Dance calls are only open to actors who have auditioned previously that day. AEA: members may audition and should request application.
Fee: $20 for Non-Equity actors.
$20 for Design/Tech applicants.
Bring at least 20 copies of resumes (photo resumes for callbacks only).
Format: 2 min. to present 1 or 2 pieces; at least one must be non-musical though musical pieces are encouraged; pianist will be provided. Callbacks same day.

MONTANA SUMMER THEATER AUDITIONS
(approximately 6–8 companies)
Dates: *early March*
Place: *rotates through Montana colleges*
Write for Application to: *Jim Bartruff, President*
                              MSTA
                              P.O. Box 1456
                              Billings, MT 59103
Registration: on day of auditions
Eligibility: Non-Equity; no residency requirements
Fee: $25
Format: 3 minutes for 2 contrasting pieces and 16 bars of a song. (Note: at least 3 of the companies are looking specifically for musical talent.)

NEW ENGLAND THEATER CONFERENCE (NETC)
(includes approximately 60 companies, from New England and the East Coast)
Audition Dates: *mid- to late March*
Place: *Tufts University, or another Boston location*
Write for Application: (Send SASE; no phone calls)
                              Marie Philips, Exec. Sec'y.
                              NETC Central
                              50 Exchange St.
                              Waltham, MA 02154
Application Deadline: mid-February
Eligibility: Non-Equity; College students must be 18 years of age or older; application form must be signed by an Instructor or Director. (About 1,350 applications are received— 650–700 applicants are auditioned.)
Fee: $15 for NETC members, $25 for non-members
Format: two audition rooms run concurrently; one for acting; one for acting/singing (/dancing); 2 min. auditions Technical & staff auditions are held Sunday or Monday afternoons. Equity auditions are held in the fall, organized by StageSource: P.O. Box 72, Essex Station, Boston, MA 02112.ʻ no phone calls.

NEW JERSEY THEATER GROUP

An association of the state's professional (AEA) theater companies. (This is a Theater Conference with a Job Fair, for interns and entry level technical and management staff in April (no auditions).

For more information, write (after Jan. 1) to: *Laura Aden, Executive Director*
New Jersey Theater Group
6 Afton Drive
Florham Park, NJ 07932
or call (201) 593-0189

NORTHWEST DRAMA CONFERENCE

(7 companies in WA, OR, AK, ID, the Northwest)
Auditions: *early February, part of regional theater conference*
Place: *rotates throughout various colleges in the Northwest*
Write for Application to: *George Caldwell, Coordinator*
Drama Dept., Washington State University
Pullman, WA 99164-2432
Application Deadline: no deadline; sign up at Conference
Eligibility: Non-Equity
Fee: none
Format: 2 pieces showing variety; 5 min. total, bring photo resume.

OHIO THEATER ALLIANCE

(30 companies attend)
Auditions: *Mid- to late February*
Place: *rotates throughout the state*
Write for Application to: (Please include SASE)
Fran Bay, Executive Director, OTA
504 N. Park St.
Columbus, OH 43215
Deadline: mid-January
Eligibility: must be OTA member, must be pre-registered Equity or Non-Equity
Fee: audition fee $10; OTA membership fee $10 for students, $20 for non-students. Fees must be paid by money order or certified check.
Format: 3 min.; must bring own accompaniment tape & player, if singing; Callbacks same day, interviews for tech and management, no separate dance auditions
Applicants who pass the audition are eligible for GLTC auditions (see above).

OUTDOOR DRAMA AUDITIONS

(Sponsor: Institute of Outdoor Drama; companies in IL, KY, MN, NC, OH, OK, TN, TX, WV)
Auditions: *mid-March*
Place: *University of North Carolina at Chapel Hill, NC.*
Write for Application to: (Enclose SASE)
Auditions Director
Institute of Outdoor Drama
CB 3240, Graham Memorial
University of North Carolina
Chapel Hill, NC 27599-3240
(919) 962-1328
Application Deadline: around March 1
Eligibility: Auditions are limited to 200 pre-registered applicants who must be at least 18 years of age and who have had previous theater training or credits. A statement of support

from a teacher or director is required.

Companies: 15 to 18 companies, majority are non-Equity, some are AEA; most casts number about 50; seasons run 12 to 14 weeks

Fee: $10 non-refundable application fee

Format: Actors—1 min. monologue; Singers—1 prepared number (accompanist provided); Dancers—group warm-up led by choreographer, combinations using modern, ballet, and folk choreography; Technicians—individual interviews.

ROCKY MOUNTAIN THEATER ASSOCIATION SUMMER THEATER AUDITIONS
(Includes ID, MT, WY, CO, UT)

Auditions: *early February (part of RMTA's "Festivention")*
Place: *University of Wyoming at Laramie*
Write for Application to: *c/o E. C. Reynolds*
                         Dept. of Theater & Dance
                         Box 3951 University Station
                         Laramie, WY 82071

Deadline: early January, or register at Festivention

Eligibility: application must include recommendation from faculty member or home institution.

Fee: $10 membership fee to join RMTA.

Fee for Festivention registration & audition before Dec. 8 is $17 for students, $25 for non-students. After Jan 4, add $3.

Format: Acting only—4 minutes, 2 contrasting monologues; Musical—6 minutes, 2 monologues plus 16 bars of song; accompaniment provided; Technical/Design/Staff interviews.

SOUTHEASTERN THEATER CONFERENCE
(Includes: AL, FL, GA, KY, MS, NC, SC, TN, VA, WV: approximately 80 companies)

Auditions: *early March, part of SETC Convention.*
Place: *rotates throughout the states*
Write for Information to: *Marian Smith, SETC*
                         311 McIver St.
                         University of North Carolina at Greensboro
                         Greensboro, NC 27412

Eligibility: Students must pass state screening; forms may be obtained from college theater department in the early fall—screening takes place in the fall at state theater meetings. Professionals write directly to SETC for applications form; deadline around February (SETC also holds AEA auditions in September; application deadline is April 15.)

Fee: students—$15 membership, $15 registration, $10 audition fee; professionals—$30 membership, $30 registration, $10 audition fee

Format: 1½ min. for acting and singing; 1 min. for acting only or singing only. Dancers audition on Thursday evening and the following Friday and Saturday. Callbacks are on the evening of the same day. Audition briefings are held at 9 AM on the day of the audition. Administrative and Tech interviews are also held during these dates, through the Job Contact Service. Jobs are listed monthly in the Job Contact Bulletin that is distributed to members.

SOUTHWEST THEATER ASSOCIATION
(Includes AR, LA, NM, OK, TX)
Auditions: *Mid- to late January*
Place: *usually held at a Texas college*
Write for Application to: *Chuck Sheffield*
                                12800 Abrams Road
                                Richland Theater Department
                                Dallas, TX 75243-2199
Application Deadline: early January
Eligibility: union and non-union.
Fee: Ranges from $15 to $20, depending on membership status in SWTA.
Format: Actors—2 minutes total. Bring 20 to 25 photo/resumes for callbacks. Dancers—
A choreographer will teach dancers a routine. Tech/Adm: Bring portfolio for interview
(3 minutes).

STRAW HAT AUDITIONS
(NYC—about 30 companies, mainly from the northeastern U.S.)
Auditions: *late March or early April.*
Place: *Manhattan*
Write for Application to: (send business size SASE: no phone calls)
                                Straw Hat
                                Box 382A, Planetarium Station
                                New York, NY 10024
Deadline: Usually 2 to 3 weeks before auditions, but appointments almost always fill up
earlier.
Eligibility: open to all non-Equity performers, some screening, no stand-by's or walk-ins',
Staff/Design open to all.
Fee: $35
Format: Performers have 2 min. to present a monologue and a musical selection—
accompanist provided. There are a limited number of non-singing appointments available.
Producers are given a bound, indexed book of performers' photo/resumes in order of
appearance. Callbacks are posted hourly. Staff/Design interviews: March 24 (Thursday
afternoon).

UNIVERSITY/RESIDENT THEATER ASSOCIATION NATIONAL UNIFIED AUDITIONS
(U/RTA)
U/RTA is an organization of professionally-oriented university and resident theaters. These
auditions may lead to summer positions with resident theater companies, or to acceptance
into a graduate program at member universities. Auditions are open to candidates in all
areas of theater. There are two stages to the auditions.
I. Preliminary Screening Auditions: Applicants must be nominated by faculty/staff of a
college/university, and must send in the required form and recommendation by the middle
of November. Preliminary screening auditions are held in early January in fourteen cities
around the country. A panel of judges makes written evaluations of each presentation
(candidates are later mailed copies), and select candidates to attend final auditions.
II. Final Auditions: If selected, applicants audition at the most convenient location (New
York City, Evanston, IL, Long Beach, CA), on a weekend in February or early March.
Applicants are seen by members of the U/RTA schools and guest theaters (there is no
guarantee that every member will attend each site). No firm offers are made until after the
last weekend of final auditions.
Acting auditions are limited to 4 min.; other auditions are 8 min. (the application form has
detailed instructions about all presentations). For information, please write to:
    University/Resident Theater Association, Inc.
    1560 Broadway, Suite 801
    New York, NY 10036

Industrial Shows

by Bill Ervolino

Do you act? Sing? Dance? Write? Stage manage? Do you want to work on your craft and make some good money in the process? Would you like to work side by side with some of the most creative people in the business? Would you like to be part of a big-budget production, one with the kind of capital behind it that utilizes state-of-the-art production techniques? If your answer to any of these questions is yes, then industrial theater may be for you. Industrial shows offer valuable training and experience in your chosen field. They pay well. And if you work in them, you will be working in the world's most advanced technology.

Larry Katen, the business representative at Actors' Equity for Off-Broadway productions, industrial shows and workshops, is high on industrials and the opportunities they offer to a wide variety of acting professionals. "I don't know why more actors don't pursue them," he says. "Industrials have become pretty open and have a good record in terms of affirmative action and nontraditional casting. I think everyone's impression of industrials used to be tall, WASPy blondes, but it's not like that at all. Today, industrials encompass a broad section of the population. And there are many opportunities for actors, singers, dancers, and spokespersons. The performers do not get seen by the general public, casting directors or agents, but the pay is great."

The current industrial contract between Actors' Equity and the Producers' Guild (an organization of industrial producers), provides minimum weekly salaries of $774 for actors, $1,092 for stage managers, and $891 for assistant stage managers. The salaries for periods of seven days to two weeks are $968 for actors, $1,355 for stage managers, and $1,112 for assistant stage managers. For periods lasting less than a week, actors receive $277 for the first day and $138 for each day thereafter; stage managers are paid $387 for the first day and $193 for each day thereafter; assistant stage managers receive $317 for the first day and $159 for each day thereafter.

Because of the high rate of pay, many performers and technicians view industrial shows as an ideal way to tide themselves over while they continue to focus on more artistic goals. There are, however, writers and performers who object to working in industrial theater—they don't want to have anything to do with dressing up like a tube of lipstick and singing "A Kiss is Still a Kiss" or jumping up on a piano and tap-dancing during a 20-gun salute to Egg McMuffins. Nevertheless, many artists do derive artistic satisfaction from working in this medium. According to Joan Marshall, head of Contempo Communications, a producer of industrial shows, and President of the Producers' Guild: "For performers, industrial theater is a lot like getting a commercial. It's not what you do for your art, but it's a way of using your art to put a roof over your head. It's an outlet for your talent, it provides a good income and some people actually find the creative challenges very stimulating. It's almost like writing a sonnet in that you are forced into a form that has certain restrictions. If you look at it that way, as many people do, it becomes a growing experience."

Sal Rasa, who is the executive producer of industrial shows for the Weiss-Watson company in Manhattan and who is also the composer of *Most of Us Are Just Angry at One or Two Things Anyway*, and *The Gospel at Colonus*, is an eloquent spokesman for the artistic merits of the form. "Theater has always been society speaking to itself about itself," Rasa says. "Rather than see theater possibilities dwindle to a few existing facilities, we should open it up. Yes, we do put on shows for sales meetings, awards ceremonies, and business meetings, but we are also attempting to go further and attack real corporate issues. For example, I am now directing a video presentation on AIDS in the workplace for the Equitable Life Insurance Company. Projects like this allow us to bring an almost journalistic and dramatic approach to real issues in the corporate world.

"Industrials truly represent the producers of today," Rasa insists. "And for serious, theatrically-minded people to avoid this arena is foolish. What we do in terms of entertainment is to create shows from start to finish. We don't specialize in star packages or ready-made acts. We create theater. We are really attempting to bring quality theater to the industrial world and this is important because our corporate clients have supported the arts enormously in this country. I don't see why they can't enjoy some of it in their own corporate sphere."

REINVENTING THE INDUSTRIAL

There was a time when industrial theater stood for slick auto pageants or lavish, Broadway-type extravaganzas touting the latest trends in the fashion industry. But cars and fashions have changed a lot in the past 20 years and so has industrial theater. And "theater" is what it's all about, according to Joan Marshall, who suggests that the term "industrial" may even be outmoded. "This is not what our basic business is about," Marshall stresses. "In fact, we are presently talking with Equity to change our classification to Business Theater. There is presently an enormous amount of this kind of theater being done and it can run the gamut."

Today, just about every major corporation in America relies on some form of theater to spice up its business meetings, motivate its sales forces, reward its top employees, or familiarize its staff with new products. And these products can run the gamut, too, whether they're as innocent as a new ruffled potato chip or as imposing as a new jetliner. Patty Soll, production manager at Caribiner, Inc., notes that in either case, the shows built around these products can be as incredible as the client wants them to be.

Soll, whose clients have included Mobil Oil, Control Data, State Farm Insurance, and CBS Television, recalls a particularly unusual show put together by Caribiner's London office: "The client was British Airways and they were looking to reveal a new plane to their people. The show was held in an airplane hangar and the audience was in seating that was designed to move up and over so that the plane could be revealed.

"Firms with the kind of funds required to put together such spectacular displays don't seem to mind spending the money. To them, a good show is an investment— something that supports their business. And whether that means using laser lights or fan-dancers, they're willing to go the distance."

As Buck Heller, senior producer and creative director of business productions at Radio City Music Hall explains it, "If you wanted to persuade someone to buy a car, just showing the tires might not sell the product. But if the whole product is well-lit and pretty, the sale is easier. A person spending five straight hours in a meeting room might not retain important information: a show breaks up all the information and makes it easier to swallow. Slides, film, video, live entertainment, guest speakers and breakout seminars are some of the ways this can be done."

While different agencies will approach an industrial assignment in different ways, there is one constant—they all need talent. A show could be a take-off on the traditional Broadway musical, with pertinent new lyrics written into well-known show tunes, or it could be a mix of comedy and drama, incorporating the latest in video technology and light effects. Whatever direction a production may take, the need for writers, performers, and technicians remains.

The Weiss-Watson company uses its own writers for industrial productions, but it does hold open calls for cast members. Spokesman Philip Weiss describes an industrial show his firm put together for the Philip Morris Company. "This particular show had two performances," Weiss notes, "one in Chicago for the Wholesale Grocers Association, and the other in Orlando, Florida for the National Association of Tobacco Distributors. It was a 40-minute live musical show with a ten-piece orchestra, a cast of 12 and it employed Carl Ballantine of 'McHale's Navy' to do his magic shtick. The primary theme of the show was that profitability is not an illusion."

The two Philip Morris shows were basically the same production with slight changes made to reflect the different needs of the grocers and the tobacco distributors. "We used the same cast for both shows," Weiss says, "so they had the opportunity to travel. We auditioned and rehearsed in New York but used local musicians in Chicago and Orlando. The set traveled with us and we had a union designer, a union light designer, and professional videotape people for the video interludes."

As for the cast, Weiss says, "We put casting announcements in the trades and the performers come down to audition. The cast loved doing it and Philip Morris is a terrific company to work for. They treat the cast like all-stars, with hospitality suites and so on. It's a terrific relationship. The cast gets to work together for about six or seven weeks. They do two actual performances plus one videotaped performance which they are paid for."

The cast also has the opportunity to work with some top-notch talent. The director for the Philip Morris productions is Crandall Diehl, who has directed Rex Harrison on Broadway in *My Fair Lady* and has staged numerous editions of The Greatest Show on Earth for Ringling Brothers. He's also the director for Siegfried and Roy at the Frontier Hotel in Las Vegas and has been involved in the theater for about 30 years.

Liza Redfield is the musical director. "She was the first female director ever on Broadway," says Weiss. "She did *The Music Man* and a couple of productions for the New York Shakespeare Festival. She has also done 17 musicals on tour and has performed as a jazz pianist."

In last year's versions of the Philip Morris shows, the stars were Patrick Quinn who appeared on Broadway in *A Day in Hollywood/A Night in the Ukraine* and at Palsson's in *Forbidden Broadway*, and Barbara Marineau who played Nellie Forbush in the recent national tour of *South Pacific*. Another member of the cast, Weiss says, was Leslie Feagan, who was in the original cast of *Anything Goes* at Lincoln Center.

NON-EQUITY PRODUCTIONS
The Philip Morris shows are pretty much the standard fare in modern industrials. They're also light years away from the type of productions that Nancy Lombardo

concocts. A comedienne, writer and actress, Lombardo fashions shows for company heads whom she describes as being tired of the same old thing. These are non-Equity productions and Lombardo makes every effort to make them as unconventional as possible.

"One I really loved doing," the actress recalls, "was a show we did in Puerto Rico for Pfizer Pharmaceuticals. The entire cast was dressed up as waiters and waitresses. The audience was made up of about 40 of Pfizer's top executives and they had no idea what was going on. We came out speaking in Spanish and gave the worst service they had ever had. And this was at the Caribe Hilton, so they were particularly horrified. At one point, for example, I brought out all their crabmeat salads. Then I left, waited until they'd all had a bite and then came back and told them in Spanish that the fish was bad. They were panicked. Plus, they were seated on the floor, Japanese-style, and we were stepping all over them. At one point I accidentally spilled a drink on one of the women but by that time she was so upset she stabbed me with her fork. Then, two other actors, Michael Schaeffer and Jane Brucker, both started flirting with the same guy. It was hysterical. We tormented them like this for about 45 minutes and then, afterwards, told them that we had been hired by the company to do this to them. Then we went into our show, which consisted of sketches and musical numbers with Pfizer products incorporated into the material."

The audience was so impressed with the show, they later hired Lombardo and one of her cast members, Joe Perce, to "get even" with the Pfizer executive who had hired the actors in the first place.

Lombardo describes her industrial projects as "high concept comedy," and says her cast members must be well-versed in improv as well as acting and singing. "For me," she explains, "versatility is the key. The more an actor can do, the better. When I look at a resume, for example, I'm especially interested in special skills—things a person can do that are beyond the norm."

REQUIREMENTS FOR THE JOB

Knowing how to break-dance isn't a requirement for most industrial work, but it certainly doesn't hurt. In fact, the more versatile you are, the better your chances are of finding work in industrial theater. In addition to acting ability, most industrial producers are looking for performers who can also sing and dance.

Can you juggle, perform magic tricks, or do you have a ventriloquism routine? There's always a need for specialty acts, according to Joan Marshall. "Not for their own sake," she says, "but we appreciate all kinds of techniques that can be worked into our concept or theme." In other words, make sure you communicate these special talents to a potential employer. You never know when they might be the hook that snares you the job."

According to Larry Katen at Actors' Equity, "You also have to be a quick study. It's a special talent and a lot of wonderful actors who can't work quickly have had problems in industrials. You have to be quick." Sal Rasa agrees: "The difference between industrials and legit theater is that there are no previews, no second chances. Things have to be right in a very short period of time."

TYPECASTING

As for type, well, the field is wide open. Although industrial work was at one time restricted to handsome leading men and bosomy showgirls, the addition of more theatrical pieces into industrial productions has led to a growing need for real people who look like real people. Most corporations are interested in making presentations that reflect either their consumers or their employees. As Caribiner's Patty Soll puts it: "For chorus work, the cast needs to look as attractive and all-American as possible. That really hasn't changed. But there are many book shows being produced and these types of shows will always need characters and types."

One thing producers do look for is performers who can convey a corporate image. This doesn't necessarily mean you have to look like Joe Yuppie or the last cover of Manhattan, Inc. It just means that you should be clean, well-manicured, and perhaps look a little more "professional" than you might for a regular audition. Your hair and makeup should be on the conservative side. Your clothes should also look suitable for an office situation. As Buck Heller explains it: "The producers and directors are theatrical folks, but the client sitting next to us may not be that astute. They have to be comfortable seeing you. They shouldn't have to imagine what you're going to look like onstage. Your appearance is very important."

ETHNICITY

Concerning ethnicity, most corporations are anxious to present shows that reflect the diversity of the general population (as well as their own pool of employees), and actively seek out minorities for their industrial productions. Notes Joan Marshall: "Ethnic types are definitely becoming more and more important in business theater. And we are certainly noticing more diverse audiences: more women, more blacks, more Hispanics. In terms of consumers, in fact, the Hispanic market is the one that is growing the most rapidly. As a result, there has been a sharp increase in clients specifically requesting more ethnically diverse performers."

For the record, the agreement between the Producers' Guild and Actors' Equity Association specifically spells out casting obligations with respect to affirmative action as follows:

"Integration is acknowledged to be a goal of Actors' Equity Association and the Producers' Guild. Each production shall be integrated with Equity ethnic minority actors, to the best of the producer's ability. . . . Recognizing the need for expanding the participation of ethnic minorities and women in the artistic process, the Producer will support a flexible and imaginative casting policy known as non-traditional casting. Non-traditional casting shall be defined as the casting of stereotypical roles (e.g., company executive, manager, salesman, spokesman, consumer, etc.) with ethnic minority and women actors. . . . Periodic meetings will be held between representatives of Equity and the Producers' Guild, Inc., to evaluate and monitor the implementation of this policy."

UNSCRIPTED PERFORMANCES—IMPROV

Interestingly, there are a growing number of companies who are finding that an evening of unscripted material can be just as valuable to them as more traditional forms of industrial theater.

Katha Feffer, creative director of the improvisational group For Play, a New York-based improvisational group, says that the demand for improv artists in industrials is on the upsurge. Caribiner creative director Mike Meth agrees: "I've used improv acts, ventriloquists, and other specialty acts and think they can bring something special to a show. I don't like gratuitous things—it has to have a reason for being there—but I've seen a lot of improv recently, and it has worked quite nicely. There are a lot of improv groups out there and it can make things a little easier for a producer because you're buying a package. You've got built-in chemistry."

For Play recently developed an industrial show for Vista International. As Feffer relates, "It was a training program for different personnel from the company on how to make working conditions better for employees. The meeting involved lots of communications seminars and problem-solving seminars and the night we were there, they had a full program that involved theater games which concentrated on communication."

Feffer says her group was well-received by the employees. "At the beginning of the evening we asked members of the audience for five topics which related to their business relationships—topics like miscommunication, and so on. We started our show off with a scenario of an office meeting in which everyone thought they were talking about the same thing, but were in fact, talking about different things. The audience enjoyed it, and at the same time we were able to make valid points that related to their jobs."

Prior to the show, Feffer says she spent three hours with Vista executives discussing problems the company was trying to solve. She was also briefed on office gossip and nicknames for key employees. "They provided us with all sorts of tidbits we could incorporate into the show," Feffer says, "and we worked them in wherever we could."

The folks at Vista, Feffer notes, "really understood what we were doing and worked with us to put together a great show. They didn't tamper with our material. They had a great stage—a great sound system. They even had someone come in that morning and make sure the piano was tuned for us. Plus—and this is usually the biggest problem—they made sure that our show did not coincide with dinner."

THE INDUSTRIAL REVOLUTION
The many professionals who have joined the ever-growing industrial revolution will tell you, for the most part, much the same thing, that business theater has been good to them. It has given them the opportunity to work, grow, and to make valuable new contacts. It could do the same for you. For further information regarding industrial shows, contact Actors' Equity Association at (212) 869-8530, the Producers' Guild at (212) 481-8001, or consult the audition notices in *Back Stage*.

Industrial Show Production Companies

ARMSTRONG WORLD
INDUSTRIES
Fred A. Stoner
150 N. Queen St.
Lancaster, PA 17603
(717) 397-0611; 396-4203

AVION
COMMUNICATIONS
Julie Sasvari
230 W. 17th St.
New York, NY 10011
(212) 807-0044

GENE BAYLISS
16 Burritts Landing
Westport, CT 06880
(203) 227-7521

BIG BROTHERS & BIG
SISTERS INC.
Margaret Lange-Lewis
324 East Wisconsin,
Suite 543
Milwaukee, WI 53202
(414) 278-7764

BOLDUC & BRADLEY
Bill Mayhew
950 Third Ave., 25th Fl.
New York, NY 10022
(212) 832-7700

MICHAEL BROWN
ENTERPRISES, INC.
Michael Brown
335 E. 50th St.
New York, NY 10022
(212) 759-2233

CTP CASTING
Lisbeth Andresen
22 W. 27th St., 10th Fl.
New York, NY 10001
(212) 696-1100

CARIBINER, INC.
Mike Meth
16 W. 61st St.
New York, NY 10023
(212) 541-5300

MICHAEL CARSON
PRODUCTIONS
Michael Carson, Pres.
250 W. 54th St.
New York, NY 10019-5515
(212) 765-2300

THE CHARTMAKERS
INC.
Steve Reiter
33 W. 60th St.
New York, NY 10023
(212) 247-7200

COMART ANIFORMS,
INC.
Gary Saltzer
360 W. 31st St.
New York, NY 10001
(212) 714-2550

CONCEPTS UNLIMITED
Richard Barclay
315 W. 57th St.
New York, NY 10019
(212) 246-9612

CONTEMPO
COMMUNICATIONS
Joan Marshall
251 W. 19th St., Suite 10D
New York, NY 10011
(212) 633-2333

CORPORATE CONCEPTS,
LTD.
Jack Schatz, Pres.
260 Fifth Ave.
New York, NY 10001
(212) 545-0933

CREATIVE
PRESENTATIONS
Gene Bullard
819 W. Lunt Ave.
Shaumburg, IL 60193
(312) 894-2248

DECOMAS INC.
Judith M. Little &
Sondra Arnold
441 Lexington Ave.
New York, NY 10017
(212) 953-9030

IMERO FIORENTINO
ASSOCIATES
Corky Thueson
44 W. 63rd St.
New York, NY 10023
(212) 246-0600

FRANK EGAN &
ASSOCIATES
c/o Leo Burnett Co., Inc.
26555 Evergreen Road
Southfield, MI 48076
(313) 355-1900
Also: c/o Leo Burnett Co.,
Inc.
950 Third Ave.
New York, NY 10022

FOURMOST
PRODUCTIONS, INC.
Paul Kastl
60 Idaho St.
Passaic Park, NJ 07055
(201) 777-8357

GINDICK PRODUCTIONS
J. Jeff Salmon
21 E. 40th St., PH
New York, NY 10016
(212) 725-2580
Casts through agents only.

GOODSIGHT/HERRMANN
Larry Goodsight
850 7th Ave., Suite 1200
New York, NY 10019
(212) 307-7377

MICHAEL JOHN
ASSOCIATES, INC.
R.M. Duffy, Chairman
39 Lewis St.
Greenwich, CT 06830
(203) 622-0777

GEORGE P. JOHNSON
COMPANY
Robert Vallee, owner
Ron Williams, VP/Nat'l. Dir.
Sales
800 Techrow
Madison Heights, MI 48071
(313) 585-5888

GRAPHIC MEDIA
COMMUNICATIONS
Julie Charles
373 Route 46 W.
Fairfield, NJ 07006
(201) 227-5000

HELLER CREATIVE INC.
Buck Heller
14 Foothill St.
Putnam Valley, NY 10579
(914) 528-6328

MARITZ
COMMUNICATIONS CO.
1515 Route 10
Parsippany, NJ 07054
(201) 540-1761

MARKETING
CONCEPTS, INC.
Neva Conley
1500 Broadway, Suite 2304
New York, NY 10036
(212) 382-0171

MEDICAL MULTI MEDIA
CORP.
Stanley Waine
211 E. 43rd St., 2302
New York, NY 10017
(212) 986-0180

MEETING
ENVIRONMENTS
Joe Iorio, Doug Speer
9 E. 19th St.
New York, NY 10003
(212) 677-3500

METROPOLITAN LIFE
INSURANCE
Beth Dembitzer
1 Madison Ave.
New York, NY 10010
(212) 578-8715

JACK MORTON
PRODUCTIONS, INC.
Bill Morton, Pres.
830 Third Ave.
New York, NY 10022
(212) 758-8400

MOTIVATION MEDIA,
INC.
Glen Peterson, Prod. Mgr.
1245 Milwaukee Ave.
Glenview, IL 60025
(312) 297-4740

NATIONAL SPEAKERS
BUREAU
John Palmer, Pres.
222 Wisconsin Ave.
Lake Forest, IL 60045
(312) 295-1122

PEPSI COLA COMPANY
Patrik J. Williams
PO Box 442
Somers, NY 10589
(914) 767-6000

RADIO CITY MUSIC
HALL PRODS.
Winnie Boone
1260 Ave. of the Americas
New York, NY 10020
(212) 246-4600

SANDY CORPORATION
1500 W. Big Beaver Rd.
Troy, MI 48084
(313) 649-0800

SECOND SIGHT INC.
Benjamin Evans
Basking Ridge, NJ 07920
(201) 822-4684

SHERIDAN JENNINGS,
LTD.
Joseph T. Jennings, Pres.
155 No. Harbor Dr.
Concourse Level
Chicago, IL 60601
(312) 565-0002

PHOEBE SNOW
PRODUCTIONS
Deborah Herr
37 W. 36th St.
New York, NY 10018
(212) 679-8756

SORGEL STUDIOS, INC.
James K. Henley, Prod./Dir.
205 W. Highland Ave.
Milwaukee, WI 53203
(414) 224-9600

TRAJECTORY
Don Doherty
140 Riverside Dr.
New York, NY 10024
(212) 724-2200

VISUAL SERVICES, INC.
Nelson Case, Jr.,
Vice Pres.
2100 N. Woodward Ave.
Bloomfield Hills, MI 48013
(313) 644-0500

VISUAL SERVICES &
INTERGROUP
PRODUCTIONS
1 W. 19th St.
New York, NY 10011
(212) 580-9551

JOHN R. WALSH &
ASSOCIATES
John R. Walsh
450 Seventh Ave.
New York, NY 10123
(212) 594-5151

WEISS-WATSON
Sal Rasa
1140 Ave. of the Americas
New York, NY 10036
(212) 753-9800

ZACKS & PERRIER
Duane Butler
96 Morton St.
New York, NY 10014
(212) 463-7308

Industrial Films

by Mike Salinas

Thousands of performers have given shape and direction to their careers by working in the little-known field of industrial and educational films. Although a good many performers assume that industrials are boring and consist mostly of non-union work, these are misconceptions which, for the most part, are not valid. While it is true that some of the films are dull beyond description, the work itself can be interesting and extremely valuable for both beginning and accomplished performers. And, industrial films are regulated by the trade unions. Both the Screen Actors Guild and the American Federation of Television and Radio Artists have union jurisdiction over industrials, each according to whether film stock or videotape is used. Joan Greenspan, national director of industrial organizing at SAG, attests to this by saying, "many people are not aware we have contracts for our members to cover these films. Actors should become acquainted with them." Indeed they should. Union figures indicate that this field grew last year by about 30 percent, and there is every indication that that kind of growth will continue indefinitely.

An industrial film helped Scott Geyer land a starring role in the Home Box Office sit-com "First and Ten." Geyer knew he was right for the role and felt that he was close to being cast for the part. But something seemed to be getting in the way. Finally, after a number of auditions, he offered the producers a tape of an industrial film he'd shot a couple of years earlier. He figured that even though the role he had played (a linoleum installer) was very different than the part for which he was being considered (a pro football player), it would still give the executives an opportunity to see how he looked on camera, and that it might help his chances. He was right. In less than 24 hours he had been cast for the role of the quarterback in "First and Ten."

WHAT ARE INDUSTRIAL FILMS?

According to the SAG handbook on industrial films there are two kinds of industrials. One kind, called Category I films, are defined as those "programs designed to train, inform, promote a product, or perform a public relations function, and are exhibited in classrooms, museums, libraries, or other places where no admission is charged." High school assembly films (on hygiene, drug abuse, how to use a slide rule, and so forth) are typical Category I films. Their counterparts in the business world are produced by corporations for the purposes of bolstering productivity and morale among their employees and to foster product knowledge.

Category II industrial films look more like commercials and are "intended for unrestricted exhibition to the general public," according to the SAG handbook. Rather than being shown on the airwaves, however, they must be shown "at locations where the product or services are sold, or . . . at public places such as coliseums, railroad stations, air/bus terminals, or shopping centers." This category includes videotapes created as promotional giveaways and "point-of-purchase" video demonstrations.

Some industrial films consist of little more than a single person droning into a camera, but the best ones are patterned after proven formats, such as television dramas or situation comedies. Industrial filmmakers believe that when dealing with complex problems like sexism or racism on the job, they are more likely to achieve their goal by imitating television, since generations that grew up with this medium are accustomed to seeing difficult issues introduced, discussed, and settled in 28 minutes. Other industrials emulate documentary films and/or news programs, and many of them go to great lengths to recreate the look and feel of the great television features, including stylish camera techniques and extensive music scores. The great bulk of industrials produced today, however, usually employ about a half-dozen contract players to act out vignettes, plus a spokesperson or narrator to drive home the all-important moral.

The main difference between a contract player and a spokesperson according to Joan Greenspan is that a " 'spokes' is one whose part is substantially in monologue, performing the preponderance of the script." Union scale for a contract player for one day's work on a Category I film is $319, whereas the spokes will make an additional $261, for a total of $580—but only for the first day. Beyond that, scale reverts to $319. For a Category II film, the figures are a little higher: $396 for a contract player and $686 for a spokes.

For a three-day contract player, the scale is $801 (or $988 for a Category II film), and a weekly player gets $1,118 (or $1,385 for a Category II film). For spokespersons, those rates are supplemented by the same one-time surcharges as above. Extras receive $106 per day, except in special circumstances (if they do a "silent bit," or if they are a photo double, they stand to make more money), and an off-camera voice-over day player makes $261 for the first hour's work and $76 for every subsequent half-hour.

Performers are usually required to provide their own costumes in industrials, for which they are paid a cleaning allowance of $15 per outfit, per two-day period "or part thereof," by the producer. They are also paid for traveling to an overnight location, and are given a meal allowance and single room accommodation. All rates are increased for weekend or holiday work.

INDUSTRIAL FILM BENEFITS
Industrials offer benefits other than just paychecks. Performers are frequently able to obtain a videotape of the performance and may have an opportunity to get their union cards. Industrial films offer good opportunities for beginning actors, too, who may be able to pick up a non-speaking role such as the part of a doorman or a clerk.

Character actors who have been frustrated in their attempts to get even minor roles on soaps may find industrials a good source of "bread and butter work." Moreover, corporations producing these films are eager to represent their companies as multi-ethnic, so a fair number of blacks, Hispanics, and Asians are able to find work in this field, often as spokespersons.

One of the greatest benefits for inexperienced performers is that industrials offer the opportunity to gain precious on-camera experience in relatively relaxed surroundings. Industrial film shoots are usually pretty calm (a far cry from the chaos of a television taping or the pressures of full-scale big-budget moviemaking), and are less constrained by time than commercials. Therefore, industrial films present an excellent way to learn the craft and mechanics of filming.

AUDITIONS—THE INDUSTRIAL FILM IMAGE

The first step for actors who want to audition for industrial films is to study the corporate look in America today. Since most of the films are set in business environments, from boardrooms to loading docks and all levels in between, it is necessary to have a feel for the people who work in these places. What distinguishes a middle-management type from a senior manager? How do men and women in corporate America dress? How do they speak? The answers to these questions can provide guidelines for the way performers should look and sound when they arrive at their auditions, and how their industrial film resume photo should look.

According to Salli Frattini, Manager of Production Services at M.J. Zink, a leading industrial production house, "For men, the look is more and more casual." However, she elaborates, casual in an industrial film means "still in a tie, but with the jacket off and the shirtsleeves rolled up." Also, she says, there are more women in industrials these days, and for them, "the look is now more business executive than secretary. For a casting session, they should wear a skirt, a nice blouse, and maybe a jacket. But the look is less conservative and more stylish than it used to be; it's not all bow ties and little high collars anymore."

Of course, for blue-collar characters like loading dock supervisors or linoleum installers, a suit is hardly a necessity. For these roles, actors should dress exactly as they would for a commercial audition. But for jacket-and-tie roles, an actor should wear something that typifies the corporate image. One way to dress for success at an industrial audition, is to wear a classic blue pinstripe suit, recently cleaned and pressed.

SPECIAL SKILLS

Performers with technical, medical, or electronic expertise are advised to list it among other special skills on their resumes. The ability to breeze through a script full of complicated assessments of cycles-per-nanosecond or meticulously detailed descriptions of eye surgery techniques will not fail to impress agents and casting directors of industrial films. Similarly, prior experience operating specialized machinery, like fork-lifts, may come in handy and should be listed as a special skill.

The majority of successful industrial performers have of, course, never had real experience in the fields portrayed in the films; what the very best spokespersons do have is authority and a clear speaking voice (and a blue pinstripe suit or two, of course). Some are very good-looking, but a high percentage are only average-looking; they range in age from mid-20s to mid-60s, with the majority somewhere in the middle.

As the field of industrial films continues to expand, more jobs are available for both novice and experienced industrial performers of all ages. "Work begets work," says one agent, "and when you've cracked the field, it's naturally easier to get the next job." And the fact is that industrials can be remunerative and can go a long way toward paying monthly bills while performers continue to work toward super-stardom, or more esthetically satisfying career goals.

Cabaret

by Bob Harrington

The world of cabaret provides performers with a milieu that is unique in the entertainment industry. The cabaret stage is usually small, and contact with the audience is intimate. To attract a following, a performer must possess that special personal magnetism called charisma. Even so, the most charismatic entertainers still know that it is not always easy to fill a house. In fact, the difficulty of bringing in an audience is one of the most troublesome problems facing cabaret artists. Whether a headliner or a novice, all cabaret entertainers share this problem. Reputation and good publicity can cushion established stars against those nights when performer and musicians outnumber patrons, but even big names find themselves occasionally playing to sparsely populated rooms. For beginners the problem is doubly acute and increases almost immediately after opening night. Once Aunt Rose and all the folks from the office have attended the big debut, who will show up for the next performance? Walk-in business cannot be relied upon—in most clubs accessible to new acts it is negligible. Audiences simply will not go to see an unknown act.

There are ways however, to build an audience, though most performers are surprisingly uninformed on the subject. Many entertainers are remarkably naive. They expect the club to provide the audience and believe that good reviews will cause audiences to magically appear; or they think people will just somehow find out about them and plunk down a cover charge. The opposite is true. No matter who you are, if you want an audience you're going to have to go out and get one, and you're going to have to work at it until you reach a level of success which allows you to hire someone else to work at it for you. You may think that big stars are able to sell out houses on the strength of their names. But when you see Barry Manilow or Patti LaBelle break box office records, you're seeing the results of a publicity blitz and hype that cost big bucks; you're seeing good management and good press relations, and you're seeing the product of years of self-promotion. It takes a monumental effort to become and remain a star, and no one is above the effort.

If you're determined to become a star, keep in mind that the first step to stardom is building an audience. A performer who fills a room never lacks bookings, and eventually attracts the right attention. And, you can approach building an audience the same way you would approach locating customers in any other business: logically, methodically, and with a plan in mind. What follows are some of the things you should be doing and some advice on how to do them to the best effect.

MAILING LISTS

The first step after you have decided to do a club act is to build (and maintain) a mailing list. Sit down and write out the names and addresses of everyone you can think of who might be interested in what you're doing. Every friend, co-worker, and relative goes on your mailing list, and you work from that core. Adding to and updating this list must become a number one priority, for how you add to your mailing list will, in many respects, determine how successful you become. After you've composed your initial list, buy a little spiral note pad. Keep it with you at all times, and jot down the name and address of any person who expresses an interest in what you are doing.

Determined performers treat their mailing lists with reverence. They use computers in some instances, and work on it for hours every week. They will add names to their lists constantly. No one walks out of one of their performances without being spoken to, thanked, and if willing, listed. They pass little guest books around before every show. The names they collect in their first runs help turn their second runs into sellouts. These performers place mailing list cards on every single table when they perform, and remind the audience of this during the performance.

You can also take a creative approach to building a mailing list. Katha Feffer of the improvisational troupe, For Play, brought the group to the Duplex from Oregon. They knew no one in the city. She built a mailing list from people back home who had friends and relatives in New York. She took yearbooks from Oregon colleges and culled out the names of the students who were from New York. She traced Oregonian graduates who had moved to New York. She invited practically everyone who had ever been passed through Oregon to see For Play—and this became her core list.

The actual mechanics of preparing a mailing list depend largely on your finances and organizational ability. A personal computer, particularly one with the capability of running off mailing labels, is, of course, ideal. The right software will make your mailing list easy to access and update, and you can use it to identify different groups within the list for targeted mailings. Even a basic system, however, can cost a lot of money, money which might be put to better use elsewhere at the beginning of a career. A computer is, after all, nothing more than an elaborate and efficient filing system, and you can do almost as well on your own. A simple, unalphabetized running list will do in a pinch when you're still addressing fliers by hand, but index cards quickly become essential. You can add to your file by simply slipping in the cards filled out by patrons at your shows. Another advantage to using index cards is that you can make notes on them to show who is responding to your mailings as you cross-reference with the people filling out new cards or signing guest books at your shows. This helps you eliminate the dead wood. Keep it simple—name, address, and zip code, affiliation if pertinent, and underneath just pencil in a date of attendance. Cards can also be rearranged by zip code quickly and easily, which simplifies things when you take them in to have address labels made.

When you are ready to have mailing labels made from your handwritten or typed list, get two copies of each address made and simply paste the extra addresses onto individual cards—the result is an instant file. You can use the same method to update your list when you're working from names scrawled on cocktail napkins, matchbook covers, and the backs of envelopes. Business cards can be taped or stapled directly to your index cards.

Those are the main details of building and maintaining a mailing list. As you can see, it's a lot of work—but it pays off. If you scrupulously keep your mailing list it will, like Mae West's diary, someday keep you.

PHOTOGRAPHS

There are pros and cons to spending heavily on good headshots for cabaret, but a good photograph can turn out to be a valuable asset. It's true that the major dailies don't like headshots, but they almost never run pictures with reviews anyway so that's not a major concern. Headshots are used in *Back Stage*, *Nightlife Magazine*, *Michael's Thing*, and other publications that cover cabaret. They are also useful for fliers, postcards, and posters.

But the headshot must be good—and that means distinctive, attractive, and slickly professional. It is not unusual for an editor to put a blurb together or ask a writer to do a piece only in order to use a particularly attractive picture. It is possible to garner an extraordinary amount of extra publicity just because of the quality and beauty of photographs. Comics who can come up with especially amusing or interesting photos will also benefit.

If you're not particularly photogenic, don't get photos taken until you can afford the best. It's amazing what a good photographer can do, and it's probably a good thing that performers aren't covered by the "truth in advertising" laws. But a bad job is worse than useless. Grainy, unflattering, blurry, or bland photographs reflect poorly on you as a performer, and are of no help in getting you any publicity.

FLIERS, POSTCARDS, POSTERS, AND ADS
A flier is essential. It is your calling card to the world of cabaret so let it represent you as a polished professional and not as a rank amateur.

Fliers designed for cabaret should be neat, clean, and simple. A headshot or publicity photo as the centerpiece, a club logo, and basic information is all that is required. Later, you may add quotes from reviews or even entire reviews (if appropriate) when you get them. It's better to spend a few dollars to get a good, basic flier professionally made (you can use this over and over by changing the dates) than to use a photocopy machine, typewriter, or crayons. Fliers can be run off on standard paper, folded in three, labeled, and mailed. They can also be distributed in piano bars, at places of employment, or anyplace that will help.

If you can afford the additional cost, postcards are an effective means of publicizing your show. For one thing, you can't throw one in the garbage without seeing who it's from. For another, postcards imply a certain amount of success and status just because they're more expensive—which is, of course, the down side—they're expensive. Generally, the guidelines for putting together a cabaret postcard are the same as they are for cabaret fliers. Keep it simple.

Posters are probably a waste of time and are certainly not cost-effective. A moderate poster campaign costs close to $1,000, and you'll never recoup that in cover charges. Posters rarely bring in much new business. All they do is notify people who already know who you are that you're around again. You can do the same thing more effectively with a good mailing list and a few well-placed ads.

What posters do accomplish is to let people in the business know that you really mean it, and again, they imply a certain status and success. If the club pays for the posters, go ahead and have them printed up. If not, don't bother unless your primary purpose is to increase your prestige and visibility within the business.

Taking out ads can cost a small fortune, and have no effect whatsoever on your audience if you don't place them correctly. For an unknown, the only affordable and sensible place for an ad is in the trade papers, where agents, colleagues and other performers will see it. After you're established and your name has been around a while, you can explore more elaborate forms of advertising.

The best way to get an ad in a paper is to find work in a club that advertises its performers on a regular basis. Most clubs will also see to it that you get listed in those publications that provide free listings. Keep your eyes open and get a feeling for the kinds of ads that work for the various clubs and performers. It doesn't work the same way for everyone. Sometimes huge ads in newspapers are not at all effective. There are many factors that determine the effectiveness of an ad, including the demographics of the publication, the day of the week, the time of performance, the type of act, and what the ad looks like.

NEWSLETTERS AND THE PERSONAL TOUCH

Performers who have a devoted, regular following might consider sending out a newsletter. If you go this route, make sure that your newsletter is interesting and informative; don't inundate your fans with homey little notes. Some performers use newsletter-type mailings to share items of special interest. This could consist of good reviews, articles of interest about them or about cabaret in general, or could describe an award or citation they've just won, and might include a short personal note. Such an approach is effective, tasteful, and appropriate. It also makes people feel that you're really trying to stay in touch. Newsletters that are filled with obviously man-ufactured information, on the other hand, are not effective and may be annoying.

The personal touch cannot be underestimated when it comes to building and maintaining a steady following. Smart performers make personal contact with every-one who comes to see them. Be accessible, be friendly, say thank you and get the names for your mailing list. It's hard to greet dozens of people and repeat yourself over and over without sounding phony. Learn how, because if you are successful in cabaret, you'll be greeting hundreds of people and repeating yourself over and over. So now is the time to cultivate a good memory for names and faces. If you are casually acquainted with a person, or if you get the feeling that the person is expect-ing more than a perfunctory thank you, make an effort to personalize the inter-change. You don't have to get into a major conversation, and you can always excuse yourself to greet other people. Countless performers muff a chance to turn a first-time patron into a steady regular by projecting wrong attitude. In cabaret, all per-formers, stars included, are accessible. Big names like Julie Wilson, Margaret Whit-ing, and Kaye Ballard still try to meet everyone who comes to one of their shows. That's one of the reasons why they're such well-loved personalities. And it's no coincidence that they also work steadily.

DEALING WITH THE CRITICS

The easiest (but not easy) publicity to get comes from critics. Critics have followings, just like performers, and their reviews can help you build an audience. A good word from a critic can also be immensely supportive and helpful to your career in other ways. Good reviews guarantee the support of the critic's publication, status within the cabaret community, and a clear validation of your talents as a performer. Such reviews can interest agents, get you jobs, and attract other critics. Reviews appear-ing while you're still performing can sell out your show, or at least increase your audience (and mailing list).

A review, however, can blow you out of the water, emotionally and career-wise, if it is a bad one. The biggest and most common single mistake made by performers is to invite critics to their shows before they're review-ready.

First, decide whether you're really ready to get reviewed. The best advice you're going to get is from the club owners, operators, and booking managers. They don't want bad reviews anymore than you do. If they're not encouraging you, take the hint. You're asking for trouble if you pressure a club owner or press agent into inviting a critic. It is not unheard of for an owner or press agent in that situation to gleefully give in and let the performer take his or her richly deserved lumps. Use your head—the people who run the club have every reason to want you to be reviewed if you're good enough. If they're not bending over backwards to get the critics out, there's a hidden message in there for you. Don't be in such a hurry.

If you decide you are ready to face the critics, and you're getting some encouragement from objective sources, then you must decide *which* critics you want to see you. *Do not think you are ready for every critic in town.* Here again, the club staff can help you. If you don't know who's who, they will. Even if you're good enough, you have to go about this carefully. You don't want a major newspaper reviewing a short one-week run that will have a much longer run later on. They won't review you again no matter how much they like you, and even a rave from the *Times* has little appreciable audience effect when your appearance has already ended. The quotes look good on your fliers and publicity, but yesterday's reviews can be as dead as yesterday's news when it comes to drawing an audience. Plan your campaign.

In reality, critics are much more aware of what's going on and far more selective than you probably think they are. If you're good enough to be reviewed by the top critics, they probably already know about you. Critics rarely see anyone they haven't already gotten at least some input on, though they occasionally respond to a particularly interesting letter or personal contact. But mostly, critics rely on feedback from club owners, press agents, bookers, waiters and waitresses, other performers, and audience members.

Critic Stephen Holden, a frequent contributor to the *New York Times*, cites the following considerations that help him decide whom to review. "I rely on publicists and on word of mouth," Holden says. "I also trust club owners. I know what to expect in different clubs and what level of professionalism to expect." To some critics, professionalism is a major factor in determining their decision to review. Others, however, will knowingly see a rank beginner. Stephen Holden will not. Holden suggests that performers "try to have some sense of whether they're really ready to be reviewed—usually they're not." Critics are also influenced by other critics' reviews (keep in mind that this is a double-edged sword), and you can build a press kit that will help you attract the major critics by building on previous reviews.

Assuming that you're ready, and that you've chosen the critics you think you're ready for, the object now becomes getting them in to see you. If you or the club you're working at has a press agent, leave it in their hands. If not, write a letter or send a flier. Every critic is different. A personal letter influences some, others prefer working off monthly club schedules and fliers. But if you choose to write, don't try to be cute. Just write a sincere letter telling why you want the critic to see you; don't try to dazzle the critic with clever *bons mots*. Avoid stridency or boastful claims and keep in mind that critics know their field, are aware of who's who, and are basically just looking for information on who's doing what and where.

Every critic operates the same way—the standard arrangement is complimentary covers and no check for drinks or food. Some clubs have a two-drink comp limit, which isn't unreasonable. But I suggest you make it your business to find out if the critic you've invited has had *three* drinks and then make sure your critic doesn't get a check for the third drink. Some clubs will comp dinners for some critics but not others, and some clubs won't comp anything but the cover. For the most part, critics know which clubs are doing what and will act accordingly. But mistakes do happen. Every critic occasionally gets a check by mistake, or gets billed without having been informed that club policy does not include comps. This can create bad feeling for the performer and for the club, and it's your responsibility to take care of this in advance. The unwritten rule is that the critic is your guest unless the club policy is otherwise. And that's something you should be aware of from the start. Some clubs have written into their contracts that critics are the guests of the club. Other clubs handle the whole thing informally, and have well-developed relationships with individual critics. It is the policy of some clubs though, to bill the performer for a critic's tab. One performer learned to her dismay that she owed a club $1,000 for food and drinks supplied to critics and agents whom she thought the club was comping. Know what you're doing before you start mailing out invitations all over town.

Most critics scrupulously avoid wearing out their welcome by running up big tabs and resent it when a club bills a performer for their dinner and drinks. Nevertheless, it is your responsibility to make arrangements for *your* critics in accordance with the policy of *your* club. Mistakes can cost you *and* the club a great deal of good will.

You'll usually find out when a critic has accepted an invitation to see you, though sometimes a club will invite one and not tell you to avoid making you nervous. If you want to keep critics happy provide them with a play list of the songs you'll be doing, including lyricist and composer. And make sure this information is accurate. If the critic coming uses photos (and again, you should know this), have one available. A short press release is all right, but don't load a critic down with tons of irrelevant information. Always include contact information (for both yourself and the club you are performing at) in your invitation to critics.

There are probably dozens of reasons why a review may not run, the most obvious one being considerations of space in the newspaper. After a review *has* run, thank-you notes are optional. No critic expects them, but all critics like them when they're thoughtfully done. They don't even have to be in response to a rave review. If a critic says something that moves you to write, then write. But never write to complain or argue, even if you think a critic is 100 percent wrong.

If you use a portion of a review in your publicity, make sure it is representative of what was actually said. You may fool some people lifting one good word or sentence out of a negative review, but you'd better believe the critic will hear about it. If you do quote, use the critic's name and not just the publication in which the review appeared.

SHOW BUSINESS IS GOOD BUSINESS

They call it show *business* for a reason. Your chance of succeeding will be greater if you master both the business and the artistic side. No one will take care of business for you in the beginning, and the more you learn at the start, the less likely it is that someone will take you for a ride later on. As in any endeavor, hard work and training will pay off if you keep at it. Stardom may may or may not come to you, but if you have the art and you take care of business, you'll always have an audience to play to.

Cabarets

NEW YORK CITY

THE BALLROOM
253 W. 28th St.
New York, NY 10001
(212) 244-3005
Established musicals acts only

THE BITTER END
147 Bleecker St.
New York, NY 10014
(212) 673-7030
Contact: Ken Gorka

BROADWAY BABY
407 Amsterdam Ave.
New York, NY 10024
(212) 724-6868
Contact: Jim Luzar (Mon. & Thurs.)

CATCH A RISING STAR
1487 First Ave.
New York, NY 10021
(212) 794-1906
Contact: Louis Faranda

CHEZ BEAUVAIS
852 Tenth Ave.
New York, NY 10019
(212) 581-6340
Contact: Joyce Beauvais

DANNYS' SKYLIGHT ROOM
at the Grand Sea Palace
346-348 W. 46th St.
New York, NY 10036
(212) 265-8133; 869-5470
Contact: Danny Apolinar or John Britton

DON'T TELL MAMA
343 W. 46th St.
New York, NY 10036
(212) 757-0788
Contact: Helen Baldassare, Michael Fogarty or Lina Koutrakos at 265-0001

THE DUPLEX
55 Grove St.
New York, NY 10014
(212) 255-5438
Contact: Bruce Hopkins or Helene Kelly

EIGHTY EIGHT'S
228 W. 10th St.
New York, NY 10014
(212) 924-0088
Contact: Erv Raible

5 & 10 NO EXAGGERATION
77 Greene St.
New York, NY 10012
(212) 925-7414
Contact: Robert Mergler

IMPROVISATION, THE
358 W. 44th St.
New York, NY 10036
(212) 765-8268
Contact: Silver Friedman

JAN WALLMAN'S RESTAURANT CABARET
49 W. 44th St.
New York, NY 10036
(212) 764-8930
Contact: Jan Wallman

JASON'S PARK ROYAL
23 W. 73rd St.
New York, NY 10023
(212) 316-4744
Contact: Larry Pellegrini

J'S
2581 Broadway, 2nd fl.
New York, NY 10025
(212) 666-3600
Contact: Mary Dyer

LESLIE'S
117 W. 58th St.
New York, NY 10019
(212) 765-1427
Contact: Karen Leslie

MICHAEL'S PUB
211 E. 55th St.
New York, NY 10022
(212) 758-2272
Established musical acts only

MONKEY BAR
at Hotel Elysee
60 E. 54th St.
New York, NY 10022
(212) 753-1066
Contact: Pat Norell at 265-0943

MOSTLY MAGIC
55 Carmine St.
New York, NY 10014
(212) 924-1472
Magicians, specialty acts
Contact: Terry Day

OAK ROOM, THE
at the Algonquin Hotel
59 W. 44th St.
New York, NY 10017
(212) 840-6800
Contact: Donald Smith at 879-4354

PALSSON'S
158 W. 72nd St.
New York, NY 10023
(212) 362-2590
Contact: Nancy McCall

SWEETWATERS
170 Amsterdam Ave.
New York, NY 10023
(212) 873-4100
Contact: Shelly Brook at above no. or at 757-6442

TROCADERO, DOWNSTAIRS AT
368 Bleecker St.
New York, NY 10014
(212) 242-0636
Contact: Mindy Martin at 473-6282

UPSTAIRS AT GREENE
STREET
105 Greene St.
New York, NY 10012
(212) 925-2415
Contact: Marlo Courtney or
Leah Sutton

WEST BANK
DOWNSTAIRS THEATER
BAR
407 W. 42nd St.
New York, NY 10036
(212) 695-6905
Contact: Rand Forrester,
Lewis Blank or Rusty
McGee

WESTBETH CABARET
THEATER CENTER
151 Bank St.
New York, NY 10014
(212) 691-2272
Contact: Arnold Engelman

WHALER BAR AND
LOUNGE
at Madison Towers Hotel
22 E. 38th St.
New York, NY 10016
(212) 685-3700
*Singing soap opera stars
only*
Contact: Paulette Weber at
787-2549 (10 A.M.–2 P.M.)

YE OLDE TRIPPLE INN
263 W. 54th St.
New York, NY 10019
(212) 245-9849
Contact: Louie, Kenny or
John

Cabarets Outside New York City

CALIFORNIA

BACKLOT CABARET
THEATRE
652 N. Lapeer Drive
West Hollywood, CA 90069
(213) 659-0472

BIG MAMA'S
22615 Mission
Hayward, CA 94541
(415) 881-9310

CARLOS 'N CHARLIE'S
8240 Sunset Blvd.
Los Angeles, CA 90046
(213) 656-8830

CINEGRILL
Hollywood Roosevelt Hotel
7000 Hollywood Blvd.
Hollywood, CA 90028
(213) 466-7000

GARDENIA
7066 Santa Monica Blvd.
Los Angeles, CA 90038
(213) 467-7444

PLUSH ROOM
York Hotel
940 Sutter St.
San Francisco, CA 94109
(415) 885-6800

ROSE TATTOO
665 N. Robertson Ave.
Los Angeles, CA 90069
(213) 854-4455

THE SALOON
718 14th St.
San Francisco, CA 94114
(415) 431-0253

CHICAGO, IL

GEORGE'S
230 W. Kinzee
Chicago, IL 60610
(312) 644-2290

RUGGLES
1633 N. Halsted St.
Chicago, IL 60614
(312) 988-9000

BOSTON, MA

CLUB CABARET
209 Columbus Ave.
Boston, MA 02116
(617) 536-0966

PHILADELPHIA, PA.

EQUUS
254 S. 12th St.
Philadelphia, PA 19107
(215) 545-8088

WASHINGTON, D.C.

ANTON'S 1201 CLUB
1201 Pennsylvania Ave. N.W.
Washington, D.C. 20036
(202) 783-1201

Stand-Up Comedy

by Bill Ervolino

There are many success stories that point to stand-up comedy as the highway to travel in search of steady work, big money, valuable exposure and stardom. Yes, even super-stardom and in some cases, mega super-stardom. For in the past six years, the burgeoning club scene has emerged as an ideal place for new talent to display its wares. And the recompense can be films, sitcoms, talk shows, television appearances, and even commercials. Stand-up, after all, is the vehicle that first brought us Woody Allen, Bill Cosby, Joan Rivers, Robin Williams, Eddie Murphy, Whoopi Goldberg, Billy Crystal, George Carlin, Roseanne Barr, and a host of other acts that learned how to stand up—and make a name for themselves.

In the comedy clubs, performers have the opportunity to learn how to handle themselves onstage and to develop their sense of timing. Perhaps more importantly, though, they learn how to shine in a blinding spotlight, one in which their talents are observed by some of the most influential people in show business.

As the editor of the comedy magazine *Comedy USA*, comic Barry Weintraub keeps a watchful eye on the stand-up comedy industry and the various film and television opportunities that continue to come out of it. "Walk into Catch a Rising Star any night of the week," Weintraub notes, "and you'll see talent scouts from MTV, the cable networks, the major networks, films . . . you name it." In Weintraub's opinion, the reason is simple: "It's easier to take a stand-up comic and teach him how to act, than it is to take an actor and teach him how to be funny."

Stanislavski might disagree with that assessment, but the fact remains that the unemployment rate among actors is very high. Among comics, however, it's virtually nil. As Weintraub explains it, "If a comic is any good at all, he (or she) is working. And if working, he (or she) has an excellent shot at being discovered and landing more work as a result of it."

"It's a situation that is accelerating at a very rapid pace," observes Cary Hoffman, owner of the uptown club Stand-Up New York, "and one which is altering stand-up tremendously. We're seeing comics today developing cleaner, more generic acts— television acts. They are also much more concerned with their acting abilities. A lot of them are even taking acting classes. By now, they are all familiar with the story of how Carl Reiner came into the Comedy Store and discovered Robin Williams. To many of them, stand-up has become a quick steppingstone to television and films."

Catch A Rising Star owner Richard Fields agrees: "We have close to 100 performers appearing regularly at 'Catch,' but I'd say only two or three of them see stand-up as a long-term goal. The rest are waiting to be discovered. And while they wait, they can earn $30,000 to $75,000 a year. Our management company currently handles some acts who are not major stars but who are earning two to four thousand per week."

Many of the clubs aggressively pursue casting people, inviting them to stop in, have a drink and check out the night's performers. "Casting people call us all the time," Cary Hoffman notes, "and yes, we do pursue them. The comedy clubs are now viscerally connected to films and just about every other medium. ABC, for example, has a pilot development program and they are always in the clubs looking for people to build pilots around. They *want* comics."

BOX OFFICE INDICATORS

Rock may still rule on the road, but according to the music trade newsletter *Pollstar*, stand-up comedy is beginning to make significant advances at concert hall box offices. *Pollstar's* 1987 list of the top 100 touring acts included five comedy headliners with average nightly grosses that *really* rocked.

Eddie Murphy, of course, was number one among comics for the year. (No surprise there—he was also 1987's top movie draw, thanks to *Beverly Hills Cop II* and his stand-up concert film *Raw*.) The "Saturday Night Live" alumnus who got his start doing stand-up at clubs in New York City and on Long Island, ranked number 28 overall among all touring acts with an average gross income per date (that's per performance) of $181,114. The other four comics on *Pollstar's* 1987 list were Howie Mandel ($73,970), Jay Leno ($44,010), Sam Kinison ($39,169) and the double bill of Louie Anderson and Roseanne Barr ($34,364). Not bad for a night's work, especially when you compare the expense of carting a comic from town to town to the expense of moving a rock act, replete with band members, instruments, sets, and tech people over the same distance.

Nowadays, there are so many rooms for young comics to play, some 500 and counting, nationwide, that at times it almost seems as if there aren't enough comics to go around. Manhattan's appetite for comedy is especially voracious. There are more than a dozen clubs that feature comedy on a regular basis, and a dozen or so more in neighboring boroughs and suburbs. Add to that list the cabarets and theaters which feature comedy and comedy troupes occasionally, the improvisational groups with their own theaters, the performance art spaces with their own comedy shows, and the list becomes quite impressive.

The club surge, once considered a fad within the entertainment industry, is now being taken very, very seriously. Catch A Rising Star, which has gone public on the New York Stock Exchange is now in the midst of a rapid nationwide expansion. During 1988–1989, according to Richard Fields, Catch will open rooms in Cambridge, MA, Princeton, NJ, Chicago, Las Vegas, Oak Brook, IL, and Reno with plans to open clubs in Los Angeles, San Francisco, Washington, D.C., and Palo Alto, CA.

TAKING A STAND

What goes into making a successful stand-up comic? There are several different factors, just as there are many different types of comedians. Most comics will tell you that they enjoy what they do, that they need to be on the stage, and that they have an overwhelming desire to make people laugh. Some of them learned early on that getting laughs was their way of fitting in—or standing out.

If you've already decided to try your hand at stand-up comedy, the next thing you have to figure out is what you're going to do while you're standing there. What are you going to say? How are you going to say it? Will you tell jokes? Stories? Play different characters? Wear funny glasses? Use props? Or just go out there and be yourself?

Comic Howie Mandel loves working with props, particularly the rubber surgical gloves he routinely slips over his head. Bob Nelson is another highly successful prop comic. Nelson incorporates characters into his act as well. Comic Stu Trivax has one character he stays with throughout his set—a sort of nerdy, discotheque-cruising loser who is the comedian's "tongue-in-cheek Humphrey Bogart alter ego." Barry Mitchell is a comic who does impressions, including an eerily on-target one of Woody Allen, but he also parodies songs on his accordion.

Clearly, different things work for different comics. Since audience tastes tend to vary, finding what works can often be a complicated procedure of trial and error. "The first night I went out onstage," Joy Behar recalls, "I did a character called Sadie Catalano. She was an Italian woman from Brooklyn who told all the news in the community." Although Behar still uses her Sadie Catalano character occasionally, she eventually decided to be more like herself onstage. Her reasoning? "In stand-up you have to be able to react. You have to ad-lib. And sometimes, with a character, that just doesn't work. For me it was just too limiting. My personality was set a long time ago and my stage persona now is pretty much the same. After all, I *am* a person. I have a lot of different things to talk about. And I have my own unique perspectives. I see things as a female, as an Italian, as someone who went to college, a mother, a working-class person—all of those things come into play. When you are basically yourself onstage you have an endless backlog of information to bring up there with you."

CREATIVITY AND EXPERIENCE

Do you think *you've* got what it takes to go out there and make people laugh? Perhaps you do. If your friends think you're funny, if your relatives think you're funny, and if the people you work with think you're funny—well, there's a good chance that you really are funny. This doesn't mean, however, that you're ready to walk out onto a stage and keep people laughing for twenty minutes. You still need an act.

Lucian Hold, who books acts for the Comic Strip, generally auditions some 30 new acts per month. "We have a call on the first Friday of every month for new comics," Hold explains, "and, of the 50 to 60 who show up, we draw numbers for about 30 of them. Those comics whose numbers are drawn are then invited back and added into our schedule. Our Mondays are audition nights, and that is when they perform. Those who do well are then invited back."

What does Hold look for in a new comic? "I like to be surprised and I like to be made to laugh," Hold says. "That's the combination. I like to see something new or different in the character or the way the joke is written. I always tell people to be original. Avoid material written by other people. And, if your friends tell you that you remind them of someone, whether it's Robin Williams or Steven Wright or whoever it is, deal with that before you come in. Try to make the act your own." Hold offers this additional piece of advice: "Don't steal material. Some auditioners will come in here using material that's been lifted from someone else's act—something they've seen in a club or on a Showtime special. Never do it. I may not recognize the material right away. But someone else will, somewhere along the way."

If you're clever enough to write your own material, smooth enough to have successful auditions, and funny enough to get regular bookings, you're just about on your way. But you will still be lacking one extremely important ingredient—experience. Without it, and without the background needed to work a crowd, to use the energy in the room and make it work for you, even the funniest act will be wildly inconsistent; your act will kill them one night and will itself be dying the next. There are more than enough comedy club-goers who are convinced that it is their responsibility, as a member of the audience, to be loud, obnoxious and abusive. They shout out punchlines, obscenities, and anything else they feel like shouting out. If they've seen your act before, they'll ask you to do a routine they've enjoyed. And if they don't like what you're doing up there, they won't have any qualms about letting you know how they feel. Working onstage, without a fourth wall to protect you, can be a formidable business. And, having to occasionally cope with rude or drunk patrons, only makes it that much trickier. To be able to handle such individuals is a skill and a talent that comes from experience—lots of experience.

HITTING THE CLUBS

If you want to be a pastry chef, you study in Paris. If you want to be a stand-up comic, you study in New York. The club scene in Manhattan, much like this city's legitimate theater, is extensive, varied and—as far as the entertainment industry is concerned—important. As just about any comedian will tell you, New York's audiences are tough, discerning and hipper than most.

Because New Yorkers *are* so demanding, it may be a good idea to start out and get your feet wet in the smaller, suburban clubs in the New York City area. At the same time you should go into the New York clubs as often as possible and see what other comics are doing and observe how audiences react and what they are reacting to. If you're ready to earn your living as a comic, though, New York clubs are not the place to be. Only "names" make good money in New York. For lesser-known acts, "on the road" is where the money is.

ENSEMBLE TROUPES

If your interests in comedy lie beyond stand-up, you may wish to check out the various local ensembles specializing in sketch comedy and improvisational theater. Your chances of walking in off the street and joining one of these ensembles is less than nil, but almost all of these groups offer improv classes which can help you gain a more well-rounded comedy background. Also, you will get to know other comics with similar interests. Perhaps you and a few of your classmates will decide to form an ensemble of your own.

Many comics appearing on such television shows as "Your Show of Shows," "Laugh-In," or "Saturday Night Live," got their start in troupes like Second City and scores of other, lesser known comedy groups throughout the United States and Canada. They learned their craft in front of live audiences, where they developed their characters and took their chances. Their subsequent success in television and films can be directly attributed to these early, valuable experiences.

There are dozens of such companies presently working in Manhattan. Some have their own spaces. Others move from place to place with every new show they put together. Among the better-known ensembles are Chicago City Limits, For Play, Interplay, Unexpected Company, Chucklehead, the Groundlings East, the Kids in the Hall, Shock of the Funny, and Artificial Intelligence.

TELEVISION INNOVATIONS

Today the bulk of stand-up comedy programming emanates from cable television, of that there can be no question. The following stand-up comedy offerings are currently airing on the cable networks: "Young Comedians," "HBO On Location," "Comedy Experiment" (Cinemax); "Comedy Cuts" (USA); and "Comedy Club Network," (Showtime). Additionally MTV has a few comedy-oriented programs in development and Arts and Entertainment continues to run the "Evening at the Improv" series.

In a recent issue of *The Cable Guide*, Dennis Miller is quoted as saying, "If you can get your hour down and get it honed enough and get some sort of reputation, you can probably get a cable deal . . . cable needs the product . . . it's big money for them. They're scouring the country looking for comics." By now there should be no question as to where *they* are looking.

PERFORMANCE OPPORTUNITIES

Certainly, stand-up comedy is not an easy career. The hours are strange. The lifestyle is fast. And the traveling—which is where most of the money is—can make you crazy. It is theater, though and it does pay. And it can help you to be seen. Stand-up comedy is also an equal opportunity profession. Though still dominated by males, a good proportion of the emerging acts are female. There are plenty of opportunities here for anyone with enough chutzpuh to climb up onstage and deliver.

There are several sources of information which can answer questions about touring, management, performance opportunities and any additional questions you may have concerning a career in stand-up comedy. One is the Professional Comedians Association, P.O. Box 222, New York, NY 10185.

The PCA was established in 1982 and, according to the organization's past president Jerry Diner, "We have currently 450 members nationwide. We are the only watchdog organization for comedians, protecting their rights in just about every avenue. Plus we also disseminate absolutely every type of information by and for professional comedians. We have a directory with an update of every booker and comedy club in the country, including one-nighters. We have a code of standards and practices, and we sponsor a player's guide for comedians which goes out to every casting agent in the country. Our newsletter, which has updates in the directory plus additional information, comes out once a month. We provide insurance for comedians. We hold seminars on writing, performing, and getting work in commercials. We held a seminar on income tax because of the many changes last year. Plus, we handle grievances for members and will step in if someone gets stiffed on a payment."

The trade publication *Comedy USA Newswire*, bills itself as "the first trade publication to take funny business seriously." For a year's subscription send $40 to: Comedy USA Newswire, 915 Broadway, Suite 1100, New York, NY 10010.

An amusing and informative glimpse into the current world of stand-up comedy appears in the book "Comic Lives" (Fireside Books) by Betsy Borns. The book contains interviews with 30 top comics as well as booking agents, club owners, and television executives.

If you are interested in a career as a comic, whether in television, films, theater, or on the comedy stage, there has never been a better time for you to get up there and take a stand. During the past decade the club scene everywhere has developed into a marvelously diverse comic landscape. The following list will give you an idea of what's going on in some of the best clubs in New York City and Los Angeles.

Stand-Up Clubs

NEW YORK CITY

CAROLINE'S AT THE
SEAPORT
89 South Street, Pier 17
New York, NY 10003
(212) 233-4900
Booking person: Campbell
McLaren

CATCH A RISING STAR
1487 First Ave.
New York, NY 10021
(212) 794-1906
Booking person: Louis
Faranda

COMIC STRIP
1568 Second Ave.
New York, NY 10028
(212) 861-9386
Booking person: Lucian
Hold

THE COMEDY ELITE
2 Bond St.
New York, NY 10012
(212) 473-1472
Booking person: David
Healy

COMEDY CELLAR
117 MacDougal St.
New York, NY 10011
(212) 254-3630
Call for booking details.

CHINA CHALET
47 Broadway
New York, NY 10012
(212) 943-4380/4428
Booking person: Tim Andre
Davis

DANGERFIELDS
1118 First Ave.
New York, NY 10021
(212) 593-1650
Call for booking details.

DUPLEX
55 Grove St.
New York, NY 10014
(212) 255-5438
Booking person: Angela
Scott

EAGLE TAVERN
355 W. 14th St.
New York, NY 10011
(212) 924-0275
Booking person: Tim Andre
Davis.

IMPROVISATION
358 W. 44th St.
New York, NY 10036
Booking person: Silver
Friedman

STAND-UP NEW YORK
236 W. 78 St.
New York, NY 10024
(212) 595-0850
Booking person: Cary
Hoffman

WHO'S ON FIRST
1205 First Ave.
New York, NY 10021
(212) 737-2772

LOS ANGELES AREA

CENTER STAGE
COMEDY CLUB
23 N. Market
San Jose, CA
(408) 298-2266

COMEDY & MAGIC CLUB
1018 Hermosa Ave.
Hermosa Beach, CA
(213) 372-1193

THE COMEDY CLUB
111 W. Pine
Long Beach, CA
(213) 437-5326

THE COMEDY STORE
9433 Sunset Blvd.
Hollywood, CA
(213) 656-6225

THE COMEDY STORE
916 Pearl
La Jolla, CA
(619) 454-9176

THE COMEDY STORE
333 Universal Terrace
  Parkway
Universal City, CA
(818) 980-1212 x 6112

HOP SINGH'S
4110 Lincoln Blvd.
Marina Del Ray, CA

IGBY'S
11637 Tennessee Place
Los Angeles, CA
(213) 477-3553

THE IMPROV
8162 Melrose Ave.
Hollywood, CA
(213) 651-2583

THE IMPROV
832 Garnet Ave.
Pacific Beach, CA
(619) 483-4520

L.A. CABARET
17271 Ventura Blvd.
Encino, CA
(213) 501-3737

THE LAFF FACTORY
8001 Sunset Blvd.
West Hollywood, CA
(213) 656-8960
Mon: Ladies Comedy Night

THE LAFF STOP
2122 SE Bristol
Newport Beach, CA
(714) 852-8762

THE LAST LAUGH
29 N. Pedro St.
San Jose, CA

94TH AERO SQUADRON
1160 Coleman Avenue
San Jose, CA
(408) 287-6150

TOPPERS
4400 Stevens Creek Blvd.
San Jose, CA
(408) 247-7795

BOB ZANY'S COMEDY
OUTLET
at Wm. Randolph's
1850 Monterey St.
San Luis Obispo, CA
(805) 543-3333

BOB ZANY'S COMEDY
OUTLET
at Bombay's
4223 State St.
Santa Barbara, CA
(805) 682-8689

BOB ZANY'S COMEDY
OUTLET
at Silver Dollar Saloon
213 E. Main St.
Santa Maria, CA
(805) 925-1193

BOB ZANY'S COMEDY
OUTLET
at Reuben's
299 S. Moorpark Rd.
Thousand Oaks, CA
(805) 495-0431

BOB ZANY'S COMEDY
OUTLET
at Club Soda
317 E. Main St.
Ventura, CA
(805) 652-1164

Afterword:
Actors Aware!

by Andrea Wolper

"Show business is a difficult and highly competitive profession . . . Even professionals have trouble finding work. So if the moment you walk in the door someone does a back flip over you—watch out. It's possible that you are about to be ripped off."

Those words are from a pamphlet published by the New York State Department of Law, Bureau of Consumer Affairs. While, hopefully, most people connected with the fashion and entertainment industries are honorable, even the most streetwise and savvy of us need to be made aware of potential problems.

Anybody can get taken if the circumstances are right. Hungry-for-work models and performers may be more vulnerable to deception than people in other professions. But this doesn't mean that you should be at the mercy of every con artist that preys on performing artists. Don't assume that someone else has all the answers just because they say they do. The best thing you can do is sharpen your instincts and learn to trust them. Keep in mind that most legitimate operations are governed by laws, union regulations, or at the very least, time-honored traditions. If you find yourself in a situation that feels dangerous, or as though it might be illegal or some kind of scam, say no thanks, and remove yourself from the situation.

SHOW BUSINESS PARENTS—VULNERABLE PREY

Show business parents are especially vulnerable to con artist schemes. What new parent doesn't consider his/her child the most adorable, winning, intelligent thing that ever lived? Unfortunately, there are people who are ready to milk such pride for all it's worth. They place ads in small "throwaway" newspapers that lure parents and their kids to a hotel where they are beguiled into spending hundreds of dollars for photographs. Such schemes work because the parents don't know that professional headshots of kids under age five are completely unnecessary. Other scams aimed at parents involve door-to-door solicitation by obscure management companies that offer to provide photographs and register the children—all for an exorbitant fee, of course.

AGENTS AND MANAGERS DIFFER

Phony managers prey on big kids as well; they get away with it, perhaps, because a lot of people don't really understand the difference between an agent and a manager. Here, from the Department of Law pamphlet, is an explanation: "Talent or model agencies are licensed by the state and their fees are limited by law. They are legally entitled to be paid a fixed commission of not more than ten percent *only* after you have landed the job and been paid for your work. There are some talent agents who are also franchised by one of more of the performers' unions [which means they agree to comply with certain union regulations]. Personal managers are not licensed by the state and their fees are not limited by law. They should provide more comprehensive services than agents, functioning perhaps as business managers and financial advisers. They may invest considerable time and money in your career."

Beware of unscrupulous managers who charge for interviews or present themselves as acting teachers who will also manage you. Joseph Rapp, executive director of the Eastern Division of the National Conference of Personal Managers asks, "What are they really doing, selling lessons or helping your career?" Rapp also warns against managers who charge for introductions to, and seminars with, agents and casting directors who give speeches on what to expect, how to behave in professional situations, etc. It is a manager's very job to provide such introductions and such information free of charge.

Another sign that things may not be on the up-and-up, suggests Rapp, is the management company name that suggests an association with the casting or talent department of, say, a motion picture studio. The association may be in name only.

CHECK REFERENCES

If you want to find out if a manager is legit, the National Conference of Personal Managers (see "Personal Managers," page 87) is a good place to start. Standards for membership are high; only a small percentage of applicants are accepted, so you can feel pretty confident that a member of the Conference is trustworthy. Rapp says, "We don't go by a manager's success, we go by his ethics and how he conducts his business." Nevertheless, Rapp continues, "there are many good managers who are not part of our organization for one reason or another. Still, sometimes we're aware of someone's reputation, good or bad. If we don't know the manager in question we'll try to direct the caller to someone who can give them further information."

Sandy Eckstein of talent agency Marcia's Kids, recommends that you ask managers for a list of agents and casting directors they have worked with, and then call those people and find out if the list is on the up-and-up.

Managers' commissions are negotiable, but the average rate is 15 percent. In a case where a manager invests in a career or advances money to the client, the commission may go as high as 25 percent. The bottom line is that the commission should bear a direct relationship to the services rendered. What are *you* getting? If you work as a day player or an extra on a soap, for example, should your manager collect 25 percent of your pay? No way.

MODELING AGENCIES—WHAT IS A REASONABLE COMMISSION?

What we know as modeling agencies are technically *model management* firms; it's a fine but important distinction. They send people out for print, or runway work, and so on; they are not licensed, nor are their commissions limited. In some cases, however, a modeling firm may have divisions that are franchised by one or more of the performers' unions.

Eileen Ford, president of Ford Models, says her modeling division collects commissions of 15 to 20 percent and, as determined by the performers' unions, Ford Talent Group collects commissions of 10 percent for television work. Adds Wilhelmina International president Bill Weinberg, the industry is competitive enough that "I don't think any of us can afford to go in with high commissions."

In the end, of course, it's up to you. If the only modeling management firm or personal manager that's interested in you takes 25 percent commissions *and* they appear to be legitimate, being represented by them might be better than no representation at all.

KICKBACK SCHEMES

Agents and managers have a lot of influence on their clients and while it's absolutely proper for them to recommend or suggest schools and photographers, there are those who get involved in kickback schemes. If someone pushes you toward one particular school, coach, or photographer, it's possible they have a direct financial interest. *If an agent or manager pushes, or says you must shoot with one particular photographer in order to work with them, think twice.*

One young woman saw an ad for shoe models, telephoned, and was told to report to the agency office that afternoon, so she could be sent on a job the following day. On arrival, she was told to hire the agency's photographer "because without these pictures I could not get a job. In short, they promised me a job that did not exist in order to trick me into purchasing the services of their photographer."

A similar scam advertised for actors and actresses for a "full-service production company." Those who responded were given an appointment. When they arrived at the designated place, they found a number of other actors had been given the same appointment time. A company representative then spoke to the assembled actors, saying the company was involved in several big projects, and dropping the names of some well-known performers. The actors were then "invited" to become part of a core unit by paying for a listing in a book called "The Producers Quick Guide to New York Talent." A contract was produced, promising that the company would "promote the artist in a very special way." The actors were urged to pay a deposit on the spot. The fee for inclusion in this book? A sum of $125 for union members, $155 for everybody else.

HEADSHEETS AND AGENCY LISTINGS

When should you pay to be included on agency headsheets and in books? It is considered legitimate for modeling and print agencies to charge for inclusion in such. The cost usually varies from year to year, depending upon printing costs, but be sure you know what you're paying for. Bill Weinberg points out that inclusion in a reputable agency's book "means you are represented on a full-time basis by that agency. Then there are those that advertise and say, 'Send a picture and $100 and we'll put you in our book and send it out to agents and casting directors.' It may or may not serve a purpose, but it does not mean representation."

Of course, there are some publications, like the *Players Guide*, that have been around for years and are established, legitimate promotional venues. On the other hand, everybody has to start somewhere, and the fact that an agency or publication is new or small or not so well-known doesn't automatically mean they're up to no good. In some cases, a smaller agency may be just the thing for an actor or model with little experience, or who has been turned down by the bigger agencies. But if you're going to spend time or money on something or someone you know little or nothing about, do some investigating. Call your local Better Business Bureau, or any comparable consumer agency, to find out if any complaints have been registered against the company. Talk to friends and other people in the business who might know something about the company in question. Ask *yourself* if it feels right.

Remember, except for inclusion on a headsheet or in the book of an agency or management firm you have reason to trust, *you should never, ever give money up front to an agent or manager. And never pay an agency or management firm any amount of money for photographs.*

When a new model comes to a legitimate modeling agency and needs pictures, explains Eileen Ford, "we have a list of 30 or 40 photographers they can test with. The model can bring the film and pay for the processing, but we provide hairstyling, makeup and wardrobe." At Wilhelmina, Weinberg says, "If we don't accept someone but feel they have potential, we suggest they go out with a friend or relative and take snapshots. If we do accept them, we hook them up with photographers who are either building their experience or who are established but like to try out new ideas. The model may pay for the film and processing. And very often makeup artists and hairstylists will come in and offer their time." With this kind of reciprocal arrangement, building a modeling portfolio should be relatively inexpensive.

RIP-OFFS AND EXPLOITATION
From the time we're very young we're taught to obey authority, that if we do what we're told, we'll be rewarded in the end. In a field where rewards come so infrequently, it's easy to turn anyone who has the power to bestow them into an authority figure to be obeyed without question. One actress reported that her nightmare began when she was cast in an Off-Off-Broadway showcase. Though she'd be paid $60 a week once the show opened, she was expected to quit the job upon which she depended for survival and devote all her time to the production. Not wanting to pass up the opportunity to be in a show, she arranged to work half-days and start rehearsals two hours later than everyone else who had, indeed, quit *their* jobs. Still, she often found herself sitting for hours waiting to rehearse and, a few days before opening she had still not received a script! When the demands on her time increased she cut her work hours to two a day. Things came to a head when, after two weeks of working sixteen-hour days on the production, she requested a night off and was refused. The show had already opened and, feeling it was time to stand up for herself, the actress skipped an extra rehearsal. A few days later she was fired. When she asked for an explanation she was verbally abused and told to get out. She did, she admits, learn a valuable lesson about putting her foot down and getting things in writing.

PAY CRISES
What do you do when you have trouble collecting your pay? When a union is involved, contact the union; otherwise, start writing letters (keep copies of all correspondence) and making phone calls. Go in person to the office of the agent or manager that sent you out or the company that hired you, and make such a pest of yourself that the person who owes you will do anything to get rid of you—that is, if they haven't skipped town.

Obviously, you can't always know who is going to cheat you, but there may be clues. An agent or manager who asks for a "registration fee," or whom you pay in order to be submitted or get cast, or who promises jobs or stardom, or who tries to pressure you into *anything*, is behaving unethically, if not illegally. If a production company can't come up with an acceptable-looking contract, if you're left with too many unanswered questions before you leave on that cross-country tour, it could be an indication that you're going to wind up in Yakutat, Alaska with no money and no way to get home.

One actor signed a contract that was handwritten on construction company letterhead (the "producer" was also president of the construction company) for a two-week job on the island of Grenada. Once there, the seven performers were housed not in a hotel, as promised, but in a two-bedroom house in the hills. Over the next few days they had little food and water, and no telephone or transportation. To add insult to injury, the show was cancelled halfway through the run and the performers were not paid the balance due them.

An actor who had a disastrous time with an overseas tour offers this advice: "Scrutinize your contract with an attorney. Frequently write your friends in the States so they'll always know where you are. If you have an accident, report it immediately. Familiarize yourself with theater law, and make friends with a family in the country you're visiting."

GET IT IN WRITING

An actress answered a casting notice for a repertory company; at the audition she was informed it was for print work. She interviewed anyway, got the job, and accepted a verbal contract of $400 for two weeks' work. After spending three days in the Poconos waiting for shooting to begin, she and three others were told they would be "paid off" in the amount of $80. They insisted on an explanation and the full $400; what they got was $80 and a lift to the bus station.

We're so sure that a sunny smile and an "I'll do anything" attitude are what the profession demands; we bend over backwards to be easygoing. As in affairs of the heart, we ignore clues that tell us something's amiss because we want so much for things to work out. Look, anyone who would fire you because you insisted on a professional contract is doing you a favor. Remember that performing is your *profession*. If it means holding out until the good guys recognize your genius, then by all means, hold out.

What would you do if you received a photocopied letter that said "stardom is within your grasp," and went on to invite you, as a "future prospective member of the cast," to send $10 to purchase a script, after which an audition could be arranged? Hopefully, you'd report it to the United States Mail Service and/or the Department of Law's Bureau of Consumer Frauds and Protection.

SCAM CITY

In another example of fraudulent use of the mails, a production company sent an actor a packet of some half a dozen pages, making an offer of employment as an extra in an unnamed Hollywood movie. Airline tickets, so the letter said, had been reserved, and a contract (with three signatures that looked as if they'd all been written by the same hand) was included. Another extraordinary feature of this contract, aside from its highly unusual use of the English language, was that the name of the president of the company was spelled differently every time it was used!

The letter stated that the company would pay all expenses including first-class airfare, limousines, hotels, meals, and a salary of $250 a day, and provide a "photographic shooting test." All that was required to be the beneficiary of this proposal was a payment of $76.87 for taxes on plane tickets and photography costs.

FAKE CASTING NOTICES

A company announced that it was accepting applications from male and female models on a particular day at a New York City hotel. Once there, the applicants learned they could pay $25 for a second interview that might lead to acceptance into a $2,500 training program! Now, many schools collect filing fees, and $2,500 is not an unusual tuition for a full-time program. But anyone seeking students by placing what looks like a casting notice is not on the level. In this instance there were some clues in the notice, but you had to know how to read between the lines. The ad implied that designer clothing and furs were to be modelled, yet it also stated that there were no height or weight requirements and that no experience was necessary. Certainly there are times when experience and a specific appearance are unimportant; just keep in mind that when non-professionals are sought, that's probably how they'll be treated.

SCHOOL SMARTS

According to the New York State Education Department, schools providing instruction in modeling or announcing must be licensed by the state. Schools that provide instruction in music, dramatic art, and dancing are exempt from licensing requirements. Naturally, the exempted categories pose the greater risk. Anybody can take out an ad, hang fliers on a telephone pole and say they're in business, and plenty of people do. Dance and music lessons, which can be paid for on a class-by-class basis most of the time, are relatively safe. But acting schools and workshops usually require a fairly hefty commitment of time and money, and it's smart to research even the more famous schools. Find out who teaches there. Does the school continue to live up to the reputation it may have earned two generations ago? Ask around. And while it is probably not wise to enroll in a class or school on the basis of name alone, neither should you reject a school or teacher simply because they're not famous. Your best sources of information are the friends and colleagues you admire and trust.

People who find they've been manipulated are often quite clear about what occurred. Usually, though they had doubts all along, they trusted the person they'd eventually call a con artist more than they did their own instincts. Well, perhaps it's not easy to recognize a snake-oil salesman when you've got stars in your eyes. If you find yourself being asked to pay for rehearsals or enroll in a workshop when nothing of the kind was mentioned in the ad or casting notice to which you have responded, watch out. Carefully read any information sheets or legal documents offered to you. Ask for explanations of anything you don't understand. Do research. When and where have previous performances taken place? Are there any reviews you can look at? Are there resumes or other credentials you can see?

SEX—OR SEXPLOITATION?

It's so hard to know how to behave sometimes, especially in a business where sex appeal is a saleable commodity. Somebody may have a job to offer me and I want that job, but why is he sitting so close?

Or you go to an audition and the fellow says he needs to see your physique because there's a locker room scene. So you strip down to your shorts and wait a minute—what's he doing with a camera?

Sometimes we want something so much that we believe we're nothing unless we get it. It's so easy to go deaf, dumb, and blind when somebody's dangling a carrot in front of your nose and that carrot has "fame," "money," "exposure" written all over it. Add to that the fact that ours is a very polite society. We're taught that to be liked is to be a success. It's not even the idea of offending that's so worrisome, it's the idea that if we don't smile a lot and act cheerful and agree with everything we're told, *we might not get the job!*

But what if there isn't any job? Remember: if you suspect even the slightest possibility of danger, forget about the job, the money, the career. Think about your safety and well-being. Think twice when someone asks you to meet them in a hotel room or apartment. Yes, a lot of people in this business work out of their apartments but before you go up, check them out. Find out if there's a good reason when an ad specifies "model-types."

THE BEST DEFENSE AGAINST VICTIMIZATION

What's really essential is that you take *you* with you—all of you: your *brains, wit, intuition, instincts,* and *self-confidence.* Learn to read casting notices with a practiced eye. If you suspect a situation could place you in danger, it's probably best to avoid it. If you are suspicious of someone for whatever reason, do a little investigating. If someone isn't willing to go through the accepted channels, think twice before getting involved. If something smells fishy, it probably is. Check it out, make some calls, do some digging. Trust your gut. Don't be afraid to ask questions for fear of losing a job. There will be many other opportunities.

Contributors

John Allen writes and publishes *The Summer Theater Guide, The Regional and Dinner Theater Guide*, and *The New Equity Audition System*. His career started in radio in the Midwest. In 1975, a series of programs he developed won an Iowa Arts Council Award. He also hosted a radio interview program on which his guests included Aaron Copland, Studs Terkel, and Hubert Humphrey. He left radio for theater in 1979 and has performed extensively. He also performs in and manages Interborough Repertory Theater, a Brooklyn-based theater company which he and his wife founded in 1985.

Jill Charles is the founding artistic director of the Dorset Theatre Festival, an Equity company which produces summer seasons at the Dorset Playhouse in Dorset, Vermont. She also edits the nationally distributed *Summer Theatre Directory, Regional Theatre Directory*, and *Directory of Theatre Training Programs*, publications which she developed as employment guides for theater professionals and guides to training and internship opportunities for students. She taught for ten years in both conservatory and liberal arts college theater departments; her last position was at Williams College in Massachusetts. She has directed over 40 productions, in Dorset and elsewhere.

Bill Ervolino is the comedy critic for the *New York Post* and a columnist and critic for *Back Stage*. He has written feature stories and interviews for the *New York Times, Daily News*, and numerous other newspapers and magazines. His first play, *The Lights on Walden Court*, was produced Off-Off-Broadway and was a 1986 co-winner of the Jane Chambers Playwriting Award.

Rorri Feinstein currently works as a comedian. Among the clubs she has appeared at are Stand-Up NY, The Comic Strip, Comedy U, as well as appearances in Chicago, San Francisco, and the Catskills. Her theater credits include a season at The Adirondack Playhouse, productions in Los Angeles, and numerous Off-Off-Broadway shows in New York. Behind the camera, she has worked as an extras casting director on several feature films, and has worked on commercials doing script/continuity, production coordination, and production managing. She is a native New Yorker and holds an MFA in Acting from UCLA.

Marje Fields has been at the head of her own agency, Marje Fields, Inc., since 1968. Her full-service agency represents writers as well as performers in TV, theater, film, and commercials. Prior to opening her own agency, she worked with Charles B. Tranum, a talent agency specializing in commercials. Before that, she worked at Air Features, where Frank and Anne Hummert wrote and produced the *original* soap operas. Ms. Fields is currently the president of the National Association of Talent Representatives, the trade organization which represents agents with SAG, AFTRA, and Equity, and assists with other industry problems.

Victor Gluck currently writes the "Notes on Theater" column in the *East Side Express,* as well as features and reviews for *Back Stage.* His theater reviews have also appeared in *Our Town, New York Guide/Wisdom's Child, Stages,* the *Brooklyn Spectator,* the *Brooklyn Times,* and the *Shakespeare Bulletin.* He has also been the dramaturge of the Soho Repertory Theatre since 1980, and has given literary advice to Manhattan Punch Line, the Hudson Guild Theatre, and the York Theatre Company. He is a member of the Drama Desk, the Outer Critics Circle, and the American Theatre Critics Association. He made his debut as a playwright at the Quaigh Theatre with the double bill *Amouresque* and *Arabesque* in 1981.

Phyllis Goldman is a dance reviewer and feature writer on dance for *Back Stage.* She has also contributed to *Elle Magazine, Interview,* and the book *Women Who Work.* She has worked as a professional dancer, a teaching assistant to Lee Theodore at the American Dance Machine Training Facility, and as a choreographer for regional theater and television. She holds a BS Degree in Education with a major in Dance from Ohio State University.

Susan Goldstein developed her "Succeeding in L.A." seminar/audio tape based on her experience as an L.A.-based producer/personal manager/publicist. Ms. Goldstein has worked in the areas of film, theater, television and music. In addition, she is a journalist, having been published in several national magazines. Her "Succeeding in L.A." seminar is offered several times a year in New York and Los Angeles, and she plans to bring it to other states and Europe.

Bob Harrington is the cabaret critic for the *New York Post* and *Back Stage,* and theater and cabaret editor for *Long Island* and *New York Nightlife* magazines. His series of educational articles on the business of cabaret in *Back Stage* garnered him a coveted Manhattan Association of Cabarets MAC Award in 1986. He is currently vice president of the Manhattan Association of Cabarets and Clubs, on the board of directors of the Outer Critics Circle and the Society of Singers, a member of the Drama Desk, and an American Theatre Wing Tony voter. He has written on cabaret and its stars for a variety of other publications, including the *Chicago Tribune* and the *Hearst Syndicate.*

Ronn Mullen, dinner theater and summer stock actor, Off-Off-Broadway director, free-lance feature writer, and theater critic, lives in New York City. He started his theater education at Ohio's Kent State University and continued at the University of California at Berkeley. He was an original member of the Obie-winning CSC Repertory Company in New York, and was a founding member of the Experimental Wing of San Francisco's improvisational group, The Committee. He is currently artistic director of the Outlaw Theatre, which performs in city shelters for the homeless and in prisons.

Joseph Rapp is now in his fifth term as president of the National Conference of Personal Managers/Eastern Division. He is an active partner in Rapp/Metz Entertainment Corporation, developing projects for motion pictures and TV. He recently completed filming "The American Dream Festival," which is set for national syndication. Mr. Rapp entered the entertainment industry in 1963 by joining Charles Rapp Enterprises, providing entertainment in clubs and resorts on the East Coast. In 1970, he formed Joseph Rapp Enterprises, a personal management company that represents variety performers and musical composers for TV and film.

Toni Reinhold is a features and entertainment writer, an investigative reporter, and an internationally syndicated columnist. She is an award-winning journalist who began her career at age 17, stringing for WHN Radio News, WNBC Radio News, and the *New York Daily News*. In 1978, Toni joined the Murdoch organization as a staff reporter for the *Star* and performed stand-in shifts at the *New York Post*. In 1985, she signed with United Features Syndicate to write two weekly entertainment Q & A columns, and a year later added a third column. Ms. Reinhold is a regular contributor to such publications as *Back Stage*, *Redbook*, and *Woman's World*.

Mike Salinas was born in Iowa and lived in Florida and Arizona before settling in New York. He is the founder of *TheaterWeek*, a consumer-oriented publication, prior to which he was a talent agent. His experience in theater encompasses both on- and back-stage work (acting, producing, designing, building, and "teching"), and he still intends to find time to write and direct musicals. Whenever possible he tips his hat to teachers who nurture theatrical ambitions, particularly Jim Erbe of Cedar Rapids, Iowa.

Joseph J. Schwartz has been employed as a writer, journalist, puppeteer, actor, college administrator, computer consultant, waiter, personal shopper, PR worker, teacher, carpenter, and janitor—among other things.

Fred Silver, a leading vocal coach, is currently an associate professor at the University of Miami's Theatre Arts department. He is a protege of the late Richard Rodgers, and his published shows include *For Heaven's Sake, Hannah, Like It Is, Exodus and Easter*, and *In Gay Company*. His latest musical, *Good Little Girls* (book, music and lyrics), originally produced by Lucille Lortel last season, is optioned for New York production. He created nightclub acts for Kaye Ballard, Lynne Carter and Hermione Gingold, and wrote "The Age of Elegance" for Nancy Dussault and Karen Morrow. His "Twelve Days After Christmas," written for Carol Burnett, has sold over a million copies. Mr. Silver is the author of *Auditioning for the Musical Theater*, published by Newmarket Press and Penguin Books.

Don Snell works in New York as an actor. Focusing on television and film, yet still managing to stay involved in theater, he has created leading roles at Playwrights Horizons and developed the lead in Amlin Gray's *How I Got That Story*. Don is what is known as a "utility player." Somewhere between leading man and character actor, the

39-year-old comedian can show up on the set, learn the scene, and get the job done. Credits: "All My Children," "Celebrity," "Dallas," "The Equalizer," *For Immediate Release*, "Guiding Light," *Places in the Heart, The Return of Donald Truslow, Rise and Shine, Time Bomb*.

Thomas Walsh is an associate editor at *Back Stage* and has been with the company in numerous capacities since 1986. He was a sports writer and editor for nearly five years with Sterling's Magazines, Inc., New York, and is the author of two recreational sports books for children. He has thrived in a broad variety of editorial positions in New York for over ten years, and his work has roamed the range from SportsChannel to *Cosmopolitan*. Among his many dreams is to really and truly see Epcot Center for himself.

Andrea Wolper works as both an actor and a free-lance writer. She has written for *New York Woman, In Fashion*, and various travel publications. She is pleased to have made numerous contributions to *Back Stage* since 1983.

Index